Pathology of Testicular and Penile Neoplasms

Maurizio Colecchia
Editor

Pathology of Testicular and Penile Neoplasms

Springer

Editor
Maurizio Colecchia
Department of Pathology
Fondazione IRCCS Istituto dei Tumor
Milan, Italy

ISBN 978-3-319-27615-1 ISBN 978-3-319-27617-5 (eBook)
DOI 10.1007/978-3-319-27617-5

Library of Congress Control Number: 2016936098

Printed on acid-free paper

This Springer imprint is published by Springer Nature
The registered company is Springer International Publishing AG Switzerland

To Mariangela and Matteo for their patient, silent, and loving support and to my parents

Preface

As editor of *Pathology of Testicular and Penile Neoplasms,* I would like to briefly explain the inspiration for this book, which came from a sentence I read in the Treasure Gallery of the British Library: "Science depends on the accurate observation, collection and recording of information." This sentence (attributed to Galileo, the father of scientific observation) is the leitmotif in this book on penile and testicular neoplasms – rare tumors which are, however, increasing in frequency and whose epidemiological implications will be illustrated here in light of the most recent knowledge in the field. Congenital testicular lesions, impaired spermatogenesis, cryptorchidism, Klinefelter syndrome, testicular dysgenesis, entities contributing to infertility and their correlation with an increased risk of cancer, and childhood and prepubertal germ cell tumors will be discussed.

The book will also describe the precursor lesions of invasive cancer as well as the staging criteria that provide the clinician with information for the correct treatment of metastatic disease. Furthermore, with the aid of summary tables, it will illustrate the main differential diagnoses between morphological entities. One chapter will be dedicated to the use of intraoperative frozen section analysis, which is increasingly being requested for the diagnosis of ultrasound-detected small testicular lesions.

As a practical handbook for pathologists, this volume will be an aid to the diagnosis of these uncommon tumors and to dealing with the diagnostic pitfalls they often present. The text will provide updates on the new editions of the classification systems for testicular and penile tumors, with a view to achieving the necessary clarity in the terminology used by the pathologist in communicating diagnostic information. It aims to familiarize also less experienced pathologists with the sampling methods for orchiectomy and penectomy specimens and with the appropriate recording of pathology findings according to the guidelines approved by the International Society of Urological Pathology (ISUP). The book is designed to provide practitioners with the tools and knowledge to formulate a complete histopathology report with all the necessary information for the clinician. Its contents reflect the experience of the authors of the various chapters (11 on testicular cancer, 3 on cancer of the penis) in light of the recent literature, documented by more than 250 photographs; we have scrutinized the currently available information in an attempt to provide valuable updates on the variants of penile carcinoma, HPV-related and unrelated penile tumors, and newly classified testicular neoplasms. The images have not been published before, and I am deeply grateful to the authors and coauthors of *Pathology of Testicular and Penile Neoplasms*, who have contributed their personal cases, giving their time and energy to the drafting of the chapters of this book, which I hope you will enjoy reading.

Milan, Italy Maurizio Colecchia

Acknowledgements

Many people have helped me get this book into shape. The contributions of Alessia Bertolotti, PhD, in all stages of its development and in the technical preparation of the slides (recutting, immunohistochemical staining, scanning of interesting cases) were irreplaceable. Biagio Paolini, MD, has improved the photomicrographs through refined color enhancement. His efforts in standardizing the appearance of the illustrations will surely be appreciated by our readers. I also gratefully acknowledge the work of Alessio Pellegrinelli, MD, who has shown surprising versatility in designing tables and drawing illustrations to make the macroscopic images of Chap. 13 easier to understand.

I thank Drs Bandieramonte, Torelli, and Catanzaro for having contributed with the macroscopic images of penile lesions from their clinical activity.

Special thanks go to Marije de Jager for meticulously correcting the manuscript. I am particularly grateful for her help in uniforming the style across chapters. Thanks go as well to Paolo Castioni and Maria Morelli, who have enthusiastically contributed to this book in various ways. I express my heartfelt appreciation to the library staff of Fondazione IRCCS Istituto Nazionale dei Tumori and in particular to Rossella Ballarini.

Finally, I gratefully remember the teachings of Professor Juan Rosai (hoping they shaped me) that directed me and many other pathologists to a methodical approach in diagnostic pathology.

Maurizio Colecchia

Contents

Contributors

Alessia Bertolotti Department of Pathology, Fondazione IRCCS Istituto Nazionale dei Tumori di Milano, Milan, Italy

Rita Canas-Marques Serviço de Anatomia Patológica, Instituto Português de Oncologia de Lisboa, Lisbon, Portugal

Liang Cheng Department of Pathology and Laboratory Medicine, Indiana University School of Medicine, Indianapolis, IN, USA

Maurizio Colecchia Uropathology Unit, Department of Pathology, Fondazione IRCCS Istituto Nazionale dei Tumori di Milano, Milan, Italy

Alessandro Conti Department of Odontostomatologic and Specialized Clinical Sciences, Section of Urology, Polytechnic University of the Marche Region, School of Medicine, United Hospitals, Ancona, Italy

Alessandro Franchi Division of Pathological Anatomy, University of Florence, Florence, Italy

Gemma Gatta Evaluative Epidemiology, Fondazione IRCCS Istituto Nazionale dei Tumori di Milano, Milan, Italy

Pilar González-Peramato Department of Pathology, Autonoma University of Madrid, Hospital Univ. La Paz., Madrid, Spain

Antonio Lopez-Beltran Department of Pathology and Surgery, Faculty of Medicine, University of Cordoba, Cordoba, Spain

Roberta Mazzucchelli Pathological Anatomy, Polytechnic University of the Marche Region, School of Medicine, United Hospitals, Ancona, Italy

Gregor Mikuz Institute of Pathology, Medical University of Innsbruck, Innsbruck, Austria

Rodolfo Montironi Pathological Anatomy, Polytechnic University of the Marche Region, School of Medicine, United Hospitals, Ancona, Italy

Gabriella Nesi Division of Pathological Anatomy, University of Florence, Florence, Italy

Nicola Nicolai Testis Surgery Unit, Fondazione IRCCS Istituto Nazionale dei Tumori di Milano, Milan, Italy

Manuel Nistal Department of Anatomy, Histology and Neuroscience, Autonoma University of Madrid, Madrid, Spain

Biagio Paolini Department of Pathology, Fondazione IRCCS Istituto Nazionale dei Tumori di Milano, Milan, Italy

Maria R. Raspollini Division of Histology and Molecular Diagnostics, University Hospital Careggi, University of Florence, Florence, Italy

Roberto Salvioni Urology Unit, Fondazione IRCCS Istituto dei Tumori di Milano, Milan, Italy

Raffaella Santi Division of Pathological Anatomy, University of Florence, Florence, Italy

Matteo Santoni Medical Oncology, Polytechnic University of the Marche Region, School of Medicine, United Hospitals, Ancona, Italy

Marina Scarpelli Pathological Anatomy, Polytechnic University of the Marche Region, School of Medicine, United Hospitals, Ancona, Italy

Valeria Sotte Medical Oncology, Polytechnic University of the Marche Region, School of Medicine, United Hospitals, Ancona, Italy

Annalisa Trama Evaluative Epidemiology, Fondazione IRCCS Istituto Nazionale dei Tumori di Milano, Milan, Italy

Part I

Testicular Tumors: Epidemiology

Epidemiology of Testicular Cancer 1

Gemma Gatta and Annalisa Trama

Descriptive Epidemiology

Introduction

Although testicular cancers are rare, accounting for only 1 % of all cancers in males, in many countries they are the most common malignancy in young men (15–35 years) [1]. Approximately 98 % of testicular cancers are germ cell tumors (GCTs); the remaining 2 % are sex cord tumors (including Leydig cell and Sertoli cell tumors), rhabdomyosarcomas, and lymphomas [1].

The age-standardized incidence rate for testicular cancers ranges widely across the world. Figure 1.1 shows the incidence of testicular cancers across different continents in 2012. White males living in Western industrialized countries, particularly in Northern and Western Europe, had the highest incidence rates of testicular tumors (12/100,000 in Denmark, Norway, and Switzerland), whereas the incidence was lowest among black males in Africa (<0.5/100,000 in the majority of African countries). In Australia and New Zealand, the incidence was 7/100,000; in North America (the USA and Canada), 5/100,000; and in South and Central America, 2/100,000, with differences between countries (Chile, 7/100,000; Uruguay, 6/100,000; Argentina and Costa Rica, 5/100,000; Mexico and Colombia, 3/100,000; Brazil, 2/100,000; and the remaining countries, <1/100,000). In Japan, the incidence was 2/100,000; in Southern, Eastern, and Central Asia, <1/100,000, while it was higher in Western Asia (1.7/100,000) with regional differences (5/100,000 in Israel, 3/100,000 in Georgia, and <1 in Oman, Qatar, Iraq, and Azerbaijan). In China, the incidence was 0.5/100,000 [2].

The testicular cancer incidence has increased in many Western countries and is still rising in most European countries [3]. By contrast, the mortality has declined since the mid-1970s; this is attributable to the development of effective treatments that are typically multidisciplinary and centered around platinum-based chemotherapy. However, recent trend analyses (1980–2010) showed a leveling-off of the rates in the most recent calendar years, suggesting that a plateau in mortality has been reached [4]. In the period 2000–2008, EUROCARE estimated the pooled 5-year relative survival to be 89 % for European testicular cancer patients, with some differences between countries including lower survival in Eastern European countries [5].

Here, we describe the epidemiology of testicular cancers on the basis of data from European population-based cancer registries (CRs) analyzed in the framework of RARECAREnet, the Information Network on Rare Cancers (www.rarecarenet.eu).

G. Gatta (✉) • A. Trama
Evaluative Epidemiology, Fondazione IRCCS Istituto Nazionale dei Tumori di Milano, Milan, Italy
e-mail: gemma.gatta@istitutotumori.mi.it; annalisa.trama@istitutotumori.mi.it

M. Colecchia (ed.), *Pathology of Testicular and Penile Neoplasms*,
DOI 10.1007/978-3-319-27617-5_1

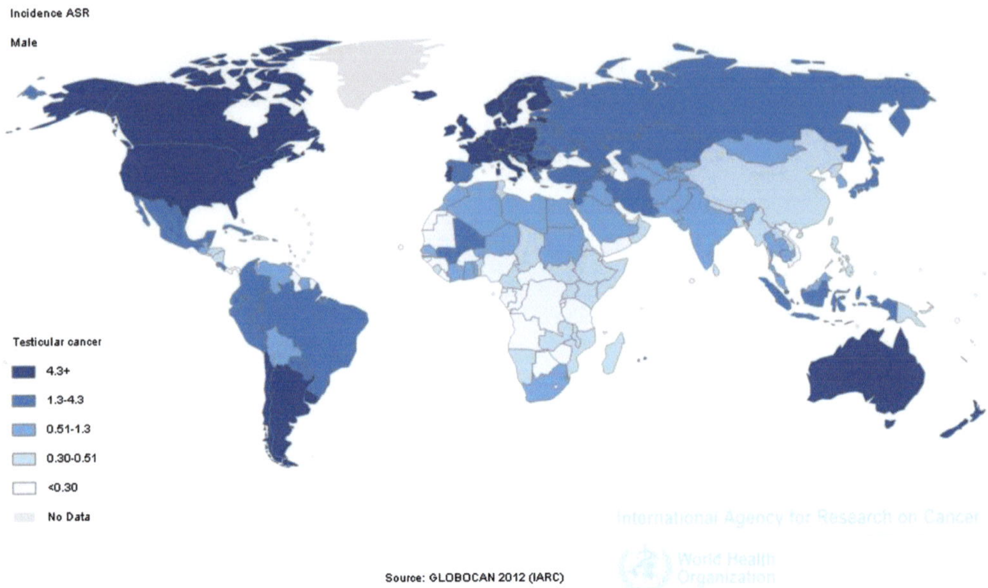

Fig. 1.1 Age-standardized world testicular cancer incidence rates per 100,000

Materials

We have chosen to use the RARECAREnet project because testicular cancer is a rare disease, and even if CRs collect data on the basis of the *International Classification of Diseases for Oncology* (ICD-O-3) [6], which includes morphology and topography, cancer statistics are usually given for broad cancer categories based on the anatomic site of the malignancies. Thus, in the current statistics, it is not possible to find information on testicular-specific histologic types. RARECAREnet, building on the experience of the previous project, RARECARE [7], classifies cancer entities on the basis of topography and morphology into a two-tier system. Tier 1 is the more general category and contains tier 2 subcategories. Tier 1 cancers are considered to involve the same clinical expertise and patient referral structure; tier 2 entities are considered to be similar from the point of view of clinical management and research. In this chapter, we investigated cancers belonging to the RARECAREnet tier 1 category "testicular and paratesticular cancers," which comprises six tier 2 entities: paratesticular adenocarcinoma, nonseminomatous testicular cancer, seminomatous testicular cancer, spermatocytic seminoma, teratoma with malignant transformation, and testicular sex cord cancer, as well as not otherwise specified (NOS) entities which cannot be assigned to a tier 2 category (Table 1.1).

RARECAREnet Project

RARECAREnet gathered European population-based CR data on patients diagnosed from 1978 up to 2007, with vital status information available up to 31 December 2008. RARECAREnet is one of the EUROCARE-related projects (www.eurocare.it). EUROCARE is the widest collaborative research project on cancer survival in Europe. The project started in 1989, and the fifth edition, EUROCARE-5, includes data on more than 21 million cancer diagnoses provided by 116 CRs in 30 European countries.

Since RARECAREnet aims to provide information on the burden of rare cancers in the European population, incidence rates were estimated as the number of new cases occurring in 2000–2007 divided by the total person-years in the general population (male and female) in each CR area over the same period.

Table 1.1 The two-tier structure of the RARECARE list of cancers illustrated for testicular and paratesticular cancers

Tier	Tumor	ICD-O-3 topography code	ICD-O-3 morphology code
1	*Testicular and paratesticular cancers*	C62, C63.0, C63.1	*C63.0, C63.1*: 8000, 8001, 8004, 8010,8011, 8012, 8120, 8123, 8140–8141, 8147, 8190, 8200, 8210–8211, 8221, 8230, 8231, 8255, 8260, 8261–8263, 8290, 8310, 8320, 8323, 8333, 8380–8384, 8401, 8430, 8440–8441, 8460–8461, 8470, 8480–8490, 8504, 8510, 8512, 8514, 8525, 8542, 8550–8551, 8560, 8562–8576 *C62*: 8000, 8001, 8590–8592, 8630–8640, 8650, 9060–9085, 9100–9102
2	Paratesticular adenocarcinoma with variants	C63.0, C63.1	8120, 8123, 8140–8141, 8147, 8190, 8200, 8210–8211, 8221, 8230, 8231, 8255, 8260, 8261–8263, 8290, 8310, 8320, 8323, 8333, 8380–8384, 8401, 8430, 8440–8441, 8460, 8470, 8480–8490, 8504, 8510, 8512, 8514, 8525, 8542, 8550–8551, 8560, 8562–8576
2	Nonseminomatous testicular cancer	C62	9080–9083, 9085, 9100–9102, 9065, 9070–9072
2	Seminomatous testicular cancer	C62	9060–9062
2	Spermatocytic seminoma	C62	9063
2	Teratoma with malignant transformation	C62	9084
2	Testicular sex cord cancer	C62	8630–8640, 8650, 8590–8592

Relative survival is the ratio between the measured survival of patients and the expected survival in the general population for the same region (or country), age, sex, and calendar year. Relative survival accounts for the mortality from causes other than the relevant cancer. Relative survival estimates were obtained using the complete approach [8], considering cases diagnosed between 2000 and 2007 and followed up to 31 December 2008.

The observed prevalence per 100,000 at the index date 1 January 2008 was estimated by the counting method [9], using data from incident cases in the period 1993–2007. CRs that started recently do not have records of longer-term cancer survivors who were diagnosed before the registry started, resulting in underestimation of the prevalence. To account for this problem, RARECARE estimated the complete prevalence using the completeness index method [10], where the estimated surviving cases diagnosed prior to 1993 were added to those counted in 1993–2007. Complete prevalence was provided at the index date of 1 January 2008. All data presented were extracted from the RARECAREnet online analysis tool.

Incidence

The total crude incidence of testicular and paratesticular cancers was 33/1,000,000 person-years, 55 % of which were seminomatous and 38 % were nonseminomatous forms. The age-adjusted incidence of these cancers in the male population was 64/1,000,000. A total of 16,061 of these cancers were estimated to be diagnosed in 2013 in the 28 EU member states. Seminomatous testicular cancer was the most common entity with a total crude incidence of

Table 1.2 Crude and age-adjusted incidence in Europe (rate per 1,000,000/year) and 95 % confidence intervals (CI) with estimated number of new cases in 2013 in EU28

Cancer entity	Incidence				Estimated new cases in 2013 in EU28
	Crude rate	95 % CI	Age-adjusted rate	95 % CI	
Testicular and paratesticular cancers	32.94	32.66–33.23	32.25	31.97–32.53	16,061
Paratesticular adenocarcinoma	0.01	0.01–0.02	0.01	0.01–0.02	8
Nonseminomatous testicular cancer	12.66	12.48–12.84	12.74	12.57–12.92	6,036
Seminomatous testicular cancer	18.20	17.99–18.41	17.55	17.35–17.76	8,961
Spermatocytic seminoma	0.32	0.29–0.35	0.29	0.26–0.32	171
Teratoma with malignant transformation	0.01	0.01–0.02	0.01	0.01–0.02	6
Testicular sex cord cancer	0.22	0.19–0.24	0.20	0.18–0.23	113

Source: RARECAREnet (www.rarecarenet.eu)
Pool of 42 European cancer registries (RARECAREnet)

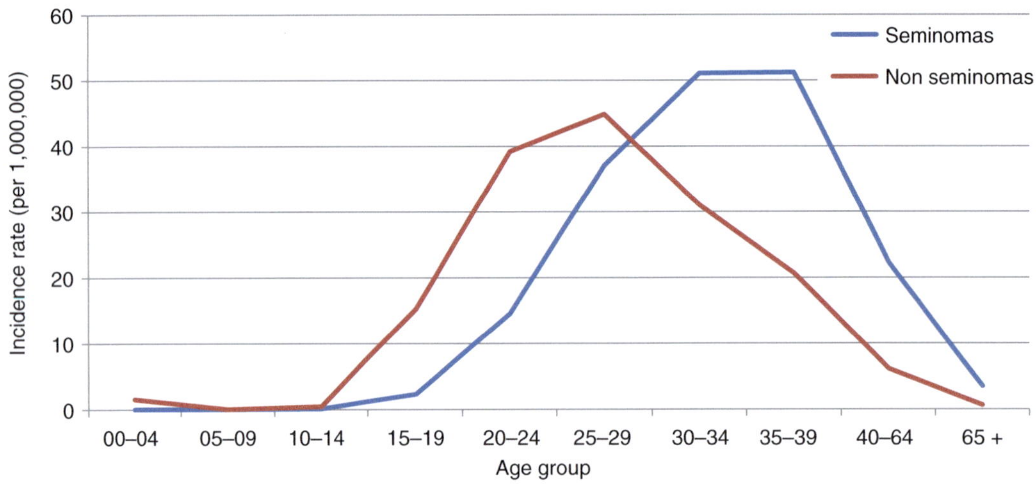

Fig. 1.2 (EUROCARE) Testicular germ cell tumor incidence per 1,000,000 by age group and histology (Source: Trama and Berrino [11])

18/1,000,000, followed by nonseminomatous testicular cancer (13/1,000,000) (Table 1.2).

GCTs have an early incidence peak in the age group 0–4 years followed by a second peak in adolescents and young adults (15–19, 25–29, and 30–34 years) (Fig. 1.2) [11]. The first peak is due to nonseminomas (incidence 1.5/1,000,000 vs. 0.07/1,000,000 for seminomas), specifically yolk sac tumors (YSTs) and teratomas, which have an incidence of 1/1,000,000 and 0.3/1,000,000, respectively. Nonseminomatous forms are more common than seminomas until the age of 30 years; however, the histologic types of patients in the age group between 15 and 30 years are mainly embryonal carcinomas and mixed GCTs and to a lesser extent teratomas and YSTs [11]. Beyond the age of 30, seminomas are predominant. Overall, seminomas present an incidence peak 10 years later than nonseminomas (Fig. 1.2) [11].

Table 1.3 shows the age-standardized incidence rates (period of diagnosis 2000–2007) by European regions. Nonseminomatous cancers

Table 1.3 Age-standardized incidence rates (per 1,000,000) for testicular and paratesticular cancers in 2000–2007 with 95 % confidence intervals (CI) by European region

	Northern Europe		Ireland and the UK		Central Europe		Southern Europe		Eastern Europe	
Cancer entity	Rate	95 % CI	Rate	95 %CI	Rate	95 % CI	Rate	95 % CI	Rate	95 % CI
Testicular and paratesticular cancers	37.75	36.40–39.14	33.11	32.61–33.61	37.96	37.39–38.54	24.72	24.02–25.32	27.41	26.81–28.02
Paratesticular adenocarcinoma	0.00	0.00–0.04	0.02	0.0–0.03	0.01	0.01–0.03	0.01	0.00–0.03	0.01	0.00–0.03
Nonseminomatous testicular cancer	16.88	15.97–17.83	12.18	11.87–12.49	14.88	14.51–15.25	10.15	9.76–10.55	11.87	11.48–12.28
Seminomatous testicular cancer	19.88	18.92–20.88	19.14	18.77–19.52	21.34	20.92–21.77	11.86	11.46–12.28	13.36	12.94–13.80
Spermatocytic seminoma	0.16	0.09–0.27	0.22	0.18–0.27	0.27	0.22–0.32	0.26	0.21–0.33	0.51	0.43–0.60
Teratoma with malignant transformation	0.07	0.02–0.15	0.00	0.00–0.01	0.02	0.01–0.04	0.01	0.00–0.03	0.01	0.00–0.03
Testicular sex cord cancer	0.15	0.08–0.25	0.22	0.18–0.27	0.22	0.18–0.27	0.21	0.15–0.27	0.15	0.11–0.20

Source: RARECAREnet (www.rarecarenet.eu)

European regions:

Northern Europe (Finland, Norway, Iceland)

Central Europe (Austria, Belgium, France, Germany, Switzerland, the Netherlands)

Southern Europe (Italy, Malta, Portugal, Slovenia, Spain)

Eastern Europe (Bulgaria, Croatia, Czech Republic, Estonia, Latvia, Lithuania, Slovakia Republic, Poland)

Ireland and the UK

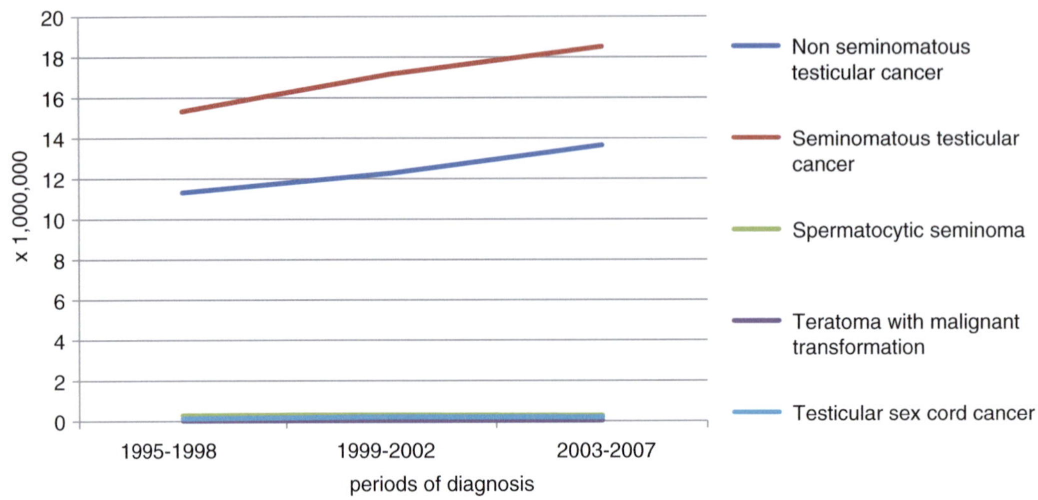

Fig. 1.3 Age-adjusted incidence rate (per 1,000,000) in Europe by cancer entity and period of diagnosis (1995–1998, 1999–2002, 2003–2007) – European standard population (Source: RARECAREnet (www.rarecarenet.eu))

had the highest incidence (17/1,000,000) in Northern Europe. The incidence of seminomatous cancers was highest in Northern and Central Europe (about 20/1,000,000) followed closely by the UK and Ireland (19/1,000,000) and more distantly by Eastern and Southern Europe. The incidence rates for the other cancers varied relatively little between regions.

Figure 1.3 shows the incidence trends for the different histologic types of testicular cancer. Seminomatous and nonseminomatous cancers have an increasing incidence trend, while no major increase is observed for the other histologies.

Several groups of investigators have reported an increasing incidence of testicular cancer over the last 20 years [12–15]. A recent population-based study from the USA revealed a significant increase in the incidence of testicular GCTs in both white and black males in the period 1973–2007. Remarkably, the incidence was much higher among whites. Because of the small sample, other ethnic origins were excluded from the study [12]. In Finland, the incidence rates of several histologic subtypes of testicular GCT have increased over the last four decades, particularly from 1990 onwards, yet the increasing trend was only seen in men aged 15–44 years [14]. In Germany, the annual incidence rate of testicular GCTs increased over the entire period (1998–2008), with seminomas accounting for most of the increase [2]. Similar results were reported by Arora et al. [15] in the UK for the period 1979–2003.

Survival

The 5-year relative survival was 95 % for testicular and paratesticular cancers (Fig. 1.4). Among these cancer types, seminomatous forms had the highest survival rate (98 %; 95 % confidence interval [CI] 97–98) followed by spermatocytic seminomas (95 %; 95 % CI 92–98) and nonseminomatous forms (93 %; 95 % CI 93–93). The 5-year relative survival was also good for sex cord tumors (82 %; 95 % CI 77–88) and paratesticular adenocarcinomas (82 %; 95 % CI 65–100), although the estimates for the latter two were based on five cases only (Fig. 1.4). Survival was consistently lower for patients aged 65 years or more than for younger patients (Table 1.4).

As regards survival by European region, the 5-year relative survival for testicular and paratesticular cancers was 97 % in Northern Europe, the UK, and Ireland, 96 % in Central Europe, 95 % in Southern Europe, and 88 % in Eastern Europe. Survival differences between the regions were

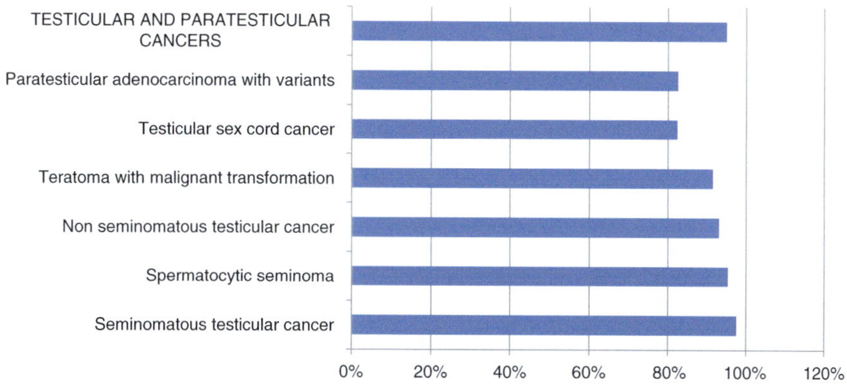

Fig. 1.4 Five-year relative survival (%) for testicular and paratesticular cancers in Europe in 2000–2007. Error bars are 95 % confidence intervals (Source: RARECAREnet (www.rarecarenet.eu))

small for seminomas, but more marked for nonseminomatous cancer, ranging from 85 % in Eastern Europe to 96 % in Northern Europe (Table 1.4).

There is little room for survival improvement among testicular seminoma patients, especially those aged <50 years. Older testicular cancer patients remain at increased risk of death, which seems mainly attributable to the lower survival of nonseminoma patients [16]. With regard to survival trends, in Europe, no major improvement in the survival of testicular cancer patients has been observed for both seminomatous and nonseminomatous forms since 1999 (Table 1.5).

A study from the Netherlands analyzing incidence and survival trends over the period 1989–2009 found significant survival changes for patients with regional lymph node involvement and distant metastases. This was attributed to improved chemotherapy, improved postchemotherapy retroperitoneal lymph node dissection, and referral of more complex patients to specialized centers [17]. Stage-related information was not systematically available from CRs and could therefore not be analyzed by RARECAREnet.

A survival improvement, from 1993 to 2007, among European and American patients with testicular cancer was observed for seminoma and nonseminoma patients in the age range 50–84 years, suggesting that increasing effectiveness of therapy was achieved among these patients [16].

Prevalence

Complete prevalence estimates in Europe point to testicular/paratesticular cancers being among the most curable solid cancers, with 475,737 prevalent cases in 2008, the majority of which surviving more than 15 years. The most prevalent testicular cancers were seminomatous forms (263,569 cases), followed by nonseminomatous forms (214,604 cases). Prevalence is pushed up by the young age of patients at diagnosis and the increasing incidence trend, but high survival (discussed above) appears as the most important contributor to the prevalence of these survivors.

Risk Factors

Descriptive epidemiology studies revealed considerable geographic, ethnic, and temporal variations in testicular cancer incidence, with an at least 30-fold variation in risk worldwide: according to *Cancer Incidence in Five Continents* (2003–2007), the annual incidence rates per 100,000 ranged from 0.1 in Congo, Ruanda, and Guinea to 12 in Chile (Valdivia) [18]. Men of European origin in the USA had rates five times higher than their African-origin counterparts [18].

In many high-risk areas, such as Europe and North America, white men have experienced greater increases in incidence throughout the late twentieth century than any other ethnic group. Uniform increases in incidence between 3 % and

Table 1.4 Five-year relative survival (number of cases and %) for testicular and paratesticular cancers with 95 % confidence intervals (CI) by age and European region for 2000–2007

		Testicular and paratesticular cancers			Nonseminomatous testicular cancer			Seminomatous testicular cancer		
		Cases (N)	Survival %	95 % CI	Cases (N)	Survival %	95 % CI	Cases (N)	Survival %	95 % CI
Age	0–14	206	97	94–100	176	97 %	94–100	9	89	71–100
	15–24	7,406	94	94–95	5,492	94	93–93	1,515	97	96–98
	25–64	42,103	96	95–96	13,889	93	92–93	26,091	98	98–98
	≥65	1,308	73	69–77	161	70	60–81	716	82	77–87
Region	Northern Europe	2,937	97	97–98	1,281	96	95–97	1,594	99	98–100
	Central Europe	16,864	96	96–96	6,347	94	94–95	9,801	98	97–98
	Eastern Europe	7,722	88	88–89	3,383	85	84–87	3,783	93	92–94
	Southern Europe	6,589	95	94–95	2,615	93	92–94	3,233	97	96–98
	Ireland and the UK	16,899	97	96–97	6,088	95	94–96	9,915	99	98–99

Source: RARECAREnet (www.rarecarenet.eu)

European regions:

Northern Europe (Finland, Norway, Iceland)
Central Europe (Austria, Belgium, France, Germany, Switzerland, the Netherlands)
Southern Europe (Italy, Malta, Portugal, Slovenia, Spain)
Eastern Europe (Bulgaria, Croatia, Czech Republic, Estonia, Latvia, Lithuania, Slovakia Republic, Poland)
Ireland and the UK

Table 1.5 Five-year relative survival (RS) with number of cases and 95 % confidence intervals (CI) in Europe by cancer entity and calendar period (1999–2001, 2002–2004, 2005–2007) – Period approach

	1999–2001			2002–2004			2005–2007		
Cancer entity	Cases (N)	RS (%)	95 % CI	Cases (N)	RS (%)	95 % CI	Cases (N)	RS (%)	95 % CI
Testicular and paratesticular cancers	13,112	94	94–95	14,046	95	94–95	14,796	95	95–96
Nonseminomatous testicular cancer	5,143	93	92–93	5,497	92	91–93	5,796	93	93–94
Seminomatous testicular cancer	7,293	97	97–98	7,844	97	97–98	8,233	98	98–98
Spermatocytic seminoma	143	95	89–100	148	99	94–100	144	96	90–100
Testicular sex cord cancer	73	86	76–96	91	86	77–94	93	79	70–89

Source: RARECAREnet (www.rarecarenet.eu)

6 % per annum have been reported in long-term trends [19]. In a number of countries, analyses of testicular cancer incidence trends have found the increases to be more consistent with a birth-cohort effect than with a calendar-period effect. For example, men born during World War II in Denmark had a lower risk of testicular cancer at all ages than men born in the preceding or subsequent periods [20].

Studies on migrants have been reported for Sweden [21], Israel [22], and the USA [23]. The cancer risk among immigrants and their offspring was analyzed from the data of the Swedish Family Cancer Database and the Swedish population-based cancer registries. First-generation immigrants to Sweden generally showed a decreased risk of testicular cancer compared with native Swedes, but the difference tended to disappear in the next generation born in Sweden [21].

Data on 1,092,373 Jewish Israeli males who underwent a general health check prior to compulsory military service at ages 16–19 between the years 1967 and 2005 were linked to the Israel National Cancer Registry to obtain the testicular cancer incidence figures up to 2006. Based on about 1,000 testicular cancer cases, the study revealed a remarkably low incidence for North African-born men (HR = 0.10) and Asian-born men (HR = 0.35), while there was an intermediate risk for men born in Israel but of North African (HR 0.48) or Asian origin (HR 0.56) compared to European origin. The risk was twice as high for men of North African or Asian origin born in Israel versus those born in North Africa or Asia [22].

Between 1992 and 2010, the annual incidence of testicular GCTs among Hispanic whites in the USA aged 15–39 years increased by 58 %, from 7.18 cases per 100,000 in 1992 to 11.34 cases per 100,000 by 2010. During the same 19-year interval the incidence among non-Hispanic white young adults increased by 7 %, from 12.41 to 13.22 per 100,000. During the 2000–2010 period, no significant incidence trends were observed among non-Hispanic whites [23].

The rapid increase in the incidence of testicular cancer over the past 50 years and the results from studies on migrants suggest that critical changes in environmental factors may contribute to the development of these tumors.

Undescended testis, or cryptorchidism, is the most recognized risk factor for testicular cancer [24]. Cryptorchidism is one of the commonest abnormalities, occurring in 2–5 % of boys born at term. [25] The risk of cancer is increased two- to eightfold in men who have had undescended testes. Five to 10 % of all men with testicular cancer have a history of cryptorchidism [25, 26].

Treatment for undescended testis before puberty can prevent testicular cancer. A cohort of about 20,000 Swedish boys treated for cryptorchidism with orchiopexy from 1964 to 1999 and followed up until the end of 2000 indicates that age at orchiopexy has an effect on the risk of testicular cancer in boys with an undescended testicle. Those treated at 13 years or older had a relative risk of 5.4 compared with the general population, about twice the risk of those treated at younger ages [27]. In the Swedish study, the risk of testicular cancer increased in the entire cohort regardless of age at surgery, supporting the hypothesis that the risk of testicular cancer is largely determined in utero and also suggesting that puberty is another crucial event in testicular carcinogenesis. Findings from a subsequent meta-analysis further support that early surgery reduces the risk of testicular cancer among cryptorchid men [28].

Other factors clearly associated with the risk of testicular cancer are prior unilateral testicular cancer and a family history of testicular cancer. From the Swedish Family Cancer Database, it appeared that the incidence ratios for familial risk were almost four- and eightfold increased when the father or a brother had testicular cancer, respectively [29].

From several studies, it emerges that a previous history of testicular cancer is strongly associated with a second cancer in the contralateral testis. Two studies from the Netherlands and New Zealand reported an increased risk of a contralateral tumor in patients who had previously had testicular cancer; the relative risk was as high as 25–28 [30, 31]. A large population-based cohort study involving about 30,000 US men estimated a lower risk: testis cancer patients had a 12 times greater risk of developing metachronous contralateral testicular cancer than men in the general population [32].

A systematic review of pre- and perinatal variables in relation to the risk of testicular cancer with a focus on maternal characteristics [33] revealed evidence for associations with maternal bleeding (odds ratio, OR = 1.33), birth order (first vs. others, OR = 1.08), and sibship size (OR ranging from 0.93 to 0.75 for 2, 3, 4 vs. 1). Three large US studies also found cesarean section to be associated with the risk of testicular cancer (OR = 1.67) [33]. The meta-analyses indicated no association with maternal age, maternal nausea, maternal hypertension, preeclampsia, and breech delivery. Bleeding is generally the result of a developmental aberration such as abnormal placental differentiation or aggressive implantation, which may be hypothesized to disrupt fetal development and increase the risk of a prenatal stem-cell progenitor of testicular cancer. Parental subfertility was suggested among the underlying causes of the association with birth order and sibship size [34]. Furthermore, all of the studied variables could theoretically be due to an altered in utero hormonal milieu [35–38] and delayed exposure to a communicable agent for the son [39, 40].

Another systematic review and meta-analysis of perinatal variables with a focus on characteristics of the son provided evidence that low birth weight, low gestational age, inguinal hernia, cryptorchidism, and twinning were associated with a higher risk of testicular cancer [24]. The ORs ranged between 1.63 and 1.22, with the exclusion of cryptorchidism, where the OR was as high as 4.3. A subsequent Swedish study confirmed that genital malformations were associated with an increased risk of testicular cancer; in addition to cryptorchidism and inguinal hernia, also hypospadias was reported, with an OR of 2.4 [41]. It should be taken into consideration that some of these factors are interconnected and could arguably be proxies of the maternal in utero environment. There is evidence that exposure to maternal hormones, particularly estrogens, is associated with testicular GCT risk (OR = 4.9) [42].

With the improvements in recent decades of the survival of premature infants, an increased frequency of testis cancers arising among survivors of premature birth may have contributed to an increase in testicular cancer rates.

Exposure to endocrine-disrupting chemicals (EDCs) during the fetal period has been postulated to be a risk factor for testicular cancer [43]. EDCs are able to interact with human endocrine systems such as the system of the sex hormones testosterone and estrogen. They can act either directly or indirectly, for example, by blocking hormone receptors or altering hormone degradation [43]. Pentachlorophenol, bisphenol A, and phthalates are examples of known EDCs to which humans are exposed via the environment. In a Swedish study, the concentrations of chlorinated biphenyls (PCBs), p,p'-dichlorodiphenyldichloroethylene, hexachlorobenzene, chlordanes, and polybrominated diphenyl ethers were higher in blood from mothers of testicular cancer patients compared with control mothers [44]. For the sum of PCBs, an OR of 3.8 was estimated. Most of the patients were born during a period with the highest concentrations of persistent organic pollutants (POPs) such as PCBs in the ecological system. Since then the concentrations have fallen substantially. In Sweden, the large difference in the increase in testicular cancer incidence between 1984–1993 and 1994–2003 supports the hypothesis that exposure to certain POPs during the fetal period is of etiologic significance in testicular carcinogenesis. EDC research will need to assess these chemicals in the most appropriate specimen to ensure accurate EDC exposure assessment during pregnancy. Currently, there are no studies evaluating the association between placental concentrations of EDCs and risk of any testicular dysgenesis syndrome (TDS) condition. Furthermore, effect modifications of the EDC–TDS associations by potential genetic factors or inflammatory processes have not been evaluated to date.

Average stature and the incidence of testicular cancer have both been increasing over several generations with strong cohort effects [45]. A systematic review and meta-analysis analyzed the relation between body size and testicular cancer, but confirmed the association with stature only, with an OR of 1.13 per 5 cm increase in height. Possible mechanisms to explain the association of stature with testicular cancer risk include childhood nutrition [46], increased levels of insulin-like growth factor [47, 48], and earlier age at puberty in those of greater height. [49, 50] As adult stature is largely determined in the period between birth and age 2 years [50], nutrition at this age may be particularly relevant to the testicular cancer risk [51].

Diet has been associated with testicular cancer in many studies. Dairy products, mainly milk and cheese, have been found to be linked with testicular cancer. These foods contain the female sex hormones estrogen and progesterone [52]. It is reasonable to hypothesize that estrogen or progesterone in milk and dairy products may be associated with the development of testicular cancer [53]. The strength of this association is further supported by the recent increasing trend in testicular cancer incidence and the increased consumption of dairy products in developed countries, which started in the 1940s and 1950s [54]. Furthermore, the level of estrogens in dairy products may be influenced by the treatment of cattle with hormones and antibiotics. A large Canadian population-based case–control study [55] involving about 600 cases investigated 21 foods or food groups and 15 nutrients and found an increased testicular cancer risk for high dairy product intake. In particular, an almost double risk was found for high intake of cheese, while no relation to milk intake was reported. However, in other studies conducted in the UK [56] and Germany [57], a relation to milk was found. The German case–control study [57] found a relative risk (RR) of 1.4 per additional 20 servings of milk per month in adolescence and a highest risk of seminoma (RR = 1.7). A subsequent American study did not find any relation between childhood dairy consumption and testicular cancer [51]. Therefore, given the contrasting evidence on whether dietary factors are associated with testis cancer, a joint review conducted by the World Cancer Research Fund and American Institute of Cancer Research in 2007 concluded that the current evidence did not warrant a thorough investigation of the potential links between food, nutrition, and testicular cancer [58].

Several occupational exposures have been suggested to be associated with testicular cancer, such as exposure to PCBs, electromagnetic fields, and pesticides. In addition, several occupations have been linked to testicular cancer: firefighters, police, military personnel, agricultural workers, and industrial workers (paper, plastic, metal) [59, 60]. Two occupations—firefighting and aircraft maintenance—are likely to be associated with testicular cancer due to environmental exposure to specific organochlorine compounds [60]. The association of testicular cancer with firefighting originates from reports of a statistically significant increased risk among firefighters in New Zealand [61, 62]. This association was supported by subsequent studies in California [63] and Florida [64] that also found significantly increased risks of testicular cancer, as well as by a study in Germany that reported a trend toward an increased risk [65]. The latest review on this topic produced a summary risk estimate of 2 [66]. The association of firefighting with the risk of testicular cancer might be related to exposure to a wide variety of carcinogenic substances, including benzene and polycyclic aromatic hydrocarbons. Mortality due to testicular cancers in a very large cohort of aircraft manufacturing workers was almost double compared to the general population, possibly due to mixed solvent exposure. An excess risk was also found among pesticide applicators in the USA [67] and the UK [68]. A study from Norway [69] reported an increased incidence of testicular cancer in farmers' sons, whereas studies from Denmark [70] and the USA [71] have not replicated this finding.

In the early 2000s, molecular epidemiologic findings of serum levels of pesticides have been made available to better assess the environmental exposure. The pesticides that have been most commonly examined to date are the organochlorine compounds. These are among the oldest pesticides used and are persistent both in the environment and in human adipose tissue [72]. In addition, organochlorine compounds can mimic sex steroid hormones and might therefore alter gene expression patterns that are important in urogenital development and homeostasis [73, 74]. Organochlorine pesticides include dichlorodiphenyltrichloroethane (DDT), its most persistent metabolite dichlorodiphenyldichloroethylene (DDE), and many others. Current evidence suggests that of the organochlorine pesticides examined, only DDE and chlordanes are associated with an increased risk of testicular cancer [60]. However, the available evidence has not permitted the identification of strong and consistent occupational risk factors for testicular cancer. Since testicular cancer occurs mainly in young adults, the potential impact of occupational exposure of mothers to endocrine disruptors during intrauterine development has to be considered [60, 75]. Other exposures – to heat, polyvinyl chloride, nonionizing radiation, heavy metals, agricultural work, and PCBs as well as marijuana use – might also have an association with testicular cancer [60].

Final Remarks

The testicular cancer incidence has increased in the past five decades and is now increasing in some countries and ethnic groups historically at low risk. Cryptorchidism is the condition most evidently related to testicular cancer. Among the potentially modifiable risk factors, studies of the age at surgery for cryptorchidism suggest that treating undescended testes before puberty reduces the risk of testicular cancer.

Cryptorchidism with hypospadias and poor semen quality together make up the TDS; they result from disrupted embryonal programming and gonadal development, possibly caused by exposures of environmental origin [75]. Several studies were conducted on diet, primarily focused on dietary patterns during early life. Although the evidence is not conclusive, diet especially in early life and puberty is likely to be very important in reducing the risk of many chronic diseases and cancers in adult life. One can further investigate these hypotheses, but from the public health point of view we believe the current state of knowledge is sufficient to implement programs to contrast the so-called Western diet.

Some occupations are likely to be associated with testicular cancer, and occupational exposure to PVC, PCBs, and organochlorine compounds requires further study. However, exposure to professional risks in agriculture and environmental exposure may occur in utero and/or act as perinatal and nonperinatal risk factors. Organochlorine compounds, especially those included in pesticides, are widely dispersed among populations and may be responsible for a large proportion of the attributable risk. In this case, the principle of precaution should be considered to promote policies of risk reduction (Table 1.6).

The low incidence of testicular cancer often constituted a barrier to conducting adequately powered epidemiologic studies. Collaborative

Table 1.6 European complete prevalence (per 1,000,000) with 95 % confidence intervals (CI) at 1 January 2008 with estimated number of prevalent cases in 2008 in EU28 by testicular cancer histology

	Complete prevalence	95 %CI	Prevalent cases by 2008 in EU28
Testicular and paratesticular cancers	93.52	92.27–94.77	475,737
Paratesticular adenocarcinoma	0.01	0.00–0.02	58
Nonseminomatous testicular cancer	42.23	40.80–43.67	214,604
Seminomatous testicular cancer	51.73	50.75–52.70	263,569
Teratoma with malignant transformation	0.04	0.01–0.08	214
Testicular sex cord cancer	0.42	0.36–0.47	2,128

Source: RARECAREnet (www.rarecarenet.eu)

investigations that pool data from a number of countries are strongly encouraged. International collaborative studies should allow more adequately powered epidemiologic studies. In order to provide new ideas and hypotheses to be examined in such studies, a survey was conducted among testicular cancer researchers on new hypotheses concerning the etiology of the malignancy [76]. Hypotheses with the highest plausibility ratings were related to prenatal exposures and exposures that might have an effect during pregnancy and in postnatal life. They included factors related to endocrine disruption, DNA damage, inflammation, and nutrition during pregnancy. The results of the survey should promote a multidisciplinary debate and enhance new etiologic research into testicular cancers.

Acknowledgments This chapter arises from the project RARECAREnet which has received funding from the European Union in the framework of the Health Programme.

References

1. Chia VM, Quraishi SM, Devesa SS, Purdue MP, Cook MB, McGlynn KA. International trends in the incidence of testicular cancer, 1973–2002. Cancer Epidemiol Biomarkers Prev. 2010;19:1151–9.
2. Ferlay J, Soerjomataram I, Ervik M, Dikshit R, Eser S, Mathers C, Rebelo M, Parkin DM, Forman D, Bray, F. GLOBOCAN 2012 v1.0, Cancer incidence and mortality worldwide: IARC CancerBase No. 11 [Internet]. Lyon: International Agency for Research on Cancer; 2013. Available from: http://globocan.iarc.fr. Accessed on 29 Dec 2014.
3. Znaor A, Lortet-Tieulent J, Laversanne M, Jemal A, Bray F. International testicular cancer incidence trends: generational transitions in 38 countries 1900–1990. Cancer Causes Control. 2015;26:151–8.
4. Bosetti C, Bertuccio P, Malvezzi M, Levi F, Chatenoud L, Negri E, La Vecchia C. Cancer mortality in Europe, 2005–2009, and an overview of trends since 1980. Ann Oncol. 2013;24:2657–71.
5. Trama A, Foschi R, Larrañagab N, Sant M, Fuentes-Raspall R, Serraino D, Tavilla A, Van Eycken L, Nicolai N, the EUROCARE-5 Working Group. Survival of male genital cancers (prostate, testis and penis) in Europe 1999–2007: results from the Eurocare-5 study. Eur J Cancer. 2015; in press.
6. Percy C, Fritz A, Jack A, Shanmugarathan S, Sobin L, Parkin DM, Whelan S. International Classification of Diseases for Oncology (ICD-O). 3rd ed. Geneva: World Health Organisation; 2000.
7. Gatta G, van der Zwan JM, Casali PG, Siesling S, Dei Tos AP, Kunkler I, Otter R, Licitra L, Mallone S, Tavilla A, Trama A. Capocaccia R; RARECARE working group. rare cancers are not so rare: the rare cancer burden in Europe. Eur J Cancer. 2011;47:2493–511.
8. Brenner H, Gefeller O, Hakulinen T. Period analysis for 'up-to-date' cancer survival data: theory, empirical evaluation, computational realisation and applications. Eur J Cancer. 2004;40:326–35.
9. Capocaccia R, Colonna M, Corazziari I, De Angelis R, Francisci S, Micheli A, Mugno E, EUROPREVAL Working Group. Measuring cancer prevalence in Europe: the EUROPREVAL project. Ann Oncol. 2002;13:831–9.
10. Capocaccia R, De Angelis R. Estimating the completeness of prevalence based on cancer registry data. Stat Med. 1997;16:425–40.
11. Trama A, Berrino F. Epidemiology of malignant germ cell tumours. The EUROCARE study. In: Nogales FF, Jimenez R, editors. The pathology and biology of germ cell tumours. New York: Springer; 2017 (in print).
12. Stang A, Trabert B, Wentzensen N, Cook MB, Rusner C, Oosterhuis JW, McGlynn KA. Gonadal and extragonadal germ cell tumours in the United States, 1973–2007. Int J Androl. 2012;35:616–25.

13. Rusner C, Trabert B, Katalinic A, Kieschke J, Emrich K, Stang A, Network of German Cancer Registries (GEKID). Incidence patterns and trends of malignant gonadal and extragonadal germ cell tumors in Germany, 1998–2008. Cancer Epidemiol. 2013;37: 370–3.
14. Pauniaho SL, Salonen J, Helminen M, Vettenranta K, Heikinheimo M, Heikinheimo O. The incidences of malignant gonadal and extragonadal germ cell tumors in males and females: a population-based study covering over 40 years in Finland. Cancer Causes Control. 2012;23:1921–7.
15. Arora RS, Alston RD, Eden TO, Geraci M, Birch JM. Comparative incidence patterns and trends of gonadal and extragonadal germ cell tumors in England, 1979–2003. Cancer. 2012;118:4290–7.
16. Verhoeven RH, Gondos A, Janssen-Heijnen ML, Saum KU, Brewster DH, Holleczek B, Crocetti E, Rosso S, Hakulinen T, Aareleid T, Brenner H, EUNICE Survival Working Group. Testicular cancer in Europe and the USA: survival still rising among older patients. Ann Oncol. 2013;24:508–13.
17. Verhoeven RH, Karim-Kos HE, Coebergh JW, Brink M, Horenblas S, de Wit R, Kiemeney BA. Markedly increased incidence and improved survival of testicular cancer in the Netherlands. Acta Oncol. 2014;53:342–50.
18. Forman D, Bray F, Brewster DH, Gombe Mbalawa C, Kohler B, Piñeros M, Steliarova-Foucher E, Swaminathan R and Ferlay J, editors. Cancer incidence in five continents, Vol. X (electronic version). Lyon: International Agency for Research on Cancer; 2013. Available from: http://ci5.iarc.fr. Accessed on 20 July 2015.
19. Bray F, Richiardi L, Ekbom A, Forman D, Pukkala E, Cuninkova M, Møller H. Do testicular seminoma and nonseminoma share the same etiology? Evidence from an age-period-cohort analysis of incidence trends in eight European countries. Cancer Epidemiol Biomarkers Prev. 2006;15:652–8.
20. Møller H. Decreased testicular cancer risk in men born in wartime. J Natl Cancer Inst. 1989;81:1668–9.
21. Hemminki K, Li X. Cancer risks in Nordic immigrants and their offspring in Sweden. Eur J Cancer. 2002;38: 2428–34.
22. Levine H, Afek A, Shamiss A, Derazne E, Tzur D, Zavdy O, Barchana M, Kark JD. Risk of germ cell testicular cancer according to origin: a migrant cohort study in 1,100,000 Israeli men. Int J Cancer. 2013;132:1878–85.
23. Chien FL, Schwartz SM, Johnson RH. Increase in testicular germ cell tumor incidence among Hispanic adolescents and young adults in the United States. Cancer. 2014;120:2728–34.
24. Cook MB, Akre O, Forman D, Madigan MP, Richiardi L, McGlynn KA. A systematic review and meta-analysis of perinatal variables in relation to the risk of testicular cancer--experiences of the son. Int J Epidemiol. 2010;39:1605–18.
25. Toppari J, Kaleva M. Maldescendus testis. Horm Res. 1999;51:261–9.
26. Dieckmann KP, Pichlmeier U. Clinical epidemiology of testicular germ cell tumors. World J Urol. 2004; 22:2–14.
27. Pettersson A, Richiardi L, Nordenskjold A, Kaijser M, Akre O. Age at surgery for undescended testis and risk of testicular cancer. N Engl J Med. 2007;356:1835–41.
28. Banks K, Tuazon E, Berhane K, Koh CJ, De Filippo RE, Chang A, Kim SS, Daneshmand S, Davis-Dao C, Lewinger JP, Bernstein L, Cortessis VK. Cryptorchidism and testicular germ cell tumors: comprehensive meta-analysis reveals that association between these conditions diminished over time and is modified by clinical characteristics. Front Endocrinol (Lausanne). 2013; 3:182.
29. Hemminki K, Chen B. Familial risks in testicular cancer as aetiological clues. Int J Androl. 2006;29: 205–10.
30. Osterlind A, Berthelsen JG, Abildgaard N, Hansen SO, Hjalgrim H, Johansen B, Munck-Hansen J, Rasmussen LH. Risk of bilateral testicular germ cell cancer in Denmark: 1960–1984. J Natl Cancer Inst. 1991;83:1391–5.
31. Colls BM, Harvey VJ, Skelton L, Thompson PI, Frampton CM. Bilateral testicular germ cell tumours in New Zealand: experience in Auckland and Christchurch 1978–94. J Clin Oncol. 1996;14:2061–5.
32. Fosså SD, Chen J, Schonfeld SJ, McGlynn KA, McMaster ML, Gail MH, Travis LB. Risk of contralateral testicular cancer: a population-based study of 29,515 U.S. men. J Natl Cancer Inst. 2005;97:1056–66.
33. Cook MB, Akre O, Forman D, Madigan MP, Richiardi L, McGlynn KA. A systematic review and meta-analysis of perinatal variables in relation to the risk of testicular cancer–experiences of the mother. Int J Epidemiol. 2009;38:1532–42.
34. Richiardi L, Akre O, Lambe M, Granath F, Montgomery SM, Ekbom A. Birth order, sibship size, and risk for germ-cell testicular cancer. Epidemiology. 2004;15:323–9.
35. Bernstein L, Depue RH, Ross RK, Judd HL, Pike MC, Henderson BE. Higher maternal levels of free estradiol in first compared to second pregnancy: early gestational differences. J Natl Cancer Inst. 1986;76:1035–9.
36. Panagiotopoulou K, Katsouyanni K, Petridou E, Garas Y, Tzonou A, Trichopoulos D. Maternal age, parity, and pregnancy estrogens. Cancer Causes Control. 1990;1:119–24.
37. Troisi R, Hoover RN, Thadhani R, Hsieh CC, Sluss P, Ballard-Barbash R, Potischman N. Maternal, prenatal and perinatal characteristics and first trimester maternal serum hormone concentrations. Br J Cancer. 2008;99:1161–4.
38. Arslan AA, Zeleniuch-Jacquotte A, Lukanova A, Afanasyeva Y, Katz J, Levitz M, Del Priore G, Toniolo P. Effects of parity on pregnancy hormonal profiles across ethnic groups with a diverse incidence of breast cancer. Cancer Epidemiol Biomarkers Prev. 2006;15:2123–30.
39. Green MS, Zaaide Y. Sibship size as a risk factor for hepatitis a infection. Am J Epidemiol. 1989;129: 800–5.

40. Ford AC, Forman D, Bailey AG, Goodman KJ, Axon AT, Moayyedi P. Effect of sibling number in the household and birth order on prevalence of helicobacter pylori: a cross-sectional study. Int J Epidemiol. 2007;36:1327–33.
41. Trabert B, Zugna D, Richiardi L, McGlynn KA, Akre O. Congenital malformations and testicular germ cell tumors. Int J Cancer. 2013;133:1900–4.
42. Weir HK, Marrett LD, Kreiger N, Darlington GA, Sugar L. Pre-natal and peri-natal exposures and risk of testicular germ-cell cancer. Int J Cancer. 2000;87:438–43.
43. Wuttke W, Jarry H, Seidlova-Wuttke D. Definition, classification and mechanism of action of endocrine disrupting chemicals. Hormones (Athens). 2010;9:9–15.
44. Hardell L, van Bavel B, Lindström G, Carlberg M, Dreifaldt AC, Wijkström H, Starkhammar H, Eriksson M, Hallquist A, Kolmert T. Increased concentrations of polychlorinated biphenyls, hexachlorobenzene, and chlordanes in mothers of men with testicular cancer. Environ Health Perspect. 2003;111:930–4.
45. Cook MB, Chia VM, Berndt SI, Graubard BI, Chanock SJ, Rubertone MV, Erickson RL, Hayes RB, McGlynn KA. Genetic contributions to the association between adult height and testicular germ cell tumors. Int J Epidemiol. 2011;40:731–9.
46. Dieckmann KP, Pichlmeier U. Is risk of testicular cancer related to body size? Eur Urol. 2002;42: 564–9.
47. Juul A, Bang P, Hertel NT, Main K, Dalgaard P, Jørgensen K, Müller J, Hall K, Skakkebaek NE. Serum insulin-like growth factor-I in 1030 healthy children, adolescents, and adults: relation to age, sex, stage of puberty, testicular size, and body mass index. J Clin Endocrinol Metab. 1994;78:744–52.
48. Khandwala HM, McCutcheon IE, Flyvbjerg A, Friend KE. The effects of insulin-like growth factors on tumorigenesis and neoplastic growth. Endocr Rev. 2000;21:215–44.
49. Hägg U, Taranger J. Pubertal growth and maturity pattern in early and late maturers. a prospective longitudinal study of Swedish urban children. Swed Dent J. 1992;16:199–209.
50. Karlberg J. Secular trends in pubertal development. Horm Res. 2002;57:19–30.
51. McGlynn KA, Sakoda LC, Rubertone MV, Sesterhenn IA, Lyu C, Graubard BI, Erickson RL. Body size, dairy consumption, puberty, and risk of testicular germ cell tumors. Am J Epidemiol. 2007;165: 355–63.
52. Hartmann S, Lacorn M, Steinhart H. Natural occurrence of steroid hormones in food. Food Chem. 1998;62:7–20.
53. Ganmaa D, Li XM, Wang J, Qin LQ, Wang PY, Sato A. Incidence and mortality of testicular and prostatic cancers in relation to world dietary practices. Int J Cancer. 2002;98:262–7.
54. Sharpe RM, Skakkebaek NE. Are oestrogens involved in falling sperm counts and disorders of the male reproductive tract? Lancet. 1993;341:1392–5.
55. Garner MJ, Birkett NJ, Johnson KC, Shatenstein B, Ghadirian P, Krewski D, Canadian Cancer Registries Epidemiology Research Group. Dietary risk factors for testicular carcinoma. Int J Cancer. 2003;106: 934–41.
56. Davies TW, Palmer CR, Ruja E, Lipscombe JM. Adolescent milk, dairy product and fruit consumption and testicular cancer. Br J Cancer. 1996;74:657–60.
57. Stang A, Ahrens W, Baumgardt-Elms C, Stegmaier C, Merzenich H, de Vrese M, Schrezenmeir J, Jöckel KH. Adolescent milk fat and galactose consumption and testicular germ cell cancer. Cancer Epidemiol Biomarkers Prev. 2006;15:2189–95.
58. World Cancer Research Fund/American Institute for Cancer Research. Food, nutrition, physical activity and the prevention of cancer: a global perspective. Washington: AICR; 2007.
59. Charbotel B, Fervers B, Droz JP. Occupational exposures in rare cancers: a critical review of the literature. Crit Rev Oncol Hematol. 2014;90:99–134.
60. McGlynn KA, Trabert B. Adolescent and adult risk factors for testicular cancer. Nat Rev Urol. 2012; 9:339–49.
61. Bates MN, Fawcett J, Garrett N, Arnold R, Pearce N, Woodward A. Is testicular cancer an occupational disease of firefighters? Am J Ind Med. 2001;40: 263–70.
62. Bates MN, Lane L. Testicular cancer in firefighters: a cluster investigation. N Z Med J. 1995;108:334–7.
63. Bates MN. Registry-based case–control study of cancer in California firefighters. Am J Ind Med. 2007;50: 339–44.
64. Ma F, Fleming LE, Lee DJ, Trapido E, Gerace TA. Cancer incidence in Florida professional firefighters, 1981 to 1999. J Occup Environ Med. 2006;48:883–8.
65. Stang A, Jöckel KH, Baumgardt-Elms C, Ahrens W. Firefighting and risk of testicular cancer: results from a German population-based case–control study. Am J Ind Med. 2003;43:291–4.
66. LeMasters GK, Genaidy AM, Succop P, Deddens J, Sobeih T, Barriera-Viruet H, Dunning K, Lockey J. Cancer risk among firefighters: a review and meta-analysis of 32 studies. J Occup Environ Med. 2006;48: 1189–202.
67. Fleming LE, Bean JA, Rudolph M, Hamilton K. Cancer incidence in a cohort of licensed pesticide applicators in Florida. J Occup Environ Med. 1999; 41:279–88.
68. Frost G, Brown T, Harding AH. Mortality and cancer incidence among British agricultural pesticide users. Occup Med (Lond). 2011;61:303–10.
69. Kristensen P, Andersen A, Irgens LM, Bye AS, Sundheim L. Cancer in offspring of parents engaged in agricultural activities in Norway: incidence and risk factors in the farm environment. Int J Cancer. 1996;65:39–50.
70. Møller H. Work in agriculture, childhood residence, nitrate exposure, and testicular cancer risk: a case–control study in Denmark. Cancer Epidemiol Biomarkers Prev. 1997;6:141–4.

71. Kardaun JW, Hayes RB, Pottern LM, Brown LM, Hoover RN. Testicular cancer in young men and parental occupational exposure. Am J Ind Med. 1991;20:219–27.
72. Jaga K, Dharmani C. Global surveillance of DDT and DDE levels in human tissues. Int J Occup Med Environ Health. 2003;16:7–20.
73. Roy JR, Chakraborty S, Chakraborty TR. Estrogen-like endocrine disrupting chemicals affecting puberty in humans--a review. Med Sci Monit. 2009;15:RA137–45.
74. Toppari J. Environmental endocrine disrupters. Sex Dev. 2008;2:260–7.
75. Skakkebaek NE, Rajpert-De Meyts E, Main KM. Testicular dysgenesis syndrome: an increasingly common developmental disorder with environmental aspects. Hum Reprod. 2001;16:972–8.
76. Stang A, Trabert B, Rusner C, Poole C, Almstrup K, Rajpert-De Meyts E, McGlynn KA. A survey of etiologic hypotheses among testicular cancer researchers. Andrology. 2015;3:19–26.

Part II

Tumors of the Testis and Paratesticular Structures

2 Congenital Lesions

Manuel Nistal and Pilar González-Peramato

Introduction

The study of disorders in sexual development, probably more than any other field, needs the collaboration of clinicians, geneticists, endocrinologists, and pathologists. There are two big improvements the Chicago 2005 Consensus Classification intended to achieve: firstly, to consider the terms pseudohermaphroditism, hermaphroditism, sex reversal, and intersex condition obsolete and, secondly, to base the classification on chromosomal constitution. The first one has generally been achieved, although telling a patient that has an ovotesticular DSD instead of a true hermaphroditism doesn't look like a real progress. The second one poses a problem for the pathologist above all regarding gonadal dysgenesis, as some of them such as 45,X Turner syndrome and variants and 45,X/46,XY mixed gonadal dysgenesis are considered under the term sex chromosome DSD just like Klinefelter syndrome (47,XXY and variants) although these entities have a very different pathological morphology. On the other hand, entities which share histological findings such as 46,XY gonadal dysgenesis and 46,XX gonadal dysgenesis are considered as different groups. The pathologist, who really is the only one that knows the type of gonad, can offer an important point of view for the diagnosis that is needed to establish a prognosis and to integrate the remaining clinical features. The undifferentiated gonad can follow different ways. In some cases, it undergoes a differentiation toward the ovary and, depending on the grade of differentiation, can result in a streak gonad consisting only of gonadal stroma, a streak gonad with ovarian follicles or a hypoplastic ovary. In other cases, the differentiation is toward the testicle and results in streak gonad with epithelial-like cords, a testis with ovarian-like cortex or a dysgenetic testis. A streak testis or an ovotestis can result when the gonad presents a differentiation in both directions. If the undifferentiated gonad disappears, the result is a true agonadism. For an adequate differentiation of fetal testes takes place, a normal synthesis and secretion of testicular hormones and a correct action of these testicular hormones on target organs has to occur. Finally, failure in testicular descent is the congenital disorder most frequently found in newborns.

M. Nistal (✉)
Department of Anatomy, Histology and Neuroscience, Autonoma University of Madrid, Madrid, Spain
e-mail: manuel.nistal@salud.madrid.org

P. González-Peramato
Department of Pathology, Autonoma University of Madrid, Hospital Univ. La Paz, Madrid, Spain
e-mail: mpilar.gonzalezperamato@salud.madrid.org

M. Colecchia (ed.), *Pathology of Testicular and Penile Neoplasms*,
DOI 10.1007/978-3-319-27617-5_2

Gonadal Dysgenesis

Gonadal dysgenesis is a disorder classically characterized by the presence of amenorrhea and streak gonads in patients that are mostly of female phenotype with hypoplastic uterus and fallopian tubes. A pathological concept as it is, the streak gonad allowed that patients with completely different phenotypes such as Turner syndrome, Swyer syndrome, and Sohval syndrome were also included as gonadal dysgenesis. Some other pathologies grouped under the term "male pseudohermaphroditism with Müllerian rests" have been reported that include the same Sohval syndrome, dysgenetic male pseudohermaphroditism, and male with uterus, all of them characterized by the presence of preferential testicular differentiation that should also be considered part of gonadal dysgenesis.

Classification of Gonadal Dysgenesis

The consensus classification of intersex disorders achieved after the International Consensus Conference held in Chicago in 2005 [1] fortunately considered obsolete some terms such as pseudohermaphroditism, hermaphroditism, sex reversal, and intersex condition and introduced the term disorders of sexual development (DSD) (Fig. 2.1). However, as this classification is based on chromosomal constitution (peripheral leukocytes karyotype), numerous criticisms have raised [2]. Specifically, in gonadal dysgenesis, some entities with completely different morphology of the gonad are considered under the term sex chromosome DSD such as Turner's syndrome and its variants, mixed gonadal dysgenesis (45X/46XY) together with Klinefelter syndrome (47XXY and variants). On the other hand, other entities with similar histological findings in the gonads are considered in different groups such as 46,XY gonadal dysgenesis and 46,XX gonadal dysgenesis. In fact, the same karyotype can give rise to different phenotypes, and it is progressively better known that gonadal dysgenesis instead of one cellular line has mosaicisms or complex chromosomal constitutions. For these reasons the problem of intersex disorder classification seems not to be solved. The approaches from different point of views genetically, endocrinologically, clinically, and pathologically have not concluded yet.

The pathologist counts on a fact that is not less real than the karyotype, which is the nature of the gonads he/she has in front of his/her. This advantage puts the pathologist in the center of the problem. On one hand, he can observe what chromosomal anomalies or genetic mutations can produce, and, on the other hand, he can explain the variability of clinical situations through the different components of the gonad.

New Nomenclature of Disorders of Sex Development (DSD)

<table>
<tr><th rowspan="3">Sex Chromosome DSD</th><th colspan="2" rowspan="1">46,XY DSD</th><th colspan="3">46,XX DSD</th></tr>
<tr><th rowspan="2">Disorders of Testicular Development</th><th rowspan="2">Disorders of Androgen Synthesis / Action</th><th rowspan="2">Disorders of Ovarian Development</th><th colspan="2">Fetal Androgen Excess</th></tr>
<tr><th>CAH</th><th>Non CAH</th></tr>
<tr><td>- 45,X Turner and variants
- 47,XXY Klinefelter and variants
- 45,X/46,XY MGD
- Chromosomal ovotesticular DSD</td><td>- Complete gonadal dysgenesis
- Partial gonadal dysgenesis
- Gonadal regression
- Ovotesticular DSD</td><td>- Androgen synthesis defect
- LH-receptor defect
- Androgen insensitivity
- 5α-reductase deficiency
- Disorders AMH
- Timing defect
- Endocrine disrupters
- Cloacal extrophy</td><td>- Ovotesticular DSD
- Testicular DSD
- Gonadal dysgenesis</td><td>- 21-OH deficiency
- 11-OH deficiency</td><td>- Aromatase deficiency
- POR gene defect
- Maternal luteoma
- Iatrogenic</td></tr>
</table>

Fig. 2.1 New nomenclature in disorders of sexual differentiation. *MGD* mixed gonadal dysgenesis, *AMH* anti-Mullerian hormone, *CAH* congential adrenal hyperplasia

Gonadal dysgenesis can be defined as an incomplete or defective differentiation of the gonads as a result of disturbance in the germ cell migration process and/or its correct organization in gonadal ridge. This anomaly is morphologically expressed as gonads with different grades of differentiation toward ovary or testis or both. The term gonadal dysgenesis includes a large spectrum of lesions such as the absence of gonad, streak gonad, and testis surrounded by an ovarian-like stroma. That is, gonadal dysgenesis includes all kind of gonads until ovarian or testicular architecture is completely established. From this moment on, we speak about ovarian hypoplasia or testicular dysgenesis. It is possible that all gonadal dysgenesis could be part of a spectrum of the same disorder [3].

Types of Gonads and Correlation with Clinical Syndromes

For a better understanding of the different types of gonads that the pathologist can observe, it is very useful to take into account that the undifferentiated gonad can give rise to different histological patterns of gonads [4, 5]. When the differentiation is toward the ovary, we can observe streak gonad only made by gonadal stroma and streak gonad with ovarian follicles or hypoplastic ovaries. When the differentiation is toward the testis, the types of gonads can be: streak gonad with epithelial cords, testis with ovarian-like cortex, and dysgenetic testis. When the gonad presents an incomplete differentiation in both ovarian and testicular directions without being ovotestes, we have a streak testis. Finally, undifferentiated gonad can also disappear as occurs in true agonadism [6] (Fig. 2.2).

In some gonads, an "undifferentiated gonadal tissue" (UGT) arrested at the fetal stage can be present (Fig. 2.3). In the literature, these gonads have been considered either as streak gonad or as ovary. This UGT can be present as a streak gonad with epithelial cord-like structures or focally in several types of gonads such as dysgenetic testis, streak testis, or ovotestis. UGT recognition is of

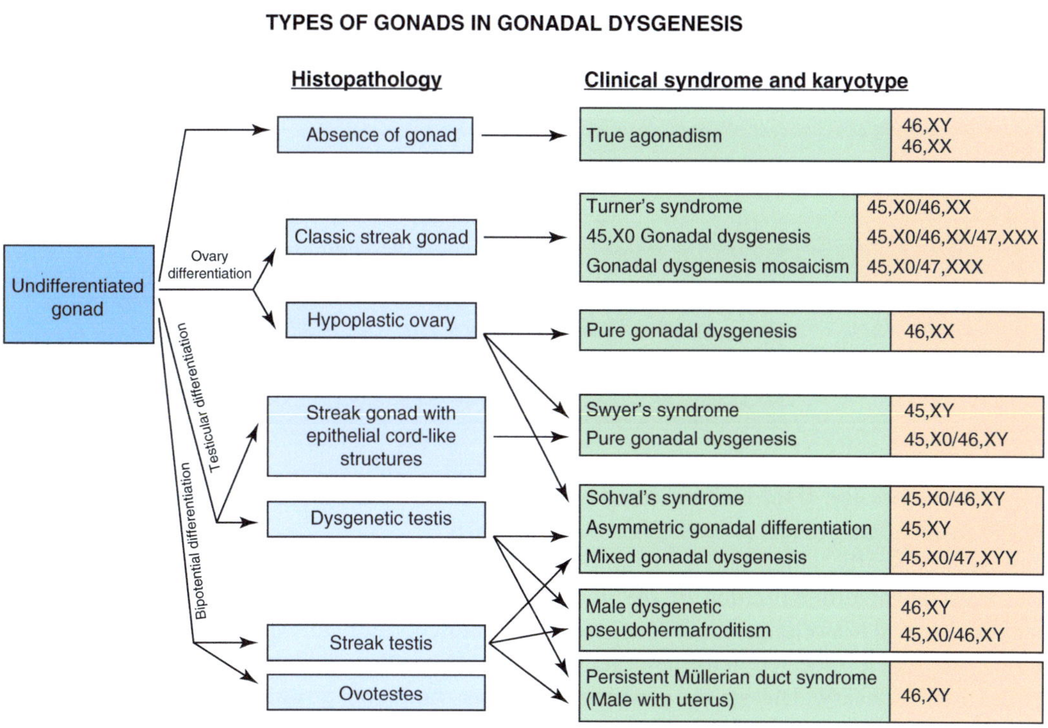

Fig. 2.2 Types of gonads and correlation with clinical syndromes in gonadal dysgenesis

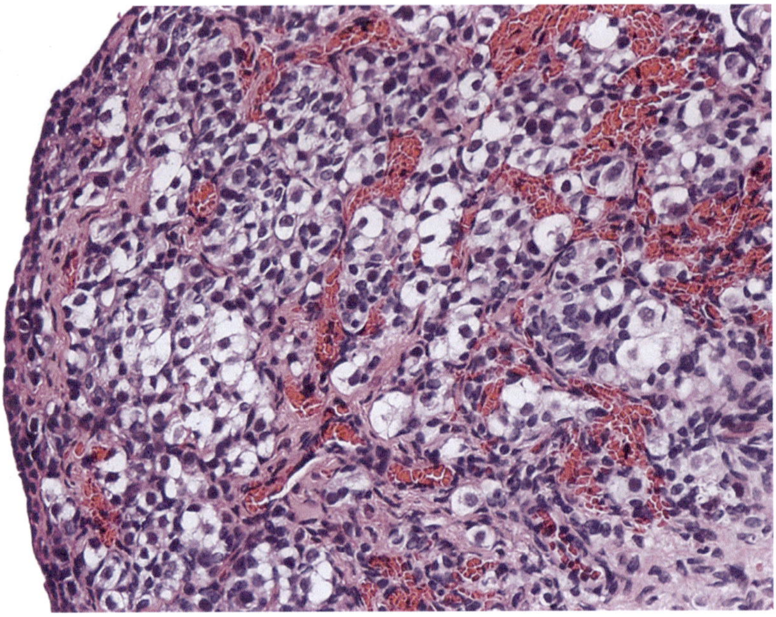

Fig. 2.3 Undifferentiated gonadal tissue. Streak gonad with undifferentiated germ cells with large pale cytoplasm arranged in nests or cords associated with smaller nongerm cells

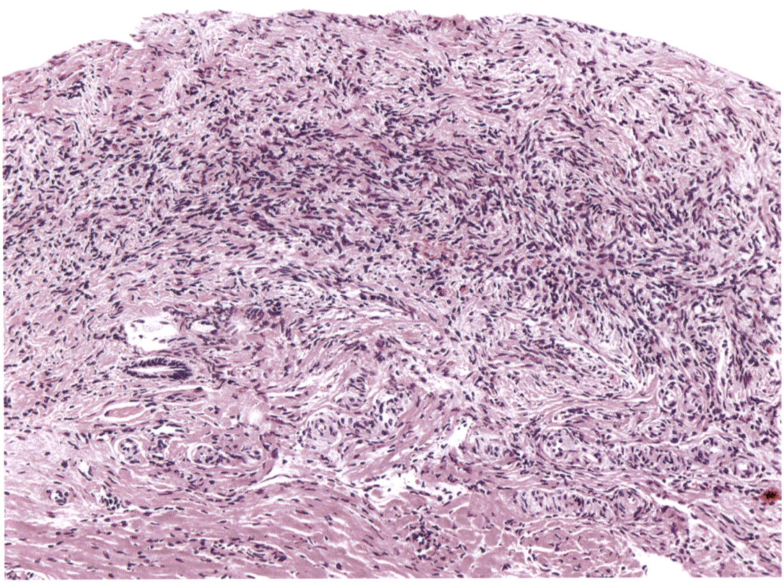

Fig. 2.4 Classic streak gonad. Elongated structure formed by whirled bundles of cells resembling ovarian stroma. Ovarian follicles are absent

great interest because of the high incidence of its transformation into gonadoblastoma [7].

Macroscopically, independent of the ovarian or testicular differentiation of the gonad, the streak gonad is an elongated, fibrous, pearly formation, which is located in the natural place of the normal ovary. The streak gonad measures 2–3 cm in length and 0.5 cm in width in the adult and can contain hilar cells or rete ovarii.

Classical Streak Gonad

Microscopically, this gonad is sometimes made up by bundles of fibrous connective tissue and other times by a whirled ovarian-like stroma (Fig. 2.4). This is the classical gonad seen in 45,X0 gonadal dysgenesis or Turner's syndrome.

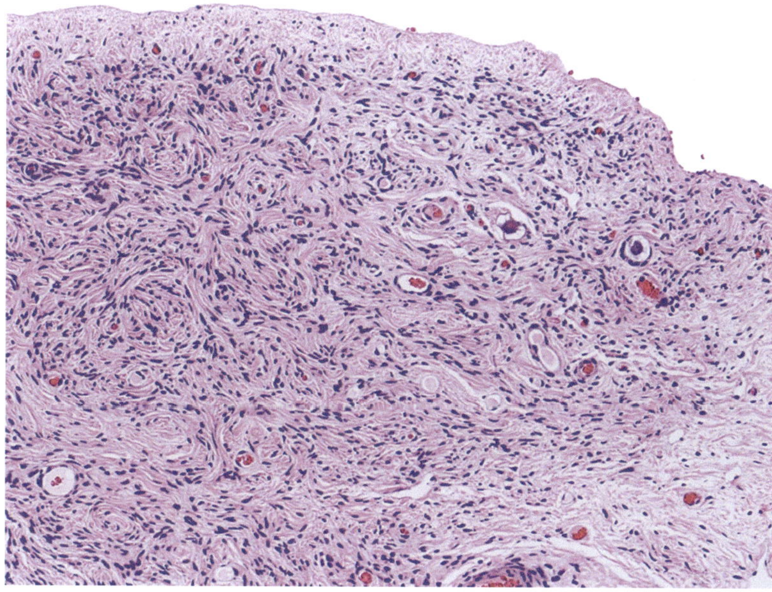

Fig. 2.5 Hypoplastic ovary. Isolated primordial follicles without any sign of maturation in a ovarian-like stroma

Occasionally, classical streak gonads may contain germ cells enclosed in primordial and eventually primary follicles [8, 9]. These germ cells have positive immunoexpression for VASA and c-Kit and are negative for OCT3/4, PLAP, and SCPY. In adult patients, atretic follicles, multiple cortical cysts, abundant hilar cells, or glandular-like groups of clear cells in the hilus can be observed. This gonad is observed in Turner's syndrome with chromosomal mosaicism and in 46,XX pure gonadal dysgenesis patients [10, 11].

Hypoplastic Ovary

This gonad is ovoid, small in size, and has a smooth surface unlike the streak gonad. Primary follicles, and occasionally follicles in development, can be conserved in the cortex with a regular pattern of distribution (Fig. 2.5). This is the characteristic gonad of 46,XX pure gonadal dysgenesis [12] and some ovotesticular dysgenesis (true hermaphrodites).

Streak Gonad with Epithelial Cord-Like Structures

The gonad consists of epithelial cord-like structures (sex cords) forming an anastomizing network that crosses in different directions an ovarian cortex-like stroma. The cord's thickness is variable, ranging from very thin to thick with coarse outlines. These cord-like structures contain two types of cells (Fig. 2.6). The most numerous ones are small cells with hyperchromatic nuclei that are considered to be pre-Sertoli cells or immature Sertoli/granulosa cells. These cells are intensely positive for AE1/AE3 and moderately positive for inhibin and D2-40, and calretinin, AMH is weakly expressed. The epithelial cord-like structures lean on a basal membrane of variable thickness. In the thickest areas, spiculated or nodular projections inside the cords can be observed. The second type of cells is germ cells. These germ cells can be located either isolated inside the stroma, forming cords or in between Sertoli/granulosa cells (Fig. 2.7). Their number is variable and in some cords can even form small nests. The immunohistochemical profile of germ cells is: OCT3/4 +, c-Kit +, PLAP +, TSPY + (testis-specific protein Y-encoded), and VASA +. In all, the histological pattern of this gonad is that of UGT. Some streak gonads with epithelial cord-like structures are devoid of germ cells, although it is probable that this gonad contained germ cells in some moment of its development but were eliminated by an apoptosis mechanism. This is the characteristic gonad of 46,XY gonadal dysgenesis [13–17].

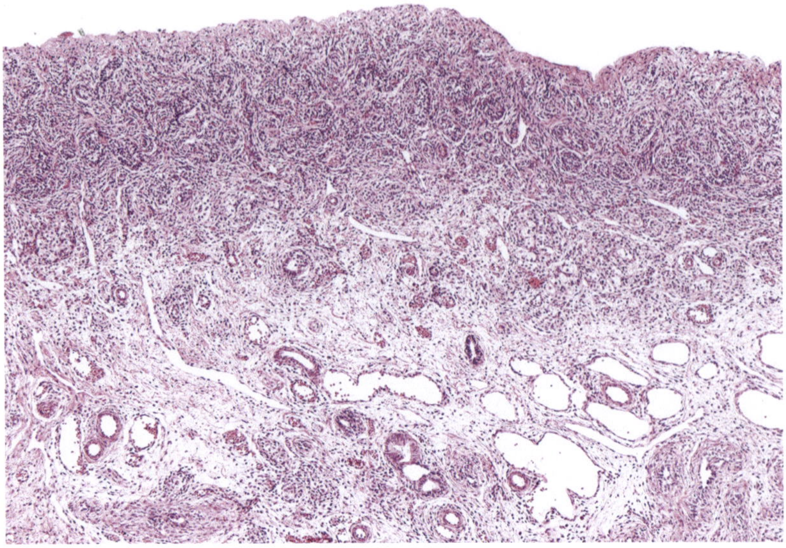

Fig. 2.6 Streak gonad with epithelial cord-like structures. Streak gonad with nests and cords of cells embedded in a stroma similar to ovarian cortex

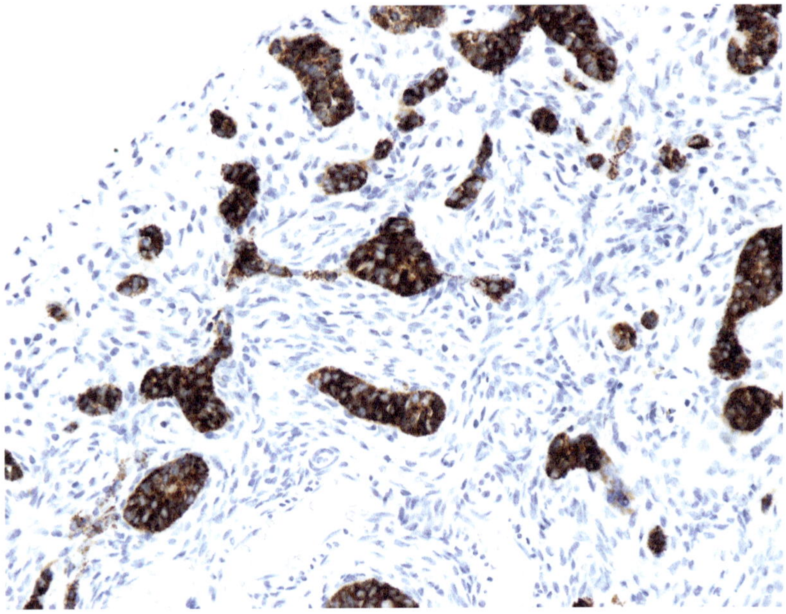

Fig. 2.7 Streak gonad with epithelial cord-like structures. The granulosa/Sertoli cells of the cords of epithelial cord-like structures shows intense calretinin immunoreactivity

Dysgenetic Testis

This gonad is usually small and cryptorchid. It consists of a compact central part containing seminiferous tubules with or without germ cells and a peripheral zone which, instead of showing a well-collagenized albuginea as occurs in normal testes, shows an ovarian stroma with or without malformed seminiferous cords. These seminiferous cords have irregular anastomosis, and their diameter vary from superficial to deep areas without an exact topography. Seminiferous tubules or cords are separated by a wide and loose stroma (Fig. 2.8). Sertoli cells express inhibin and AMH. They also express calretinin, like Leydig cells, preferably in the more superficial seminiferous cords. In the central areas of the testis, calretinin is only expressed in the smaller tubules, usually devoid of germ cells, and in Leydig cells. The image of seminiferous tubules formed by calretinin positive Sertoli cells that

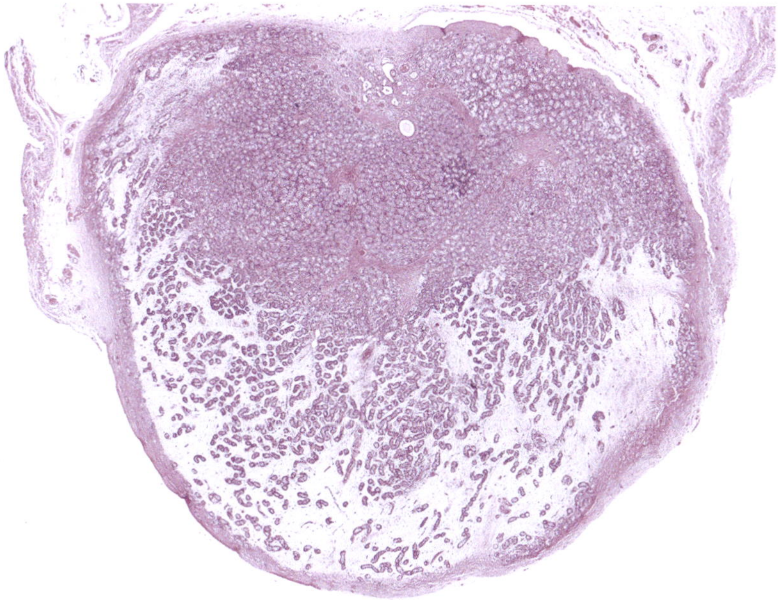

Fig. 2.8 Dysgenetic testis. The gonad shows a central part with compact packing of seminiferous tubules surrounded by an outer part with seminiferous tubules in a loose stroma reaching the surface

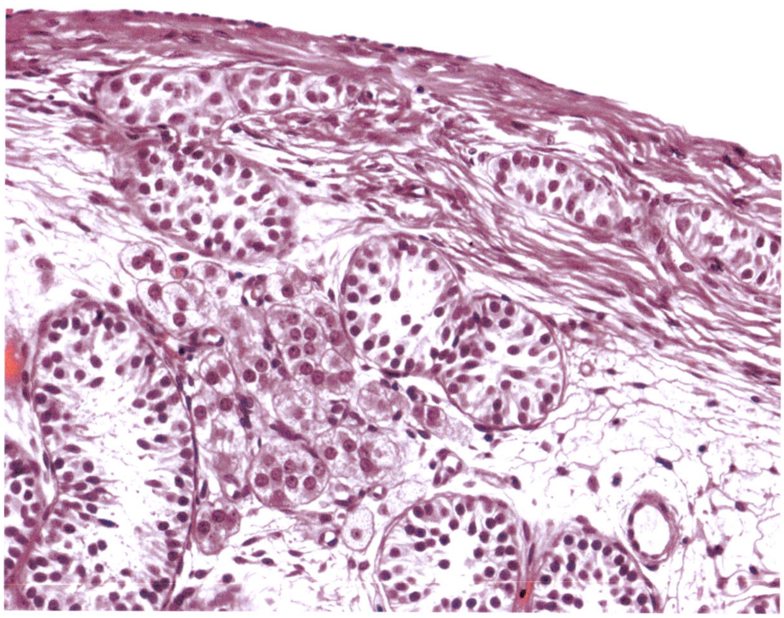

Fig. 2.9 Dysgenetic testis. Seminiferous tubules with delayed development inside the albuginea which has an ovarian cortex-like structure

surrounds other negative cells as half moon is a frequent finding. Germ cells are found both in the seminiferous tubule lumen and over the basal membrane. The germ cell phenotype is: VASA+, TSPY +, and D2-40+ and a subpopulation is OCT3/4 +, c-Kit +, and PLAP+.

Studies of dysgenetic testes in pubertal and adult patients are scanty. The irregular contour with strange shapes of the seminiferous tubules and the whirled stroma in the albuginea are conserved (Fig. 2.9). Maturation of Sertoli cells is incomplete as expressed by tubular lumen absence and nuclear characteristic of dysgenetic cell (round or ovoid nuclei instead of triangular nuclei with deep grooves of adult Sertoli cell). Most tubules are devoid of germ cells. The interstitium shows an apparent Leydig cell hyperplasia, both diffuse and peritubular. Immunohistochemical techniques allow a better understanding of the peculiar relationship among Leydig cells, peritubular cells, and Sertoli cells. Calretinin and inhibin immunostainings show many Leydig cells forming concentric circles in the tubular wall. These Leydig cells are located either among peritubular cells or between peritubular cells and the basal membrane. Some groups of tubules with germ cell neoplasia in situ (Genis) can be observed in spite of the fact that most of the tubules are devoid of germ cells.

This type of gonad was described by Jirasek [18] as "testicular dysgenesis," and it can be observed in the three syndromes that are classically included in male pseudohermaphroditism with Müllerian rests: (a) mixed gonadal dysgenesis (Sohval syndrome or asymmetric gonadal differentiation [19]), whose more frequent karyotypes are 45,X0/46,XY, 46,XY, and 45,X0/47,XYY [20–23]; (b) male dysgenetic pseudohermaphroditism, which usually shows the karyotypes 46,XY or 45,X0/46,XY [24–26]; and (c) Müllerian duct persistence syndrome (male with uterus), which has the 46,XY karyotype [27–31].

Streak Testis

This gonad has two intimately joined zones. The most voluminous part is formed by a dysgenetic testis with an ovarian cortex-like stroma close to the tunica albuginea. This stroma is in continuity with a streak gonad usually containing epithelial cords or some ovarian follicles. This gonad is observed in the three previously reported syndromes: mixed gonadal dysgenesis, dysgenetic male pseudohermaphroditism, and Müllerian duct persistence syndrome [32].

In summary, gonadal dysgenesis includes the following situations: 45,X0 gonadal dysgenesis, 46,XX pure gonadal dysgenesis, 46,XY gonadal dysgenesis, mixed gonadal dysgenesis, dysgenetic male pseudohermaphroditism, and Müllerian duct persistence syndrome.

Male Undervirilization

Normal male development needs an adequate differentiation of fetal testes, a normal synthesis and secretion of testicular hormones, and a correct action of these testicular hormones on target organs. Anti-Müllerian hormone secreted by Sertoli cells inhibits the Müllerian duct development toward uterus and fallopian tubes. Testosterone secreted by Leydig cells virilizes wolffian ducts. The transformation of testosterone into dihydrotestosterone by 5-α reductase enzyme induces male external genitalia development. A failure in any of these steps can determine male undervirilization (male pseudohermaphroditism).

Defective Leydig Cell Function

A defective Leydig cell function groups two different conditions: the variable enzymatic deficit that leads to insufficient androgens synthesis and the absence or hypoplasia of Leydig cells.

Defective Androgen Synthesis

Defective androgen synthesis comprises several autosomal recessive syndromes secondary to an error in the testosterone biosynthesis that leads to incomplete or absent virilization [33, 34]. Five enzymes are responsible for testosterone synthesis (Fig. 2.10). The absence or decrease in any of them determines a decrease in androgens production.

Lipoid Congenital Adrenal Hyperplasia

Lipoid congenital adrenal hyperplasia is the most severe form of congenital adrenal hyperplasia (CAH) [35, 36]. It is a disorder characterized by impaired synthesis of all adrenal and gonadal steroid hormones, resulting in phenotypical females with a 46,XY karyotype with a severe salt-losing syndrome. Most of the cases are due to a defect in the steroidogenic acute regulatory (StAR) protein. A defect in P450 scc causes the remaining cases. Patients usually present in the first 2 months of life with a salt-losing crisis [37, 38]. Most males have female external genitalia reflecting the absence of testosterone synthesis between 6th and 12th weeks of gestation. A small group of patients have female or ambiguous external genitalia with blind-ended vagina, hypoplasia of wolffian derivatives, absence of Müllerian structures, and cryptorchidism in most of the cases [39]. Fetal adrenal glands are enlarged in most cases and show accumulation of

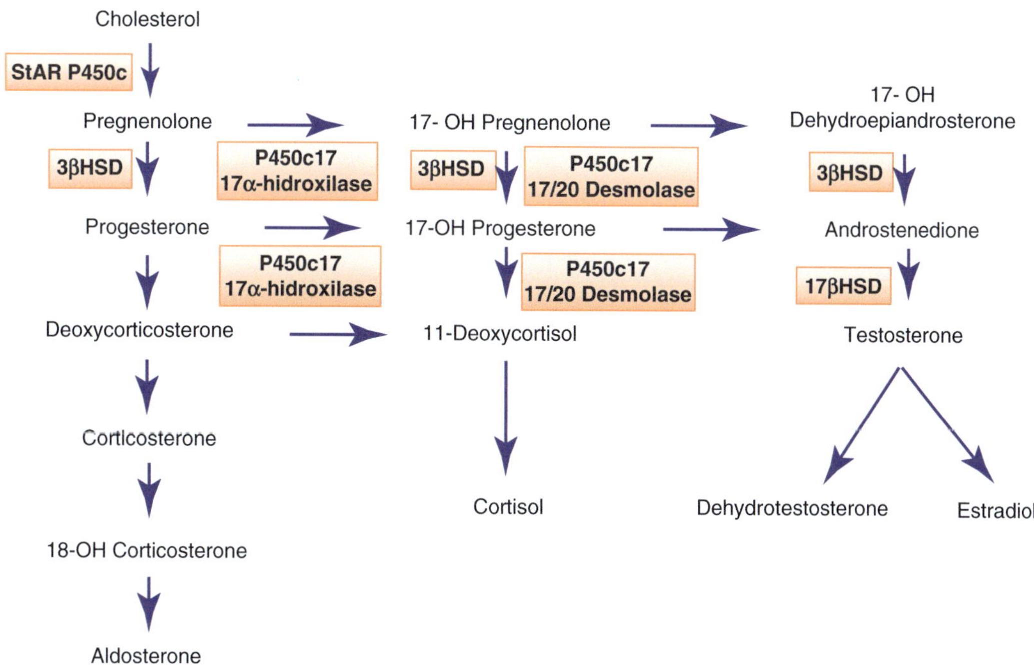

Fig. 2.10 Enzymatic defects in impaired testosterone biosynthesis

large lipid droplets [40, 41]. The adrenal glands decrease with age to nearly complete disappearance, resulting in adrenal glands of small size. In childhood, seminiferous tubules usually show both Sertoli and germ cells or Sertoli-only tubules [42, 43]. Testis of pubertal patients have usually been reported as normal for the age [44, 45] or with lipid accumulation in Sertoli cells [46].

Deficiency of 3-b Hydroxysteroid Dehydrogenase/17,20-Lyase

There is a classical form of deficiency of 3-BHSD with salt losing that presents in the first months after birth due to insufficient aldosterone synthesis, and another clinical presentation in which no loss of salt occurs, whose diagnosis is usually delayed until puberty. Both forms are due to mutations in type-2 *3BHSD* gene located in chromosome 1 [47]. Some patients present only with hypospadias [48] or micropenis [49].

Deficiency of 17-α Hydroxylase/17,20-Lyase

Deficiencies of 17-α hydroxylase and 17,20-lyase are due to mutations of the *CYP17* gene that encodes cytochrome P450c17 [50]. The enzymatic defect of 17-α hydroxylase concerns both cortisol and testosterone synthesis [51]. The alteration in the testosterone secretion in fetal testes leads to male undervirilization. Patients are raised as girls. At puberty they may show amenorrhea, scanty axillary and pubic hair, eunuchoid appearance [52], and gynecomastia [53].

Deficiency of 17,20 Desmolase

The gene that codifies this enzyme has been mapped on chromosome 10. Variable degrees of 17,20 desmolase deficit have been observed, explaining the variability of external genitalia ranging from a female phenotype to minimally virilized males with micropenis, bifid scrotum, perineal hypospadias, and cryptorchidism. This is a result of insufficient testosterone production during fetal life [54]. Histological studies of these testes in infants show decreased numbers of spermatogonia [55, 56]. At puberty, patients show incomplete virilization without gynecomastia.

Deficiency of 17-B Hydroxysteroid Dehydrogenase

The enzyme 17-BHSD transforms androstenedione to testosterone and estrone to estradiol. Its deficiency is due to mutations in the *HSD17B3* gene, at locus 9q22 [57, 58]. Its deficiency leads to sex-linked familial presentation pictures. Most patients have a female phenotype at birth and are raised as females but undergo virilization at puberty [59, 60]. Patients may show cryptorchidism. Most frequent histological patterns are hypospermatogenesis, mixed atrophy, or Sertoli-cell-only tubules [61, 62].

Leydig Cell Hypoplasia

The classical features of this autosomal recessive male undervirilization include: (a) predominantly female external genitalia; (b) no pubertal development of secondary sexual characteristics (males or females) (c) absence of uterus and fallopian tubes, presence of epididymis and vas deferens; (d) 46XY karyotype; (e) low serum testosterone levels associated with markedly increased gonadotropin levels; (f) no response to hCG stimulation; (g) no enzymatic defect in testosterone biosynthesis; and (h) undescended and small testes, which on section appear grayish and mucous [63–65]. The age of diagnosis ranges from 4 months to 35 years, although most patients are diagnosed at puberty.

In 50 % of cases, the defect seems to be caused by inactivating mutations in the gene receptor LH/CG (*LHCGR*), although isolated cases show mutations only in certain exons [66]. In the remaining cases no mutations have been found, suggesting defects in other genes or in non-studied regions of *LHCGR* [67].

Biopsies of patients with Leydig cell hypoplasia show seminiferous tubules with reduced diameter, thickened basal membrane, and presence of both Sertoli cells and spermatogonia. In the interstitium, Leydig cells may be absent, scanty, or appear immature [68]. These characteristic findings of this variant of male undervirilization contrast with the hyperplasia of Leydig cells frequently observed in most syndromes of male undervirilization, including those due to defective androgen synthesis or to deficiencies in the peripheral action of androgens on target organs.

Defective Peripheral Action of Androgens

Deficiencies in the peripheral action of androgens comprise the syndromes of androgen insensitivity (complete and incomplete testicular feminization syndrome) and 5-α reductase deficiency.

Syndromes of Androgen Insensitivity (AIS)

The syndromes of resistance to androgens comprise a group of patients with male genotype (46,XY) whose phenotype ranges from female (testicular feminization) to normal male that present clinically with infertility and intermediate degrees of undervirilization [69]. AIS syndromes result from total or partial resistance of target organs to androgen action [70, 71]. Different clinical presentations result from mutations of the *AR* gene [72–77]. The frequency of androgen insensitivity syndromes is estimated in 1/20,000 newborns, and the transmission is recessive X linked in 2/3 of cases.

There are several phenotypes associated with AIS that are grouped under the following three terms: complete testicular feminization (CAIS); partial testicular feminization (PAIS) that includes Lubs' syndrome, Gilbert-Dreyfus' syndrome, Reifenstein's syndrome, and Rosewater's syndrome; and slight or minimal androgen insensitivity (MAIS), that present by infertility or Kennedy's diseased.

Complete Androgen Insensitivity Syndrome (CAIS)

CAIS syndrome is rarely diagnosed in infancy unless patients present with hernia, as from 0.8 to 2.4 % of females with inguinal hernia have CAIS [78], and a testis is unexpectedly discovered during the surgical procedure of hernia repair [79, 80]. Sometimes a tumor develops in an inguinal testis, or there is a family history that leads to a karyotype study that usually is 46,XY. In adults, primary amenorrhea is a frequent presenting sign. Patients have delayed onset of puberty and above average stature.

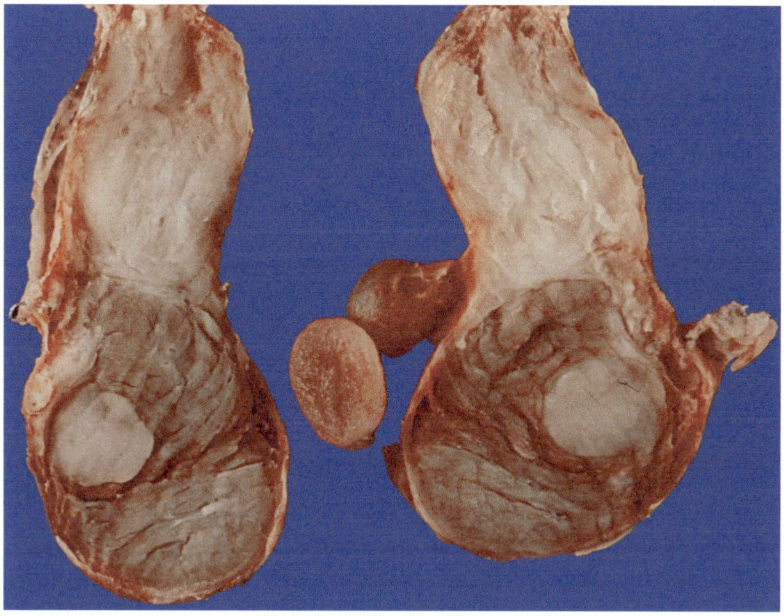

Fig. 2.11 Complete androgen insensitivity syndrome. Right gonad showing a trabecular appearance and a whitish lobulated nodular formation associated with a fasciculate gray-white mass in one pole of the testis

Testes in CAIS patients may be located in the abdomen, inguinal canal, or labia majora. The incidence of abdominal testes is higher in patients with complete female phenotype and absence of pubic hair. In the first year of life, testes show a nearly normal pattern, except for a slight decrease in seminiferous tubular diameter and fertility index. After the first year of age, germ cell depletion is remarkable, and the few remaining germ cells concentrate in some isolated seminiferous tubules that remain together [81]. These testes differ from cryptorchid testes by showing a more cellular testicular interstitium with spindle cell bundles reminiscent of ovarian stroma among seminiferous tubules. During the first year of life, Leydig cells with wide, eosinophilic, or microvacuolated cytoplasm can be observed.

At puberty, CAIS patients show female external genitalia, short vagina, adequate breast development, and presence or absence of pubic and axillary hair [82, 83].

Adults with CAIS or PAIS show testes with variable size, from small to voluminous. On section, testes are brown gray with yellowish areas (Fig. 2.11). Histologically, these testes contain seminiferous tubules with small diameter (cords), devoid of lumen, lined only by Sertoli cells [84, 85]. One third of patients show isolated germ cells [86]. Leydig cells are numerous. The testicular interstitium shows a fibrous tissue (Fig. 2.12). Two thirds of patients develop Sertoli-Leydig cell hamartomas (Figs 2.13 and 2.14). Less than one fourth of testes have Sertoli cell adenomas that consist of fetal- or infantile-like seminiferous tubules, devoid of germ cells and peritubular myofibroblasts.

80 % of patients show thick bundles of smooth muscle in paratesticular location (smooth muscle hamartomas).

Partial Androgen Insensitivity Syndrome (PAIS)

Patients with an incomplete or partial form of AIS may show a phenotype that varies from female to male [87]. Several intermediate forms have been reported under the following syndromes: Lubs' syndrome [88], Gilbert-Dreyfus'syndrome [89], Reifenstein's syndrome [90], and Rosewater's syndrome [91].

The correlation between genotype and phenotype in patients with AIS shows no phenotype variation in CAIS families, while the phenotype in PAIS is extremely variable and rarely predicted by the AR genotype [92].

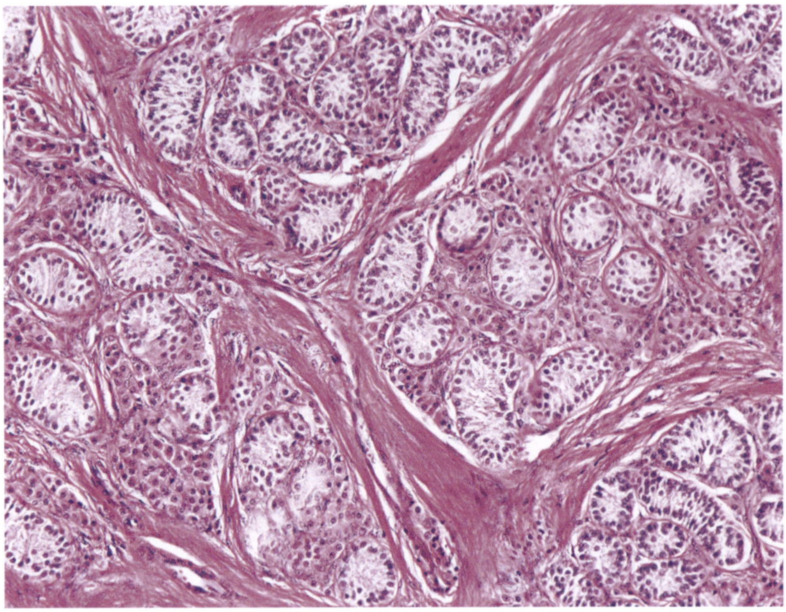

Fig. 2.12 Complete androgen insensitivity syndrome. Seminiferous tubules with prepubertal maturation in an adult patient are surrounded by numerous Leydig cells and separated by thick septa of hyalinized stroma

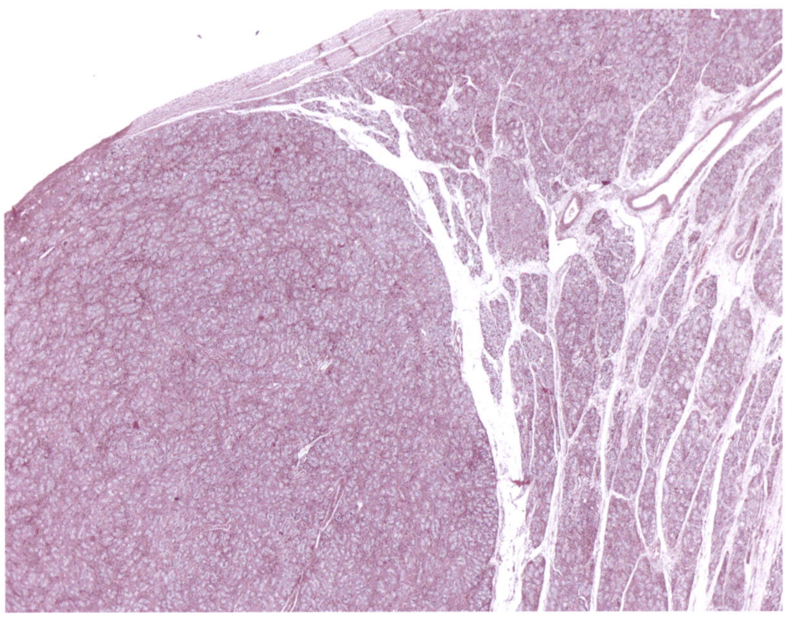

Fig. 2.13 Sertoli-Leydig hamartoma in a patient with complete androgen insensitivity syndrome. The nodular formation is well delimited from the surrounding parenchyma and consists of both immature seminiferous tubules and Leydig cells

Mild Androgen Insensitivity Syndrome (MAIS)

There is a minor form of AIS that is observed in some patients with male phenotype that consult due to infertility [93]. The frequency is lower than 19 % [94]. Other form of AIS is Kennedy disease that consists of X-linked spino-bulbo-muscular atrophy (SBMA). This is a motor neuron disease with a recessive pattern of inheritance that affects adult males [95]. Most patients show an abnormal reproductive system [96–98]. Testes are initially normal, and many patients with SBMA have fathered children. As the disease evolves, patients develop progressive testicular atrophy and gynecomastia.

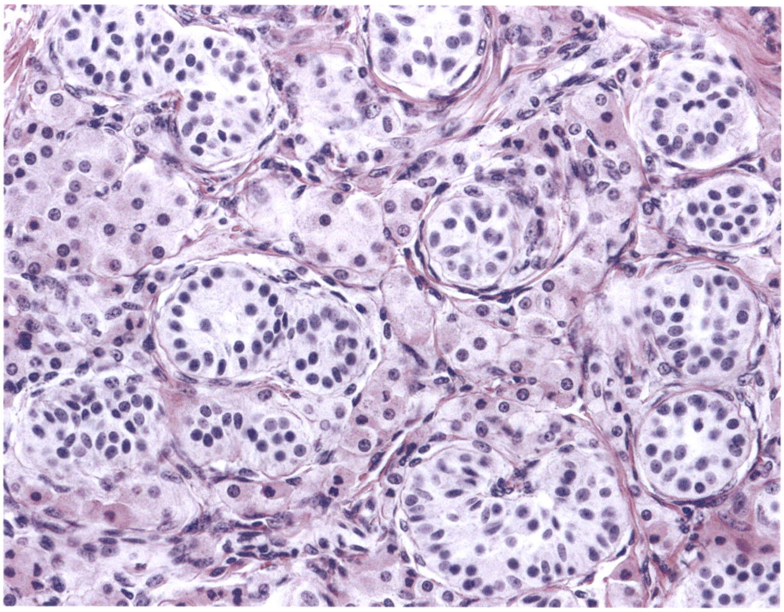

Fig. 2.14 Detail of a Sertoli-Leydig hamartoma in a patient with complete androgen insensitivity syndrome showing immature seminiferous tubules surrounded by hypertrophic Leydig cells

Defect in 5α-Reductase

It is a rare variant of male undervirilization characterized by a defect in conversion of testosterone to dihydrotestosterone in peripheral tissues such as external genitalia and prostate due to a defect in 5-α reductase in 46,XY patients. The disease is autosomal recessive. The isoforms of 5-α reductase are encoded by two corresponding genes: *SRD5A*, at 5p15 for isoenzyme 1, and *SRD5A2*, at 2p23 for isoenzyme 2 [99]. Infants with this disorder show a clitoriform penis, bifid scrotum, and a vagina opening onto the urethra or a urogenital sinus. The ejaculatory ducts open onto the vagina, and the testes are located in the inguinal duct or labioscrotal folds. Many patients are raised as girls. At puberty, the most striking feature is the marked virilization [100]. These patients develop a male phenotype with penis enlargement and a wrinkled and pigmented scrotum. This is accompanied by deepening of the voice tone. Adults have penile erections and ejaculations, normal libido, scanty vellus and beard, and absence of the temporal line recession of hair.

In the first years of life, testes may show reduced mean tubular diameter and decreased number of germ cells as well as groups of xanthomized leydig cells [101]. At puberty, significant changes occur; seminiferous tubules show reduced caliber, and most lack a lumen. The only components of the seminiferous epithelium are numerous Sertoli cells, showing incomplete maturation [101, 102]. Spermatogenesis is exceptional. Interstitium shows an increased numbers of morphologically normal Leydig cells.

Other Forms of Male Undervirilization

A large number of dysmorphologic syndromes are associated with incomplete masculinization of external genitalia. These include Smith-Lemli-Opitz syndrome (initially called "RSH" syndrome after the initials of the first three patients), Opitz syndrome (G/BBB syndrome), ATR-X syndrome, Gardner-Silengo-Wachtel syndrome, Meckle syndrome, branchioskeletal-genital syndrome, Down syndrome, and other trisomies. All these syndromes are directly associated with mutations in genes that regulate different steps of sexual differentiation.

True Hermaphroditism (Ovotesticular Disorder)

Ovotesticular disorders of sex development (ovotesticular DSD) is a disorder of gonadal differentiation, characterized by the presence of testicular and ovarian parenchyma in the same individual. It is a rare disorder as it occurs in less than 10 % of the population with ambiguous external genitalia [103–105]. Most hermaphrodites are sporadic.

Karyotype and Phenotype

The most frequent *karyotype* of patients with ovotesticular DSD is 46,XX (60 %), followed by chromosomal mosaicisms which in decreasing order of frequency include 46,XXl46XY, 46,XY/47,XXY, 45,X0/46,XY, 46,XX/45,X0, 46,XX/47,XXY (33 %), and finally 46,XY karyotype (7 %). These global figures do not express the actual incidence of karyotypes in some places of the world. In Europe chromosomal mosaicism is found in 40.5 % of cases, while only in 21 % of cases in North America. Most African patients with true hermaphroditism (96.6 %) show a 46,XX karyotype [106, 107].

Pathogenetic theories explaining ovotesticular DSD start from the premise that if the patient has testes, the testicular-determining factor (TDF) produced by the *SRY* gene is present. This is easy to explain when the karyotype is 46,XY, mosaicism 46,XX/4,5XY, or chimera 46,XY. Finding testicular parenchyma in a patient with a 46,XX karyotype (the most common situation) is more difficult to understand and has been explained by four pathogenetic mechanisms: (1) a hidden mosaicism including a cell line carrying the Y chromosome [108], (2) translocation of paternal Y chromosomal material that includes the *SRY* gene to the X chromosome, (3) an autosomal mutation with variable penetrance, and (4) by X-linked chromosome mutations, either coupled with a rare X chromosome inactivation [109], allowing testicular differentiation in the absence of *SRY* [110], or mutations in genes such as *SOX9* and *FGF9* that regulate the action of *SRY* [111]. Molecular studies have revealed that only a few 46,XX patients with ovotesticular DSD show Y-DNA chromosome sequences [112]. This is in contrast with the so-called XX males (46,XX testicular DSD) who show Y chromosome material including TDF in 80 % of cases [113].

The *phenotype* of hermaphrodites varies from female to normal male. Most patients consult for the first time at puberty. Phenotypical males consult by breast development (95 % ovotesticular DSD patients show some degree of gynecomastia) [114] or periodical hematuria [115] or cryptorchidism [116]. Patients with female phenotype present with menstrual disorders or clitoromegaly and more rarely with cyclic pain in a descended or undescended gonad [117]. True hermaphroditism should be suspected in every infant, showing sexual ambiguity [118].

Types of Gonads

The types of gonads observed in ovotesticular DSD patients are: ovotestis (44 %), ovary (33 %), and testis (22 %). The degree of gonadal descent is directly proportional to the amount of testicular tissue present [119].

- The *ovotestis* is predominantly seen on the right side and abdominal in half of the cases and inguinal, scrotal, or labial in the remaining cases. Only 5 % of patients with bilateral ovotestes show complete gonadal descent [120, 121]. Grossly, ovotestes can be bilobed or ovoid. If bilobed, testicular and ovarian tissues are joined by a pedicle. If ovoid, the ovarian tissue forms a cap on the testicular parenchyma. The limits between testicular and ovarian parenchyma may be well defined in some cases (Fig. 2.15), while in others the oocytes are spread among seminiferous cords/tubules (Fig. 2.16) or even inside the tubules. The ovarian/testicular proportion of tissue varies widely from one patient to another [122]. In adults, several degrees of follicular maturation, corpora lutea or corpora albicantia, can be observed. The seminiferous tubules rarely develop spermatogenesis, often show a Sertoli-only dysgenetic appearance, and frequently undergo hyalinization. The interstitium contains numerous Leydig cells.
- The *testis* is preferentially located on the right side (60 %) at any level from the abdomen to

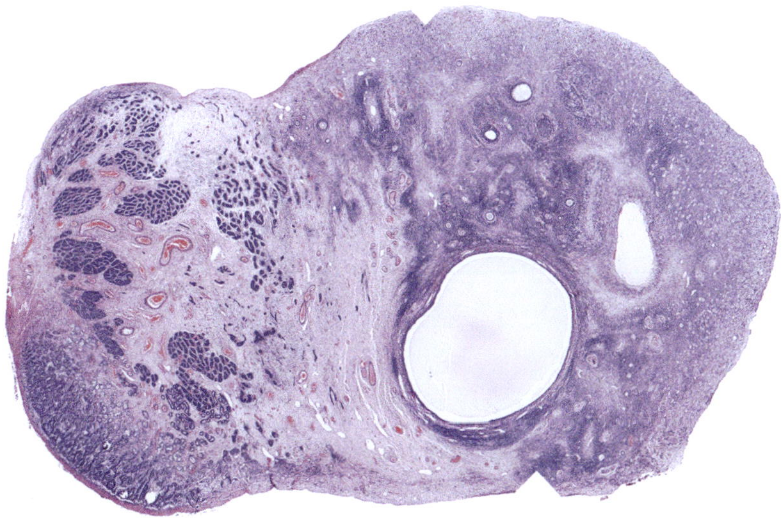

Fig. 2.15 Ovotestes of a prepubertal patient showing an ovary with several follicles in development in one pole. In the opposite pole there is a testicular parenchyma with seminiferous tubules in a wide stroma. In the periphery undifferentiated tissue

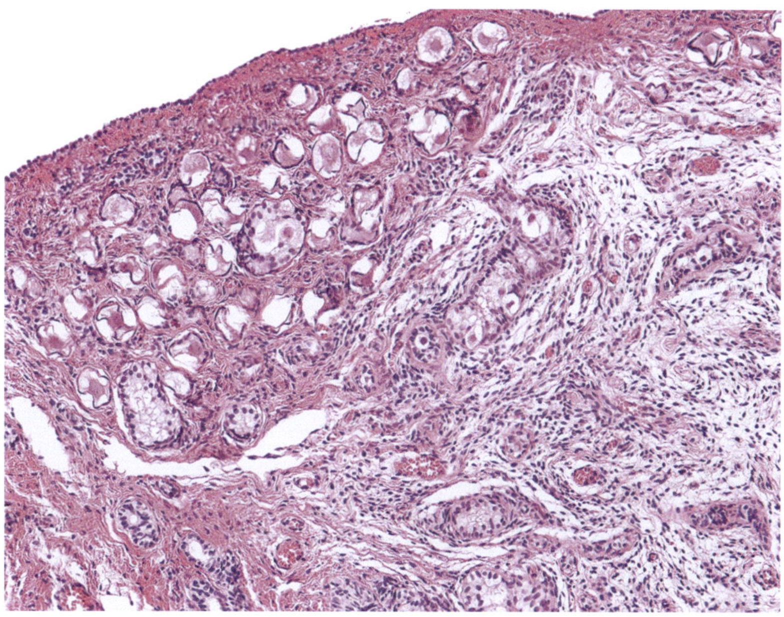

Fig. 2.16 Ovotestes showing numerous primordial follicles and isolated seminiferous tubules with germ cells within an abundant stroma

the scrotal pouch or labia. From infancy, a low tubular fertility index is remarkable in the testis. At puberty, the seminiferous tubules do not reach a normal diameter and often consist only of dysgenetic Sertoli cells, similar to those observed in many cryptorchid testes. Incomplete spermatogenesis can be observed in some cases, but complete spermatogenesis is exceptional [123].

- The *ovary* is most frequently found on the left side (63 %) and nearly always in the abdomen. In most instances, the ovary is hypoplastic and shows scanty primordial follicles (Fig. 2.17). In a few patients, the ovary is histologically and functionally normal. More than two dozen pregnancies in patients with ovotesticular DSD have been reported [124–126]. This is in contrast with the exceptional cases of paternity [127]. The origin of oocytes might be an ovotestis [128] or an ovary [129]. Most patients develop hypergonadotropic hypogonadism.

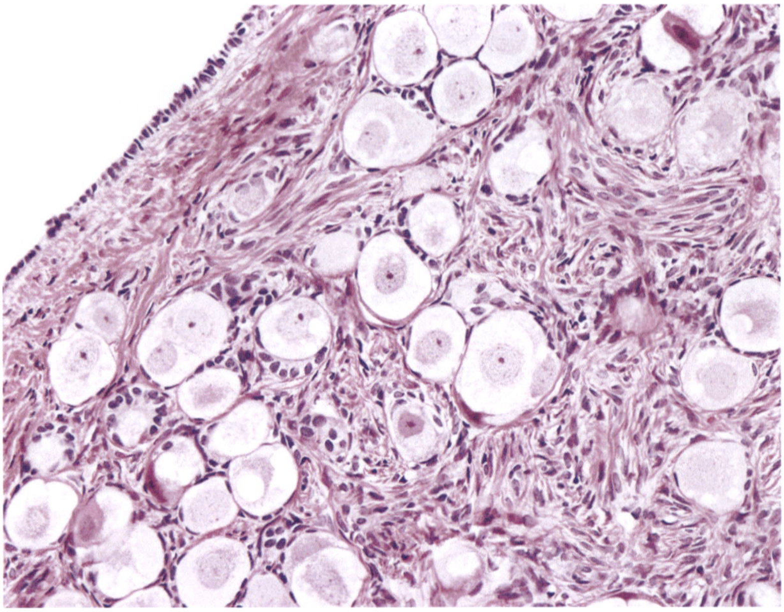

Fig. 2.17 Abundant primordial follicles in an infantile ovary contralateral to the ovotestis

Undescended Testes

Failure in testicular descent is the congenital disorder most frequently found in newborns. Testicular descent is not always complete at birth. Between 4 and 5 % of newborns have incompletely descended testes. This percentage is higher in premature newborns, reaching 100 % in those weighing less than 900 g at birth [130, 131]. Testes usually descend in the first 3 months of postnatal life, and by 1 year of age, only 0.96–1.58 % of testes remain undescended. After the first year of life, spontaneous descent is exceptional. The incidence of cryptorchidism seems to have risen in recent years, with the last reported figures around 1.8 % of all boys [132–134].

Types of Undescended Testes

True Cryptorchidism

True cryptorchidism defines testes in the abdomen, inguinal duct, or high in the scrotum that cannot be moved into the scrotum during physical exploration [135]. *Ectopic testes* are those testes located outside the normal pathway of testicular descent. This group includes the classic ectopies: interstitial (superficial inguinal), femoral (crural), perineal, transverse (crossed testicular ectopia), pubopenile, pelvic, and other more rare ectopies such as testes in the abdominal wall. Patients with *retractile testes* represent between 1/4 and 1/3 of patients clinically diagnosed as undescended testes [136]. Retractile testes can be mobilized to the bottom of the scrotum with adequate gentle manipulation. There are two types of true cryptorchidism: congenital and acquired.

Congenital Cryptorchidism

From an epidemiological point of view, the following situations are considered to have a high risk of congenital cryptorchidism: increased maternal age, maternal obesity, toxemia of pregnancy, alcohol consumption, bleeding during late pregnancy, exposure phthalates during fetal development, smoking during pregnancy, high maternal stature, history of subfertility, birth by cesarean section, low weight at birth, prematurity, twinning, intrauterine growth restriction, hypospadias [137], other congenital malformations, and births occurring between September and November or during May and June [138, 139]. The highest risk of cryptorchidism is associated with low weight at birth [140]. Causes of congenital cryptorchidism may be hormonal dysfunction involving testosterone, anti-Müllerian hormone (AMH), epidermal growth factor (EGF), and estrogens. Mechanical causes include anatomical anomalies of the gubernaculum, insufficient abdominal pressure, short spermatic cord, underdeveloped vaginal process, and maldeveloped epididymis. Neuromuscular causes include abnormalities in the calcitonin gene-related peptide (CGRP) and the cremaster nucleus. Genetic causes are mutations in the insulin-like factor 3 or its receptor [141]. Other hereditary [142, 143] or acquired conditions may also produce cryptorchidism.

Acquired Cryptorchidism

This term refers to descended scrotal testes that, during postnatal life, can ascend and be lodged even in the abdominal cavity [144]. Two types of acquired undescended testes have been considered:

1. The so-called postoperative "trapped testis" [145] is a normally descended testis that "escapes" from the scrotum after surgery for inguinal hernia or hydrocele [146–148]. This iatrogenic complication may occur in 1.2 % of children who undergo hernia repair. An adherence of the testis or the cremaster muscle to the surgically incised zone causes upward displacement of the testis by myofibroblastic contraction during wound healing.
2. The *spontaneously ascended testis*. The etiology of spontaneously ascended testis is not known, but several hypotheses have been proposed: failure in postnatal spermatic cord elongation [149, 150], inadequate growth of spermatic vessels [151], failure in reabsorption of the vaginal process [152, 153], permanent spasm of the cremaster muscle [154], and abnormal insertion of the gubernaculum [155].

Histological Lesions in Undescended Testes

In Childhood

The existence and severity of congenital lesions in cryptorchid testes cannot be known by any functional studies. Therefore, the histological study of a testicular biopsy is required to evaluate the presence and severity of testicular parenchyma lesions in cryptorchidism. In this evaluation one should have in mind that, from birth to puberty, the testis is a dynamic structure with waves of proliferation and differentiation. At birth, testicular volume is approximately 0.5 ml. At 3 years of age, it increases slightly to about 0.6 ml, rising up in prepubertal boys to about 1–2 ml, and at the end of puberty, it reaches 20 ml. In the undescended testes a decreased volume and lesser and slower growth are observed. This difference is already significant at 6 months of age [156].

The pathologist should evaluate both semiquantitative and qualitative parameters in order to obtain as much information as possible from the histological study of the testicular biopsies from undescended testes [157]. The semiquantitative morphometric parameters are: mean tubular diameter (MTD), tubular fertility index (TFI), number of germ cells per cross-sectioned tubule, the Sertoli cell index (SCI), and the number of Leydig cells in the interstitium. The qualitative findings include: the pattern of germ cell distribution in the testicular parenchyma (regular or irregular), the presence of abnormal spermatogonia (multinucleated, hypertrophic, and/or atypical) and gonocytes, focal granular changes in Sertoli cells, abnormal tubules (megatubules, ring-shaped tubules), microliths, and androgen receptors in children older than 4-year-old.

Most cryptorchid testes also present lesions in the first year of life, suggesting primary rather than acquired lesions as a consequence of long-standing cryptorchidism. Patients fail to undergo the increased pituitary levels of gonadotropins that induce a peak of testosterone between 3 and 6 months of age in a process known as minipuberty [158]. This lack of hormonal stimulation has four important consequences: (1) an incomplete migration of gonocytes and fetal spermatogonia from the center of the seminiferous tubules to the periphery where they lay over the basal membrane, (2) defective transformation of gonocytes into type A dark spermatogonia (Ad), (3) persistence of gonocytes after the first year of life, and (4) failure of primary spermatocytes to appear in the first 4 years of age [159].

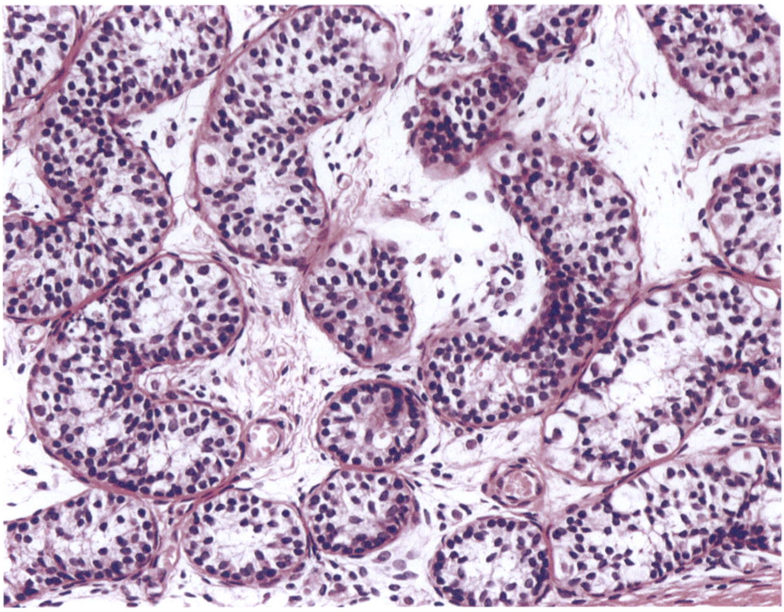

Fig. 2.18 Undescended testes with type II lesions. Seminiferous tubules with germ cells next to other tubules devoid of germ cells

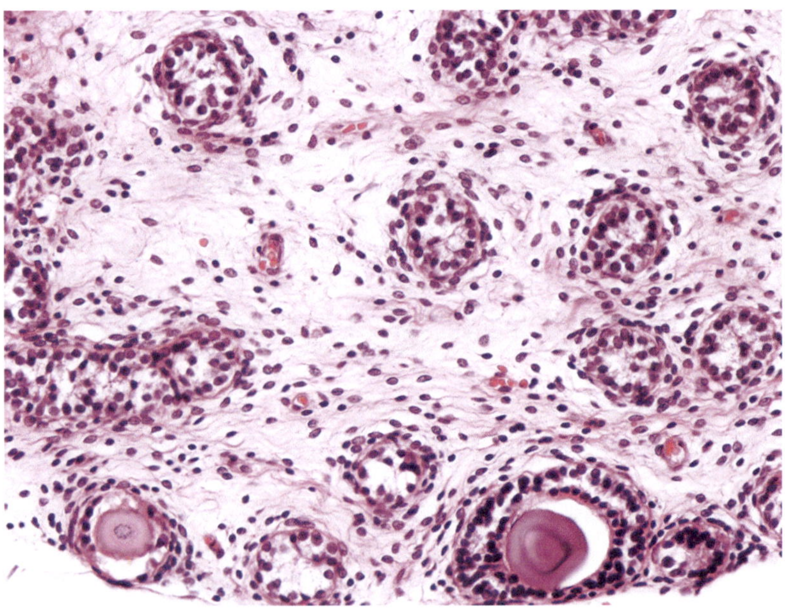

Fig. 2.19 Undescended testes with type III lesions. Tubular hypoplasia with the absence of germ cells, testicular microlithiasis, and abundant loose stroma

The most frequent histological findings during infancy are decreased germ cell number and reduction in tubular diameter, both in congenital and acquired cryptorchidism [160]. Based on four parameters (TFI, MTD, SCI, and the spermatogonial distribution pattern), most testicular biopsies from cryptorchid testis of children less than 4 years of age can be classified into three groups: type I (testes with slight alterations, 31 % of undescended testes), type II (testes with marked germinal hypoplasia, 29 %) (Fig. 2.18), and type III (testes with severe germinal hypoplasia, 40 %) [161] (Fig. 2.19).

About 8 % of the testes with type I lesions show many multinucleated spermatogonia (with three or more nuclei) [162], and both c-kit and

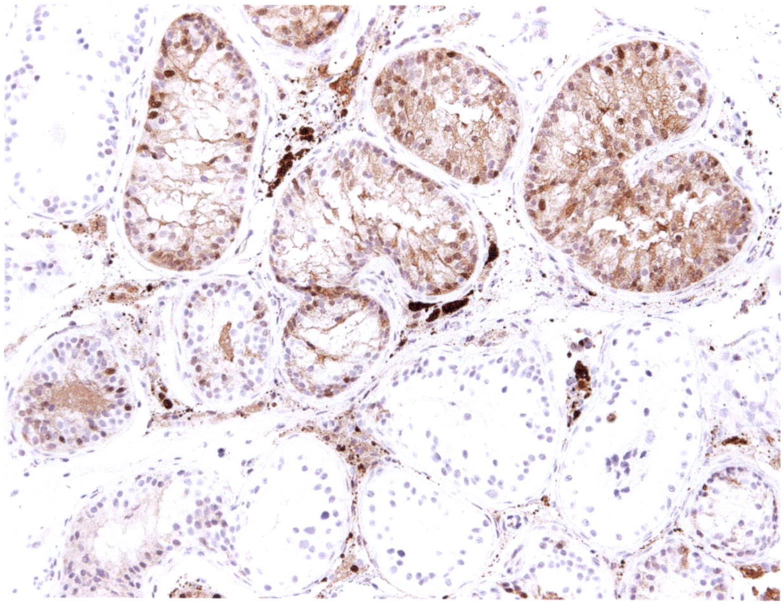

Fig. 2.20 Postpubertal cryptorchid testes. Group of seminiferous tubules with delayed maturation in an adult patient (calretinin)

PLAP expressions persist in about 5 % of immature germ cells. The seminiferous tubules of testes with type II or III lesions show a thickened lamina propria during childhood and, at puberty, Sertoli cell hyperplasia; and more than 30 % of these testes present microliths, ring-shaped tubules, and granular change in Sertoli cells. Type I lesions are comparable to the lesions seen in experimental cryptorchidism and also in normal testes with lesions induced by increased temperature [163].

Patients with bilateral cryptorchidism have a higher incidence of type II and III lesions than those with unilateral cryptorchidism. The bilateral cryptorchid testes bear variable degrees of abnormalities that, in addition to germ cells, involve Sertoli cells, peritubular myofibroblasts, and Leydig cells; these lesions become evident only after puberty [164] and are more severe in intraabdominal testes [165].

In unilateral cryptorchidism, the contralateral scrotal testis also displays histologic lesions of variable severity with an incidence that varies from 23 to 60 % in the different series. Usually these lesions are less severe than those of their counterpart cryptorchid testis, although lesions can also be equal or even more severe. These findings support the hypothesis of a bilateral defect in many cases of unilateral cryptorchidism.

Lesions in cryptorchid testes that underwent spontaneous ascent are developed later and are similar to those found in congenital cryptorchidism [166], whereas patients with cryptorchidism following herniotomy show less important germ cell number decreases [167], which are only evident after the fifth year of age [168].

At Pubertal Age

During puberty, undescended testes show a severe maturation delay in both tubular and interstitial components [169]. Seminiferous tubules display an apparent Sertoli cell hyperplasia per cross-sectioned tubule, as a result of the failure in lengthening and coiling of the seminiferous tubule during pubertal development, and also show decreased diameters and a delayed germ cell proliferation when these cells are present. Frequently, as puberty progresses, testicular development is very irregular, varying from one lobule to another. Seminiferous tubules that have initiated spermatogenesis are next to other tubules, showing a prepubertal maturative pattern. A careful study reveals a delay in Sertoli cell maturation (Fig. 2.20), estimated by nuclear morphology. Irregular expressions of androgen receptor have been detected by immunohistochemical methods in these Sertoli cells [170]. The tubules with

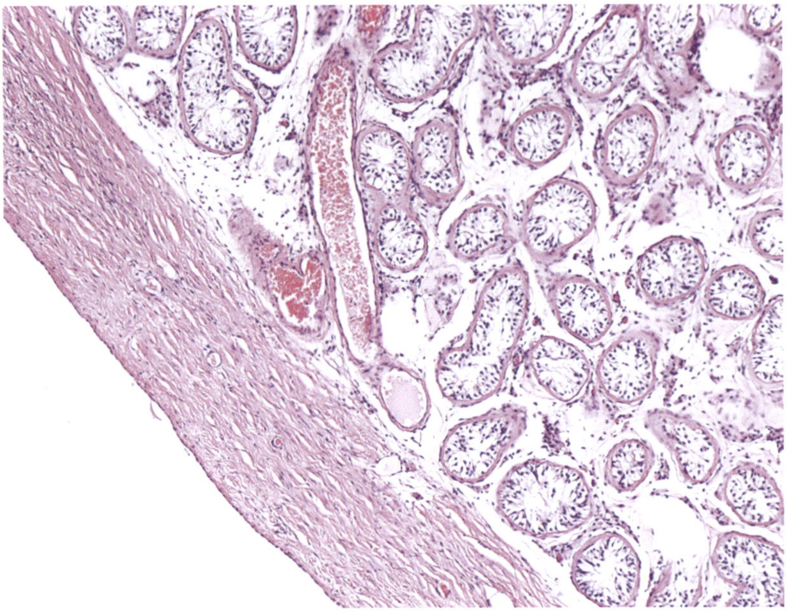

Fig. 2.21 A 27-year-old patient with cryptorchidism. Testicular parenchyma showing seminiferous tubules with thickened basement lamina lined by immature Sertoli cells and scanty Leydig cells in the interstitium

prepubertal pattern also show a delayed maturation in the tubular wall myofibroblasts, which are unable to express muscle-specific actin.

In Adulthood

Testicular biopsies of the removed cryptorchid testes from adults have revealed that most these testes show histological lesions in all their structural components, as well as in the rete testis and epididymis. The seminiferous tubules present a reduced diameter and deficient spermatogenesis. The most frequent germ cell pattern is spermatogonial maturation arrest, followed by Sertoli-cell-only tubules with dysgenetic Sertoli cells, mixed atrophy, and diffuse tubular sclerosis (Fig. 2.21). Only in tubules with advanced spermatogenesis, the morphology of Sertoli cell nuclei is normal [171]. The dysgenetic Sertoli cells in Sertoli-cell-only tubules, in addition to show immunoreaction to vimentin as the normal adult Sertoli cells do, can immunoexpress cytokeratins and desmin in the basal cytoplasm (Fig. 2.22). These immunoreactions are also positive in intraluminal accumulates of sloughed Sertoli cells [172].

The tubular wall shows decreases amounts of elastic fibers [173], increased collagenization, and irregular deposits of collagen IV and laminin in the basal lamina [164]. Peritubular myoid cells in experimental cryptorchidism show disorganization of actin filaments [174].

The undescended testes removed at adult age often present straight or slightly coiled tubules that frequently branch; hypoplastic tubules showing a small lumen and a thick wall lined by a tall columnar epithelium, formed only by Sertoli cells of eosinophilic cytoplasm; Sertoli cells nodules, seminiferous tubules with granular changes in Sertoli cells [175, 176]; and Leydig cell ectopy. Interstitial Leydig cells often exhibit cytoplasmic vacuolation, and their number is truly increased in some cases and only apparently increased in others. The testicular parenchyma adjacent to the rete testis often shows foci of adipose metaplasia. Most cryptorchid testes, and especially those with Sertoli-only-cell tubules, show an underdeveloped rete testis, whose epithelium has not differentiated squamous and columnar cells (conversely to that normally occurs along the puberty) and remains with the infantile pattern. This rete testis pattern has been called “dysgenetic rete testis.” Other rete testis anomalies such a hypoplasia, cystic hypoplasia, and adenomatous hyperplasia are also frequent [177, 178] (Fig. 2.23).

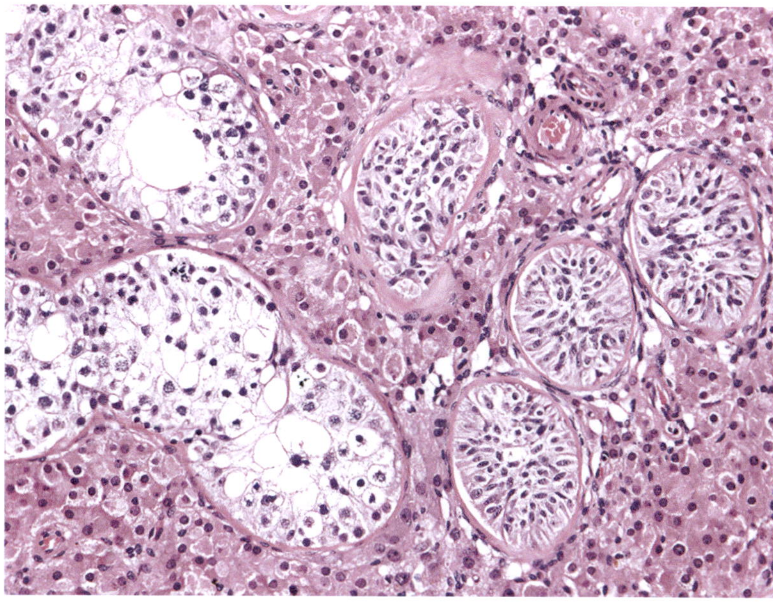

Fig. 2.22 Diffuse hyperplasia of Leydig cells in an adult testis with mixed atrophy

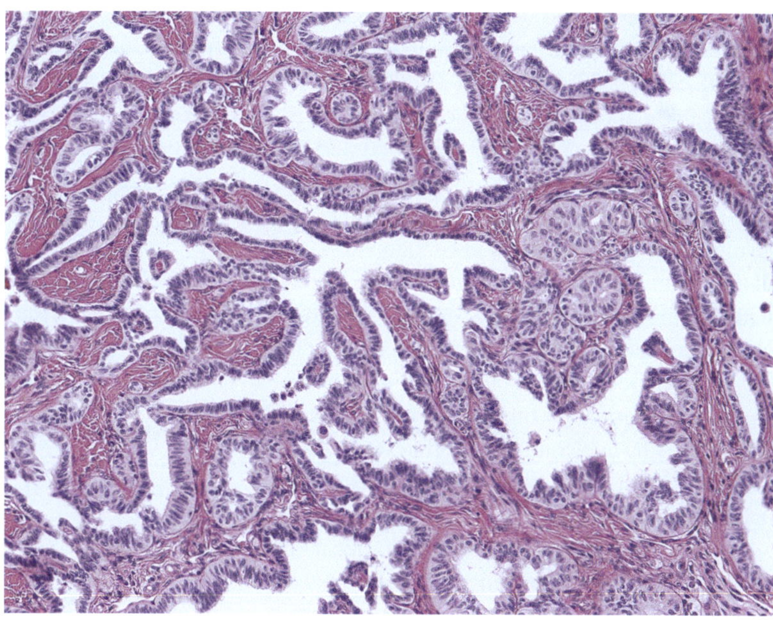

Fig. 2.23 Adenomatous hyperplasia of the rete testis with glandular and papillary areas

Correlation Between Lesion Pattern in Infancy and Morphological Findings in Adult Testes

It is of great importance to be able to predict the histological lesions that will have the testicular parenchyma in postpubertal ages from the study of the elemental lesions observed in biopsies of cryptorchid testes performed in infancy [179].

The comparison between the histologic findings from bilateral testicular biopsies performed at the time of orchidopexy in cryptorchid children with those obtained from the same patients in adulthood (performed for evaluation of infertility) can be carried out in institutions which have studied a large number of pediatric testicular biopsies. A 21 patients' series compares histological findings in prepubertal and postpubertal testicular biopsies in the same patient group of cryptorchid men [180]. The authors found that those testes with higher tubular fertility index (normal testis and those with type I lesions) developed diffuse and complete spermatogenesis in more than 2/3 of the cases, although it was quantitatively abnormal. The other third developed mixed atrophy of the testis (MAT). MAT is defined as the synchronous occurrence of tubules containing germ cells (showing variable degrees of spermatogenesis) and Sertoli-cell-only tubules. All the type II lesions and 85 % of the type III lesions developed MAT, leading to the conclusion that MAT is the most frequent lesion in adulthood (68.29 %) in cryptorchid patients presenting with infertility. MAT was observed in both the undescended testis and contralateral descended testis of the same patients, even if the surgical correction occurred at an early age. A positive correlation was found between the severity of the testicular lesions in childhood and the amount of spermatogenesis in adulthood. The type III lesions resulted most frequently in the development of MAT with less than 50 % of tubules with complete spermatogenesis, incomplete spermatogenesis, lesions of the basal compartment of seminiferous tubules, and testes with 100 % Sertoli-cell-only tubules. Prepubertal testes with clustering of tubules containing germ cells usually have incomplete spermatogenesis or less than 50 % of tubules with complete spermatogenesis at adulthood.

Sperm excretory duct anomalies occur in 9–36 % of cryptorchid patients. These anomalies can cause in adults obstruction of the excretory ducts; thus, testicular biopsies can also show an obstructive pattern of lesion superimposed [181].

In summary, the classification of testicular lesions in childhood into three types (I, II, and III) correlates with the amount of spermatogenesis found in postpubertal biopsies. The most important parameter is TFI. The spermatogenesis can also be impaired by an obstructive process, complete or incomplete, functional or organic. The testicular biopsy not only allows adequate evaluation of the either congenital or obstructive lesions, but also detects testes with focal spermatogenesis in order to establish the possibility of treatment with assisted reproductive techniques.

Cryptorchidism as a Manifestation of Malformative or Endocrinological Syndromes

Although cryptorchidism usually appears as an isolated anomaly, it is often associated with congenital endocrine or chromosomal disorders and DSD [182, 183]. Cryptorchidism has been reported in patients with GnRH deficit, as Kallmann syndrome and in Prader-Willi syndrome; androgen-receptor anomalies characteristically of testicular feminization syndromes; 5-α-reductase deficiency; several types of undermasculinization caused by absent anti-Müllerian hormone; and Klinefelter and Noonan syndromes. The association of impalpable testes with hypospadias suggests a DSD, disorder that is confirmed in 27–30 % of cases [184, 185]. Cryptorchidism also occurs in patients with the following syndromes: caudal regression, prune belly, Smith-Lemli-Opitz, Aarkog-Scott (also called Rubinstein-Taybi syndrome or CHARGE association), and trisomies 13, 18, and 21.

References

1. Lee PA, Houk CP, Ahmed SF, Hughes IA, International Consensus Conference on Intersex organized by the Lawson Wilkins Pediatric Endocrine Society and the European Society for Paediatric Endocrinology. Consensus statement on management of intersex disorders. International Consensus Conference on Intersex. Pediatrics. 2006;118:e488–500.
2. Damiani D, Guerra-Júnior G. New definitions and classifications of the intersexual states: in which the Chicago Consensus has contributed to the state of the art? Arq Bras Endocrinol Metabol. 2007;51:1013–7.
3. Canto P, De La Chesnaye E, Lopez M, Cervantes A, Chavez B, Vilchis F, Reyes E, Ulloa-Aguirre A, Kofman-Alfaro S, Mendez JP. A mutation in the 5′non-high mobility group box region of the SRY gene in patients with Turner syndrome and Y mosaicism. J Clin Endocrinol Metab. 2000;85: 1908–11.

4. Nistal M, Garcia-Fernández E, Mariño-Enríquez A, Serrano A, Regadera J, González-Peramato P. Diagnostic value of the gonadal biopsy in the disorders of sex development. Actas Urol Esp. 2007; 31:1056–75.
5. Nistal M, González-Peramato. Las disgenesias gonadales. Aproximación a través de la anatomía patológica al diagnóstico. Rev Horm Crecim. 2010;XIII:1–11.
6. Silengo M, Del Monaco A, Linari A, Lala R. Low birth-weight, microcephalic malformation syndrome in a 46, XX girl and her 46, XY sister with agonadism: third report of the Kennerknecht syndrome or autosomal recessive Seckel-like syndrome with previously undescribed genital anomalies. Am J Med Genet. 2001;101:275–8.
7. Cools M, Stoop H, Kersemaekers AM, Drop SL, Wolffenbuttel KP, Bourguignon JP, Slowikowska-Hilczer J, Kula K, Faradz SM, Oosterhuis JW, Looijenga LH. Gonadoblastoma arising in undifferentiated gonadal tissue within dysgenetic gonads. J Clin Endocrinol Metab. 2006;91:2404–13.
8. Parmley T. The histologic morphology of gonadal dysgenesis: early premature gonadal failure. Semin Reprod Endocrinol. 1983;1:121–7.
9. Modi DN, Sane S, Bhartiya D. Accelerated germ cell apoptosis in sex chromosome aneuploid fetal human gonads. Mol Hum Reprod. 2003;9:219–25.
10. Boczkowski K. Pure gonadal dysgenesis and ovarian dysplasia in sisters. Am J Obstet Gynecol. 1970;106: 626–8.
11. Marrakchi A, Belhaj L, Boussouf H, Chraibi A, Kadiri A. [Pure gonadal dysgenesis XX and XY: observations in fifteen patients]. Ann Endocrinol (Paris). 2005;66:553–6.
12. Meyers CM, Boughman JA, Rivas M, Wilroy RS, Simpson JL. Gonadal (ovarian) dysgenesis in 46, XX individuals: frequency of the autosomal recessive form. Am J Med Genet. 1996;63:518–24.
13. Berkovitz GD, Fechner PY, Zacur HW, Rock JA, 3rd Snyder HM, Migeon CJ, Perlman EJ. Clinical and pathologic spectrum of 46,XY gonadal dysgenesis: its relevance to the understanding of sex differentiation. Medicine (Baltimore). 1991;70:375–83.
14. Scherer G, Held M, Erdel M, Meschede D, Horst J, Lesniewicz R, Midro AT. Three novel SRY mutations in XY gonadal dysgenesis and the enigma of XY dysgenesis cases without SRY mutations. Cytogen Cell Genet. 1998;80:188–92.
15. Crone J, Amann G, Gheradini R, Kirchlechner V, Fekete CN. Management of 46, XY partial gonadal dysgenesis-revisited. Wien Klin Wochenschr. 2002; 114:462–7.
16. Yoon KH, Lee YJ. A case of 46, XY pure gonadal dysgenesis with loss of the sex-determining region of Y chromosome. Korean J Lab Med. 2008;28:151–4.
17. Gwin K, Cajaiba MM, Caminoa-Lizarralde A, Picazo ML, Nistal M, Reyes-Múgica M. Expanding the clinical spectrum of Frasier syndrome. Pediatr Dev Pathol. 2008;11:122–7.
18. Jirasek J. Principles of reproductive embryology. In: Simpson JL, editor. Disorders of sexual differentiation. New York: Academic Press; 1976. p. 51–111.
19. Sohval AR. Hermaphroditism with "atypical" or "mixed" gonadal dysgenesis. Am J Med. 1964;36: 281–92.
20. Nonomura N, Nakamura M, Namiki M, Kiyohara H, Mizutani S, Okuyama A, Sonoda T. Mixed gonadal dysgenesis: case reports and a review of 65 Japanese cases. Arch Androl. 1991;26:15–9.
21. Alvarez-Nava F, Soto M, Borjas L, Ortiz R, Rojas A, Martinez S, Revol A, Barrera H, Alvarez Z. Molecular analysis of SRY gene in patients with mixed gonadal dysgenesis. Ann Genet. 2001;44:155–9.
22. Chemes H, Muzulin PM, Venara MC, Mulhmann MC, Martinez M, Gamboni M. Early manifestations of testicular dysgenesis in children: pathological phenotypes, karyotype correlations and precursor stages of tumor development. APMIS. 2003;111: 12–23.
23. Caglayan AO, Demiryilmaz F, Kendirci M, Ozyazgan I, Akalin H, Bittmann S. Mixed gonadal dysgenesis with 45, X/46, X, idic(Y)/46, XY, idic(Y) karyotype. Genet Couns. 2009;20:173–9.
24. Ribeiro Scolfaro M, Aparecida Cardinalli L, Gabas Stuchi-Perez E, Palandi De Mello M, De Godoy Assumpcao J, Matias Baptista MT, Bustorff Silva JM, Trevas Maciel-Gerra A, Jr. Guerra G. Morphometry and histology of gonads from 13 children with dysgenetic male pseudohermaphroditism. Arch Pathol Lab Med. 2001;125:652–6.
25. Slowikoska-Hilczer J, Szarras-Czapnik M, Kula K. Testicular pathology in 46, XY dysgenetic male pseudohermaphroditism: an approach to pathogenesis of testis cancer. J Androl. 2001;22:781–92.
26. Nishina-Uchida N, Fukuzawa R, Hasegawa Y, Morison IM. Identification of X monosomy cells from a gonad of mixed gonadal dysgenesis with a 46,XY karyotype: case report. Medicine (Baltimore). 2015;94:e720.
27. Nistal M, Paniagua R, Isorna S, Mancebo J. Diffuse intratubular undifferentiated germ cell tumor in both testes of a male subject with a uterus and ipsilateral testicular dysgenesis. J Urol. 1980;124:286–9.
28. Josso N, Belville C, di Clemente N, Picard JY. AMH and AMH receptor defects in persistent Müllerian duct syndrome. Hum Reprod Update. 2005;11:351–6.
29. Wuerstle M, Lesser T, Hurwitz R, Applebaum H, Lee SL. Persistent mullerian duct syndrome and transverse testicular ectopia: embryology, presentation, and management. J Pediatr Surg. 2007;42: 2116–9.
30. Carcavilla A, Alonso M, Ezquieta B, García-Galloway E, Barrio R, Nistal M. An XX male with an intratubular undifferentiated germ cell neoplasia. Fertil Steril. 2008;90:2005.
31. Belville C, Maréchal JD, Pennetier S, Carmillo P, Masgrau L, Messika-Zeitoun L, Galey J, Machado G, Treton D, Gonzalès J, Picard JY, Josso N, Cate

RL, di Clemente N. Natural mutations of the anti-Mullerian hormone type II receptor found in persistent Mullerian duct syndrome affect ligand binding, signal transduction and cellular transport. Hum Mol Genet. 2009;18:3002–13.

32. Nistal M, Paniagua R, González-Peramato P, Reyes-Múgica M. Perspectives in pediatric pathology, chapter 5. Gonadal dysgenesis. Pediatr Dev Pathol. 2015;18:259–78.
33. Job J, Canlorbe P, Job J, Person M, editors. Pediatric endocrinology. 2nd ed. New York: Wiley Medical; 1981. p. 347.
34. Grumbach MM, Conte FA. Disorders of sex differentiation. In: Wilson JD, Foster DW, editors. Williams textbook of endocrinology. 8th ed. Philadelphia: Saunders Co; 1992. p. 916–21.
35. Prader A, Gurtnen HP. Das Syndrom des Pseudohermaphroditismus Masculinus bei kongenitaler Nevennierenrinden-Hyperplasie ohne Androgenüberproduktion. Helvet Paediatr Acta. 1955;10: 397–412.
36. Prader A, Siebenmann RE. Nebenniereninsuffizienz bei kongrnitaler Lipoihyperplasie der Nebennieren. Helv Paediatr Acta. 1957;12:569–95.
37. Chen X, Baker BY, Abduljabbar MA, Miller WL. A genetic isolate of congenital lipoid adrenal hyperplasia with atypical clinical findings. J Clin Endocrinol Metab. 2005;90:835–40.
38. Bhangoo A, Anhalt H, Ten S, King SR. Phenotypic variations in lipoid congenital adrenal hyperplasia. Pediatr Endocrinol Rev. 2006;3:258–71.
39. Saenger P, Klonari Z, Black SM, Compagnone N, Mellon SH, Fleischer A, Abrams CAL, Shackelton CHL, Miller WL. Prenatal diagnosis of congenital lipoid adrenal hyperplasia. J Clin Endocrinol Metab. 1995;80:200–5.
40. Saenger P. Abnormal sex differentiation. J Pediatr. 1984;104:1–17.
41. Caron KM, Soo SC, Wetsel WC, Stocco DM, Clark BJ, Parker KL. Targeted disruption of the mouse gene encoding steroidogenic acute regulatory protein provides insights into congenital lipoid adrenal hyperplasia. Proc Natl Acad Sci U S A. 1997;94:11540–5.
42. Kirkland RT, Kirkland JL, Johnson CM, Horning MG, Librik L, Clayton GW. Congenital lipoid adrenal hyperplasia in a eight-year- old phenotype female. J Clin Endocrinol. 1973;36:488–96.
43. Kim SO, Choi C, Kim CJ, Kim JS, Kwon D, Kang TW, Park K, Ryu SB, Jung SI, Oh KJ, Im CM. Lipoid congenital adrenal hyperplasia: pathologic features of the testis. Urology. 2010;75:176–8.
44. Dhom G. Zur Morphologie und Genese der kongenitalen Nebennierenrindenhyperplasie beim männlichen scheinzwitter. Z Allg Pathol Anat. 1958;97:346–57.
45. Ogata T, Matsuo N, Saito M, Prader A. The testicular lesion and sexual differentiation in congenital lipoid adrenal hyperplasia. Helv Paediatr Acta. 1989;43:531–8.
46. Hauffa BP, Miller WL, Grumbach MM, Conte FA, Kaplan SL. Congenital adrenal lipoid hyperplasia due to deficient cholesterol side-chain cleavage activity (20,22-desmolase) in a patient treated for 18 years. Clin Endocrinol (Oxf). 1985;23:481–93.
47. Zhang L, Mason JI, Naiki Y, Copeland KC, Castro-Magana M, Gordon-Walker TT, Chang YT, Pang S. Characterization of two novel homozygous missense mutations involving codon 6 and 259 of type II 3beta-hydroxysteroid dehydrogenase (3betaHSD) gene causing, respectively, nonsalt-wasting and salt-wasting 3betaHSD deficiency disorder. J Clin Endocrinol Metab. 2000;85:1678–85.
48. Aaronson IA, Carkmak MA, Key LL. Defects of the testosterone biosynthetic pathway in boys with hypospadias. J Urol. 1997;157:1884–8.
49. Sapunar J, Vidal T, Bauer K. Abnormalities of adrenal steroidogenesis in Chilean boys with micropenis. Rev Med Chil. 2003;131:46–54.
50. Lam CW, Arlt W, Chan CK, Honour JW, Lin CJ, Tong SF, Choy KW, Miller WL. Mutation of proline 409 to arginine in the meander region of cytochrome p450c17 causes severe 17 alpha-hydroxylase deficiency. Mol Genet Metab. 2001;72:254–9.
51. Auchus RJ, Gupta MK. Towards a unifying mechanism for CYP17 mutations that cause isolated 17,20-lyase deficiency. J Clin Endocrinol Metab. 2006;91:2428–31.
52. Monno S, Mizushima Y, Toyoda N, Kashii T, Kobayashi M. A new variant of the cytochrome P450c17 (CYP17) gene mutation in three patients with 17 alpha-hydroxylase deficiency. Ann Hum Genet. 1997;61:275–9.
53. Savage MO. Ambiguous genitalia, small genitalia and undescended testes. Clin Endocrinol Metab. 1982;11:127–58.
54. Kaufman FR, Costin G, Goebelsmann U, Stanczyk FZ, Zachmann M. Male pseudohermaphroditism due to 17,20-desmolase deficiency. J Clin Endocrinol Metab. 1983;57:32–6.
55. Goebelsmann U, Davajan V, Isreal R, Mestman JH, Mishell DR, Zachmann M. Male pseudohermaphroditism consistent with 17-20-desmolase deficiency. Gynec Invest. 1974;5:60–4.
56. Zachmann M. Endocrine findings in male pseudohermaphroditism. Eur J Pediatr. 1993;152:S58–61.
57. Geissler WM, Davis DL, Wu L, Bradshaw KD, Patel S, Mendonca BB, Elliston KO, Wilson JD, Russell DW, Andersson S. Male pseudohermaphroditism caused by mutations of testicular 17 beta-hydroxysteroid dehydrogenase 3. Nat Genet. 1994;7:34–9.
58. Faienza MF, Giordani L, Delvecchio M, Cavallo L. Clinical, endocrine, and molecular findings in 17beta-hydroxysteroid dehydrogenase type 3 deficiency. J Endocrinol Invest. 2008;31:85–91.
59. Gross DJ, Landau H, Kohn G, Farkas A, Elrayyes E, El- Shawwa R, Lasch EE, Rösler A. Male pseudohermaphroditism due 17B-hydroxysteroid dehydrogenase deficiency: gender reassignment in

early infancy. Acta Endocrinol (Copenh). 1986;112: 238–46.

60. Twesten W, Johannisson R, Holterhus PM, Hiort O. Severe 46, XY virilization deficit due to 17beta-hydroxysteroid dehydrogenase deficiency. Klin Padiatr. 2002;214:314–5.
61. Longo FJ, Coleman SA, Givens JR. Ultrastructural analysis of the testes in male pseudohermaphroditism due to deficiency of 17-ketosteroid reductase. Am J Clin Pathol. 1975;64:145–54.
62. Ademola Akesode F, 3rd Meyer WJ, Migeon CJ. Male pseudohermaphroditism with gynaecomastia due to testicular 17-ketosteroid reductase deficiency. Clin Endocrinol (Oxf). 1977;7:443–52.
63. Brown DM, Markland C, Dehner LP. Leydig cell hypoplasia: a cause of pseudohermaphroditism. J Clin Endocrinol Metab. 1978;45:1–7.
64. Eil C, Austin RM, Sesterhenn I, Dunn JF, Cutler Jr GB, Johnsonbaugh RE. Leydig cell hypoplasia causing male pseudohermaphroditism: diagnosis 13 years after prepubertal castration. J Clin Endocrinol Metab. 1984;58:441–8.
65. Arnhold IJ, Mendonça BB, Bloise W, Toledo SP. Male pseudohermaphroditism resulting from Leydig cell hypoplasia. J Pediatr. 1985;106:1057.
66. Kossack N, Simoni M, Richter-Unruh A, Themmen AP, Gromoll J. Mutations in a novel, cryptic exon of the luteinizing hormone/chorionic gonadotropin receptor gene cause male pseudohermaphroditism. PLoS Med. 2008;5:e88.
67. Richter-Unruh A, Martens JW, Verhoef-Post M, Wessels HT, Kors WA, Sinnecker GH, Boehmer A, Drop SL, Toledo SP, Brunner HG, Themmen AP. Leydig cell hypoplasia: cases with new mutations, new polymorphisms and cases without mutations in the luteinizing hormone receptor gene. Clin Endocrinol (Oxf). 2002;56:103–12.
68. Toledo SPA, Arnhold IJP, Lunthold W, Russo EMK, Saldanha PH. Leydig cell hypoplasia determining familial hypergonadotropic hypogonadism. In: Papadatos CJ, Bartsocas CS, editors. Endocrine genetics and genetics of growth, Progress in clinical and biological research, vol. 200. New York: Alan R Liss; 1985. p. 311–4.
69. Brinkmann AO. Molecular basis of androgen insensitivity. Mol Cell Endocrinol. 2001;179:105–9.
70. Rutgers JL, Scully RE. The androgen insensitivity syndrome (testicular feminization): a clinicopathologic study of 43 cases. Int J Gynecol Path. 1991;10:126–44.
71. Imperato-McGinley J, Canovatchel WJ. Complete androgen insensitivity: pathophysiology, diagnosis and management. Trends Endocrinol Metab. 1992;3:75–81.
72. Quigley CA, De Bellis A, Marschke KB, El-Awady MK, Wilson EM, French FS. Androgen receptor defects. Historical, clinical and molecular perspectives. Endocr Rev. 1995;16:271–321.
73. Radmayr C, Culig Z, Glatzl J, Neuschmid-Kaspar F, Bartsch G, Klocker H. Androgen receptor point mutations as the underlying molecular defect in 2 patients with androgen insensitivity syndrome. J Urol. 1997;158:1553–6.
74. Jukubiczka S, Nedel S, Werder EA, Schleiermacher E, Theile U, Wolff G, Wieacker P. Mutations of the androgen receptor gene in patients with complete androgen insensitivity. Hum Mutat. 1997;9:57–61.
75. Gottieb B, Pinsky L, Beitel LK, Trifiro M. Androgen insensitivity. Am J Med Genet. 1999;89:210–7.
76. Zhu Y-S, Cai L-Q, Cordero JJ, Canovatchel WJ, Katz MD, Imperato-McGinley J. A novel mutation in the CAG triplet region of exon 1 of androgen receptor gene causes complete androgen insensitivity syndrome in a large kindred. J Clin Endocrinol Metab. 1999;84:1590–4.
77. Singh R, Shastry PK, Rasalkar AA, Singh L, Thangaraj K. A novel androgen receptor mutation resulting in complete androgen insensitivity syndrome and bilateral Leydig cell hyperplasia. J Androl. 2006;27:510–6.
78. Sarpel U, Palmer SK, Dolgin SE. The incidence of complete androgen insensitivity in girls with inguinal hernias and assessment of screening by vaginal length measurement. J Pediatr Surg. 2005;40:133–6.
79. Van Zijl JA, Evers JLH, Gerver WJM. Testicular feminization syndrome in the neonate. Gynecol Obstet Invest. 1990;29:161–4.
80. Viner RM, Teoh Y, Williams DM, Patterson MN, Hughes IA. Androgen insensitivity syndrome: a survey of diagnostic procedures and management in the UK. Arch Dis Child. 1997;77:305–9.
81. Regadera J, Martinez-García F, Paniagua R, Nistal M. Androgen insensitivity syndrome. An immunohistochemical, ultrastructural, and morphometric study. Arch Pathol Lab Med. 1999;123:225–34.
82. Morris JM. The syndrome of testicular feminization in male pseudohermaphrodites. Am J Obstet Gynecol. 1953;65:1192–211.
83. Boehmer AL, Brinkmann O, Brüggenwirth H, van Assendelft C, Otten BJ, Verleun-Mooijman MC, Niermeijer MF, Brunner HG, Rouwé CW, Waelkens JJ, Oostdijk W, Kleijer WJ, van der Kwast TH, de Vroede MA, Drop SL. Genotype versus phenotype in families with androgen insensitivity syndrome. J Clin Endocrinol Metab. 2001;86:4151–60.
84. Müller J. Morphometry and histology of gonads from twelve children and adolescents with the androgen insensitivity (testicular feminization) syndrome. J Clin Endocrinol Metab. 1984;59:785–9.
85. Rutgers JL. Advances in the pathology of intersex conditions. Hum Pathol. 1991;22:884–91.
86. Nistal M, De La Roza C, Cano J. Síndrome de feminización testicular completa. Patología. 1979;12:119–25.
87. Wilson JD, Harrod MJ, Goldstein JL, Hemsell DL, MacDonald PC. Familial incomplete male pseudohermaphroditism, type 1. Evidence for androgen resistance and variable clinical manifestations in a family with the Reifenstein syndrome. N Engl J Med. 1974;290:1097–103.

88. Lubs Jr HA, Vilar O, Bergenstal DM. Familial male pseudohermaphroditism with labial testes and partial feminization: endocrine studies and genetic aspects. J Clin Endocr Metab. 1959;19:1110–20.
89. Gilbert-Dreyfus S, Sebaoun CL, Belaisch J. Étude d'un cas familial d'androgynoidisme avec hypospadias grave, gynecomastie et hyperoestrogenie. Ann Endocr. 1957;18:93–101.
90. Reifenstein Jr EC. Hereditary familial hypogonadism. Proc Am Fed Clin Res. 1947;3:86.
91. Rosewater S, Gwinup G, Hamwi GJ. Familial gynecomastia. Ann Inter Med. 1965;63:377–85.
92. Deeb A, Mason C, Lee YS, Hughes IA. Correlation between genotype, phenotype and sex of rearing in 111 patients with partial androgen insensitivity syndrome. Clin Endocrinol (Oxf). 2005;63:56–62.
93. Lombardo F, Sgro P, Salacone P, Gilio B, Gandini L, Dondero F, Jannini EA, Lenzi A. Androgens and fertility. J Endocrinol Invest. 2005;28:51–5.
94. Morrow AG, Gyorki S, Warne GL, Burger HG, Bangah ML, Outch KH, Mirovics A, Baker HW. Variable androgen receptor levels in infertile men. J Clin Endocrinol Metab. 1987;64:1115–21.
95. Finsterer J, Stöllberger C. Quinine-responsive muscle cramps in X-linked bulbospinal muscular atrophy Kennedy. J Neurol. 2009;256:1355–6.
96. Stefanis C, Papapetropoulos T, Scarpalezos S, Lygidakis G, Panayiotopoulos CP. X-linked spinal and bulbar muscular atrophy of late onset. A separate type of motor neuron disease? J Neurol Sci. 1975;24:493–503.
97. Harding AE, Thomas PK, Baraitser M, Bradbury PG, Morgan-Hughes JA, Ponsford JR. X-linked recessive bulbospinal neuronopathy: a report of ten cases. J Neurol Neurosurg Psychiatry. 1982;45:1012–9.
98. Arbizu T, Santamaria J, Gomez JM, Quilez A, Serra JP. A family with adult spinal and bulbar muscular atrophy, X-linked inheritance and associated testicular failure. J Neurol Sci. 1983;59:371–82.
99. Russell DW, Berman DM, Bryant JT, Cala KM, Davis DL, Landrum CP, Prihoda JS, Silver RI, Thigpen AE, Wigley WC. The molecular genetics of steroid 5 alpha-reductase. Recent Prog Horm Res. 1994;49:275–84.
100. Peterson RE, Imperato-McGinley J, Gautier T, Sturla E. Male pseudohermaphroditism due to steroid 5 alpha-reductase deficiency. Am J Med. 1977;62:170–91.
101. Fernández-Cancio M, Nistal M, Gracia R, Molina MA, Tovar JA, Esteban C, Carrascosa A, Audí L. Compound heterozygous mutations in the SRD5A2 gene exon 4 in a male pseudohermaphrodite patient of Chinese origin. J Androl. 2004;25:412–6.
102. Okon E, Livni N, Rösler A, Yorkoni S, Segal S, Kohn G, Schenker JG. Male pseudohermaphroditism due to 5 alpha-reductase deficiency. Ultrastructure of the gonads. Arch Pathol Lab Med. 1980;104:363–7.
103. Damiani D, Fellous M, McElreavey K, Barbaux S, Barreto ES, Dichtchekenian V, Setian N. True hermaphroditism: clinical aspects and molecular studies in 16 cases. Eur J Endocrinol. 1997;136:201–4.
104. Krstic ZD, Smoljanic Z, Vukanic D, Varinac D, Janjic G. True hermaphroditism: 10 years' experience. Pediatr Surg Int. 2000;16:580–3.
105. Wettasinghe KT, Sirisena ND, Andraweera PH, Jayasekara RW, Dissanayake VH. A case series of five sri lankan patients with ovotesticular disorder of sex development. Clin Pediatr Endocrinol. 2012;21:69–73.
106. Van Niekert WA. True hermaphroditism. Clinical morphological and cytogenetic aspects. New York: Harper and Row; 1974.
107. Krob G, Braun A, Kuhnle U. True hermaphroditism: geographical distribution, clinical findings, chromosomes and gonadal histology. Eur J Pediatr. 1994;153:2–10.
108. Kojima Y, Hayashi Y, Asai N, Maruyama T, Sasaki S, Kohri K. Detection of the sex-determining region of the Y chromosome in 46, XX true hermaphroditism. Urol Int. 1998;60:235–8.
109. Kolon TF, Ferrer FA, Mckenna PH. Clinical and molecular analysis of XX sex reversed patients. J Urol. 1998;160:1169–72.
110. Berkovitz GD, Fechner PY, Marcantonio SM, Bland G, Stetten G, Goodfellow PN, Smith KD, Migeon CJ. The role of the sex-determining region of the Y chromosome (SRY) in the etiology of 46, XX true hermaphroditism. Hum Genet. 1992;88:411–6.
111. Kojima Y, Hayashi Y, Mizuno K, Sasaki S, Fukui Y, Koopman P, Morohashi K, Kohri K. Up-regulation of SOX9 in human sex-determining region on the Y chromosome (SRY)-negative XX males. Clin Endocrinol (Oxf). 2008;68:791–9.
112. Abbas NE, Toublanc JE, Boucekkine C, Toublanc M, Affara NA, Job J-C, Fellous M. A possible common origin of "Y-negative" human XX males and XX true hermaphrodites. Hum Genet. 1990;84:356–60.
113. Fechner PY, Marcantonio SM, Jaswaney V, Stetten G, Goodfellow PN, Migeon CJ, Smith K, Berkovitz GD, Amrhein JA, Bard PA, Lee PA, Reid C, Tsalikian E, Urban MD. The role of the sex-determining region Y gene in the etiology of 46,XX maleness. J Clin Endocrinol Metab. 1993;76:690–5.
114. Ouhilal S, Turco J, Nangia A, Stotland M, Manganiello PD. True hermaphroditism presenting as bilateral gynecomastia in an adolescent phenotypic male. Fertil Steril. 2005;83:1041.
115. Osorio Acosta VA, Alonso Dominguez FJ. True hermaphroditism. Arch Esp Urol. 2004;57:856–60.
116. Morel Y, Rey R, Teinturier C, Nicolino M, Michel-Calemard L, Mowszowicz I, Jaubert F, Fellous M, Chaussain JL, Chatelain P, David M, Nihoul-Fekete C, Forest MG, Josso N. A etiological diagnosis of male sex ambiguity: a collaborative study. Eur J Pediatr. 2002;161:49–59.
117. Olsson CA, Tessier PA, Brown ML, Austen Jr G. True hermaphroditism. J Urol. 1971;105:586–90.
118. Luks FI, Hansbrough F, Klotz Jr DH, Rottmeier PK, Tolete-Velcek F. Early gender assignment in true hermaphroditism. J Pediatr Surg. 1988;23:1122–6.
119. Van Niekert WA, Retief AE. The gonads of human true hermaphrodites. Hum Genet. 1981;58:117–22.

120. Kropp BP, Keating MA, Moshang T, Duckett JW. True hermaphroditism and normal male genitalia: an unusual presentation. Urology. 1995;46: 736–9.
121. McDaniel EC, Nadel M, Woolverton WC. True hermaphrodite with bilaterally descended ovotestes. J Urol. 1968;100:77–81.
122. Wiersma R, Ramdial PK. The gonads of 111 South African patients with ovotesticular disorder of sex differentiation. J Pediatr Surg. 2009;44:556–60.
123. Aaronson IA. True hermaphroditism. A review of 41 cases with observations on testicular histology and function. Br J Urol. 1985;57:775–9.
124. Williamson HO, Phansey SA, Mathur RS. True hermaphroditism with term vaginal delivery and a review. Am J Obstec Gynecol. 1981;141:262–5.
125. Tanaka Y, Fujiwara K, Yamauchi H, Mikami Y, Kohno L. Pregnancy in a woman with a Y chromosome after removal of an ovarian dysgerminoma. Gynecol Oncol. 2000;79:519–21.
126. Schultz BA, Roberts S, Rodgers A, Ataya K. Pregnancy in true hermaphrodites and all male offspring to date. Obstet Gynecol. 2009;113:534–6.
127. Younis JS, Radin O, Kerner H, Ben-Ami M. Successful monozygotic twin pregnancy fathered by a male 46, XY true hermaphrodite. Reprod Biomed Online. 2011;22:80–2.
128. Tiltman AJ, Sweerts M. Multiparity in a covert true hermaphrodite. Obstet Gynecol. 1982;60:752–4.
129. Minowada S, Fukutani K, Hara M, Shinohara M, Kamioka J, Isurugi K, Nijima T. Childbirth in true hermaphrodite. Eur Urol. 1984;10:414–5.
130. Scorer CG. The descent of the testis. Arch Dis Child. 1964;39:605–9.
131. Thonneau PF, Gandia P, Mieusset R. Cryptorchidism: incidence, risk factors, and potential role of environment; an update. J Androl. 2003;24:155–62.
132. JOHN RADCLIFFE Hospital Cryptorchidism Study Group. Cryptorchidism: an apparent substantial increase since 1960. Br Med J. 1986;293:1401–4.
133. OHN RADCLIFFE Hospital Cryptorchidism Study Group. Cryptorchidism: a prospective study of 7.500 consecutive male births. 1984–1988. Arch Dis Child. 1992;67:892–9.
134. Storgaard L, Bonde JP, Olsen J. Male reproductive disorders in humans and prenatal indicators of estrogen exposure. A review of published epidemiological studies. Reprod Toxicol. 2006;21:4–15.
135. Scorer CG, Farrington GH. Congenital deformities of the testis and epididymis. New York: Appleton – Century – Crofts; 1971. p. 136–46.
136. Nistal M, Paniagua R. Infertility in adult males with retractile testes. Fertil Steril. 1984;41:395–403.
137. Akre O, Lipworth L, Cnattingius S, Sparén P, Ekbom A. Risk factor patterns for cryptorchidism and hypospadias. Epidemiology. 1999;10:364–9.
138. Hjertkvist M, Dauber JE, Berhg A. Cryptorchidism: a registry based study in Sweden on some factors of some possible etiological importance. J Epidemiol Community Health. 1989;43:324–9.
139. Berkowitz GS, Lapinski RH, Godbold JH, Dolgin SE, Holzman IR. Maternal and neonatal risk factors for cryptorchidism. Epidemiology. 1995;6:127–31.
140. Weidner IS, Moller H, Jensen TK, Skakkebaek NE. Risk factors for cryptorchidism and hypospadias. J Urol. 1999;161:1606–9.
141. Ferlin A, Zuccarello D, Zuccarello B, Chirico MR, Zanon GF, Foresta C. Genetic alterations associated with cryptorchidism. JAMA. 2008;300:2271–6.
142. Pardo Mindan FJ, Vargas Torcal F, García Julian G, Virto Ruiz MT. Familial cryptorchidism. Pediatrics. 1975;56:616.
143. Hutson JM, Hasthorpe S, Heyns CF. Anatomical and functional aspects of testicular descent and cryptorchidism. Endocr Rev. 1997;18:259–80.
144. Guven A, Kogan BA. Undescended testis in older boys: further evidence that ascending testes are common. J Pediatr Surg. 2008;43:1700–4.
145. Eardley KC, Saw KC, Whitaker RH. Surgical outcome of orchidopexy II. Trapped and ascending testes. Br J Urol. 1994;73:204–6.
146. Kaplan GW. Iatrogenic cryptorchidism resulting from hernia repair. Surg Gynecol Obstet. 1976;142: 671–2.
147. Surana R, Puri P. Iatrogenic ascent of the testIs: an under-recognized complication of inguinal hernia operation in children. Br J Urol. 1994;73:580–1.
148. Colodny AH. Iatrogenic ascent of the testis: an underrecognized complication of inguinal hernia operation in children. Br J Urol. 1994;74:531–2.
149. Myers NA, Officer CB. Undescended testis: congenital or acquired? Aust Paediatr J. 1975;11:76–80.
150. Gracia J, Navarro E, Guirado F, Pueyo C, Ferrandez A. Spontaneous ascent of the testis. Br J Urol. 1997;79:113–5.
151. Docimo SG. Testicular descent and ascent in the first year of life. Urology. 1996;48:458–60.
152. Atwell JD. Ascent of the testis: fact or fiction. Br J Urol. 1985;57:474–7.
153. Clarnette TD, Rowe D, Hasthorpe S, Hutson JM. Incomplete disappearance of the processus vaginalis as a cause of ascending testis. J Urol. 1997;157:1889–91.
154. Wright JE. Testes do ascend. Pediatr Surg Int. 1989;4:269–72.
155. Rabinowitz R, Hulbert Jr WC. Late presentation of cryptorchidism: the etiology of testicular re-ascent. J Urol. 1997;157:1892–4.
156. Jedrzejewski G, Wozniak MM, Madej T, Kryza R, Zielonka-Lamparska E, Wieczorek AP. The differences in testicular volumes in boys 8–36 months old with undescended, retractile and hydrocele testis – usefulness of scrotal screening ultrasound. Early Hum Dev. 2012;88:185–9.
157. Nistal M, Paniagua R. Testicular biopsy. Contemporary interpretation. Urol Clin North Am. 1999;26:555–93.
158. Hadziselimovic F, Hocht B, Herzog B, Buser MW. Infertility in cryptorchidism is linked to the stage of germ cell development at orchidopexy. Horm Res. 2007;68:46–52.

159. Huff DS, Hadziselimovic F, Snyder 3rd HM, Duckett JW, Keating MA. Postnatal testicular maldevelopment in unilateral cryptorchidism. J Urol. 1989;142:546–8.
160. Rusnack SL, Wu H-Y, Huff DS, Snyder III HM, Zderic SA, Carr MC, Canning DA. The ascending testis and the testis undescended since birth share the same histopathology. J Urol. 2002;168:2590–1.
161. Nistal M, Paniagua R, Díez-Pardo JA. Histologic classification of undescended testes. Hum Pathol. 1980;11:666–74.
162. Cortes D, Thorup J, Visfeldt J. Multinucleated spermatogonia in cryptorchid boys: a possible association with an increased risk of testicular malignancy. APMIS. 2003;111:25–30.
163. Huff DS, Fenig DM, Canning DA, Carr MG, Zderic SA, Snyder 3rd HM. Abnormal germ cell development in cryptorchidism. Horm Res. 2001;55:11–7.
164. Santamaría L, Martinez-Onsurbe P, Paniagua R, Nistal M. Laminin, type IV collagen, and fibronectin in normal and cryptorchid human testes. An immunohistochemical study. Int J Androl. 1990;13:135–46.
165. Abouzeid AA, Mousa MH, Soliman HA, Hamza AF, Hay SA. Intra-abdominal testis: histological alterations and significance of biopsy. J Urol. 2011;185:269–74.
166. Yoshida T, Ohno K, Morotomi Y, Nakamura T, Azuma T, Yamada H, Hayashi H, Suehiro S. Clinical and pathological features of ascending testis. Osaka City Med J. 2009;55:81–7.
167. Mayer J, Rune GM, Holas A, Schimpl G, Schmidt B, Haberlik A. Ascent of the testis in children. Eur J Pediatr. 1995;154:893–5.
168. Imthurn T, Hadziselimović F, Herzog B. Impaired germ cells in secondary cryptorchid testis after herniotomy. J Urol. 1995;153:780–1.
169. Nistal M, Paniagua R, Abaurrea MA, Santamaria L. Hyperplasia and the immature appearance of Sertoli cells in primary testicular disorders. Hum Pathol. 1982;13:3–12.
170. Regadera J, Martínez-García F, González-Peramato P, Serrano A, Nistal M, Suárez-Quian C. Androgen receptor expression in Sertoli cells as a function of seminiferous tubule maturation in the human cryptorchid testis. J Clin Endocrinol Metab. 2001;86:413–21.
171. Läckgren G, Plöen L. The morphology of the human undescended testis with special reference to the Sertoli cell and puberty. In J Androl. 1984;7:23–38.
172. Rogatsch H, Jezek D, Hittmair A, Mikuz G, Feichtinger H. Expression of vimentin, cytokeratin, and desmin in Sertoli cells of human fetal, cryptorchid, and tumour-adjacent testicular tissue. Virchows Arch. 1996;427:497–502.
173. Gotoh M, Miyake K, Mitsuya H. Elastic fibers in tunica propria of undescended and contralateral scrotal testes from cryptorchid patients. Urology. 1987;30:359–63.
174. Maekawa M, Kazama H, Kamimura K, Nagano T. Changes in the arrangement of actin filaments in myoid cells and Sertoli cells of rat testes during postnatal development and after experimental cryptorchidism. Anat Rec. 1995;241:59–69.
175. Nistal M, Garcia-Rodeja E, Paniagua R. Granular transformation of Sertoli cells in testicular disorders. Hum Pathol. 1991;22:131–7.
176. Nistal M, Regadera J, Winitzky P, Tejerina E, Chemes H. Granular changes in Sertoli cells in children and pubertal patients. Fertil Steril. 2005;83: 1489–99.
177. Nistal M, Jiménez-Heffernan JA. Rete testis dysgenesis. A characteristic lesion of undescended testes. Arch Pathol Lab Med. 1997;121:1259–64.
178. Nistal M, Castillo MC, Regadera J, García-Cabezas MA. Adenomatous hyperplasia of the rete testis. A review and report of new cases. Histol Histopathol. 2003;18:741–52.
179. Nistal M, Riestra ML, Paniagua R. Correlation between testicular biopsies (prepubertal and postpubertal) and spermiogram in cryptorchid men. Hum Pathol. 2000;31:1022–30.
180. Nistal M, Paniagua R, Riestra ML, Reyes-Múgica M, Cajaiba MM. Bilateral prepubertal testicular biopsies predict significance of cryptorchidism-associated mixed testicular atrophy, and allow assessment of fertility. Am J Surg Pathol. 2007;31:1269–76.
181. De Miguel MP, Mariño JM, Gonzalez-Peramato P, Nistal M, Regadera J. Epididymal growth and differentiation are altered in human cryptorchidism. J Androl. 2001;22:212–25.
182. Sasagawa I, Yamaguchi O, Shiraiwa Y, Nakada T. Klinefelter's syndrome associated with unilateral cryptorchidism in childhood. Urol Int. 1991;47: 178–80.
183. Yamaguchi T, Kitada S, Osada Y. Chromosomal anomalies in cryptorchidism and hypospadias. Urol Int. 1991;47:60–3.
184. Rajfer J, Walsh PC. The incidence of intersexuality in patients with hypospadias and cryptorchidism. J Urol. 1976;116:769–70.
185. Kaefer M, Diamond D, Hendren WH, Vemulapalli S, Bauer SB, Peters CA, Atala A, Retik AB. The incidence of intersexuality in children with cryptorchidism and hypospadias: stratification based on gonadal palpability and meatal position. J Urol. 1999;162: 1003–7.

Entities Contributing to Infertility and Their Relationship to Oncogenic Risk

3

Manuel Nistal and Pilar González-Peramato

Introduction

Infertility is defined as the inability of a couple to conceive naturally after 1 year of regular nonprotected sexual intercourse. It affects about 15 % of couples. The male factor alone is responsible for at least 20 % of a couple's infertility and contributes either alone or associated with the female factor in up to 50 % of infertile couples. The incidence of male infertility is increasing. Its etiology is considered to be secondary to genetic factors in 15 % of cases and secondary to vasectomy, varicocele, hormonal dysfunction, testicular trauma, genitourinary infections, obesity, diabetes, chemotherapy, radiotherapy, or sexual dysfunction in another 15 % [1]. The etiology is unknown in 60–70 % of cases and these cases are referred to as "idiopathic male infertility."

Male infertility is considered a risk factor for the development of testicular cancer [2, 3]. Current studies are focusing on the identification of genetic links between impaired spermatogenesis and testicular cancer. The most studied pathologies are chromosomal anomalies, defects in DNA repair mechanisms, and testicular dysgenesis syndrome [4].

Chromosomal Anomalies

The frequency of chromosomal aberrations is approximately 0.6 % in the general population, 5 % in infertile men, and up to 15 % in azoospermic patients [5]. Anomalies in karyotype are directly related to the severity of the spermatogenesis impairment. However, it should be taken into account that the same chromosomal abnormalities can be found in normozoospermic men. Chromosomal abnormalities can be homogeneous or in mosaic, and they can affect sex chromosomes as well as autosomes. The most frequent chromosomopathies are 47,XXY, 47,XYY, 46,XX, and 45,X/46,XY. Other anomalies in sex chromosomes include structural aberrations in the Y chromosome and autosomal aberrations.

Klinefelter Syndrome

The incidence of Klinefelter syndrome in the infertile population is 3 %, increasing to 11 % in patients who are azoospermic [6]. The extra X chromosome in patients with Klinefelter syn-

M. Nistal (✉)
Department of Anatomy, Histology and Neuroscience, Autonoma University of Madrid, Madrid, Spain
e-mail: manuel.nistal@salud.madrid.org

P. González-Peramato
Department of Pathology, Autonoma University of Madrid, Hospital Univ. La Paz., Madrid, Spain
e-mail: mpilar.gonzalezperamato@salud.madrid.org

M. Colecchia (ed.), *Pathology of Testicular and Penile Neoplasms*,
DOI 10.1007/978-3-319-27617-5_3

drome can result from paternal nondisjunction meiosis I, which occurs in approximately 50 % of cases. Focal spermatogenesis can be found not only in mosaicisms (46,XY/47,XXY) but also in the classical form of Klinefelter syndrome (47,XXY) in spite of testicular atrophy, hypogonadism, and marked elevation of serum gonadotrophins. The histologic picture varies from diffuse hyalinization of seminiferous tubules with pseudoadenomatous hyperplasia of Leydig cells to a mixture of tubular hyalinization, tubules with spermatogenesis, and Sertoli cell-only tubules (Fig. 3.1).

Karyotype 47,XYY

The extra Y chromosome in patients with a 47,XYY karyotype can be originated by two mechanisms: paternal nondisjunction at meiosis II after normal chiasmata in meiosis I (84 %) or postzygotic mitotic errors (16 %) [7]. These patients usually do not have alterations in fertility as the extra Y chromosome is often lost in the premeiotic stages. In some cases testicular biopsies show mixed atrophy characterized by tubules with spermatogenesis along with Sertoli cell-only tubules.

46,XX Karyotype with Normal Male Phenotype

The 46,XX karyotype with a normal male phenotype is always associated with azoospermia. Testicular biopsies show either Sertoli cell-only tubules or tubular hyalinization with moderate Leydig cell hyperplasia reminiscent of the classical picture of Klinefelter syndrome [8].

In patients with Klinefelter syndrome and individuals with 47,XYY or 46,XX karyotype, no increased incidence of testicular tumors has been observed. This is particularly remarkable in patients with Klinefelter syndrome, as more than 27 % of these patients have cryptorchidism [9] and a high incidence of extratesticular germ cell tumors. The low incidence of testicular germ cell tumors in patients with Klinefelter syndrome is probably related to the absence of germ cells in the testes of most cases.

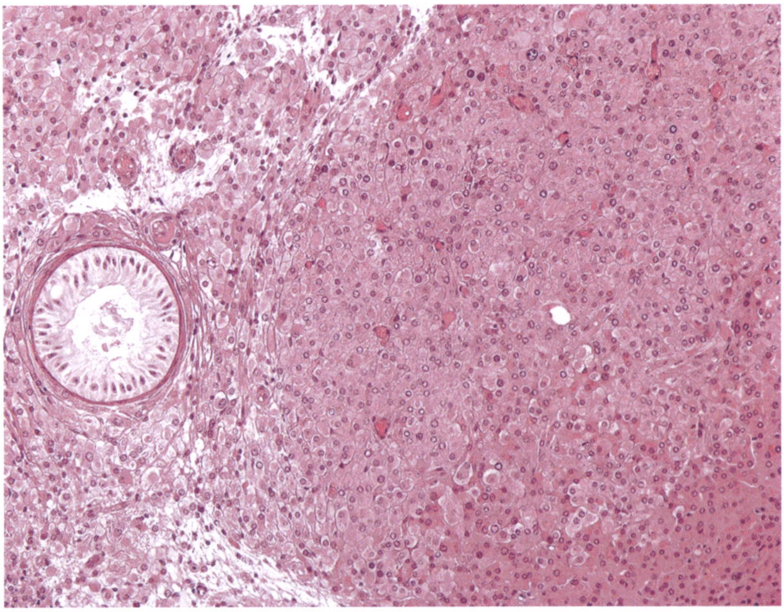

Fig. 3.1 Klinefelter syndrome. Leydig cell pseudoadenomatous hyperplasia and isolated Sertoli cell-only tubules

Karyotype 45,X0/46,XY

A 45,X0/46,XY karyotype is associated with a wide spectrum of disorders in sexual differentiation including complete XY gonadal dysgenesis (Swyer syndrome), 45,X0/46,XY in females, 45,X0/46,XY Turner syndrome, pure gonadal dysgenesis, Sohval syndrome, dysgenetic male pseudohermaphroditism, ovotesticular disorder, and hypospadias. Most patients are infertile and have a variable risk of developing germ cell tumors including gonadoblastomas (Fig. 3.2), dysgerminomas, teratomas, and choriocarcinomas. The risk of testicular germ cell tumor development in individuals with complete XY gonadal dysgenesis and 45,X0/46,XY females is 15–45 %. In general, the risk of tumors is higher in persons with ambiguous external genitalia and intra-abdominal gonads [10, 11].

SRY Gene Mutations

Patients with SRY gene mutations frequently show complete gonadal dysgenesis. Their phenotypes vary from the presence of Turner features to ambiguous genitalia. More than half of the patients develop germ cell tumors [12, 13].

Structural Anomalies of the Y Chromosome

The most frequent structural anomalies of the Y chromosome include deletions, ring chromosomes, inversions, and translocations [6]. Partial deletion of the distal portion of the Yq euchromatic region is associated with azoospermia secondary to loss of the AZF region. The most frequent picture in testicular biopsies of patients with structural Y chromosome anomalies is Sertoli cell-only tubules. A higher incidence of testicular tumors has not been observed in this group of patients.

Autosomal Anomalies

The most frequent anomalies are chromosome 21 trisomy, translocations, inversions, and extra nonsatellite marker chromosomes. Translocations

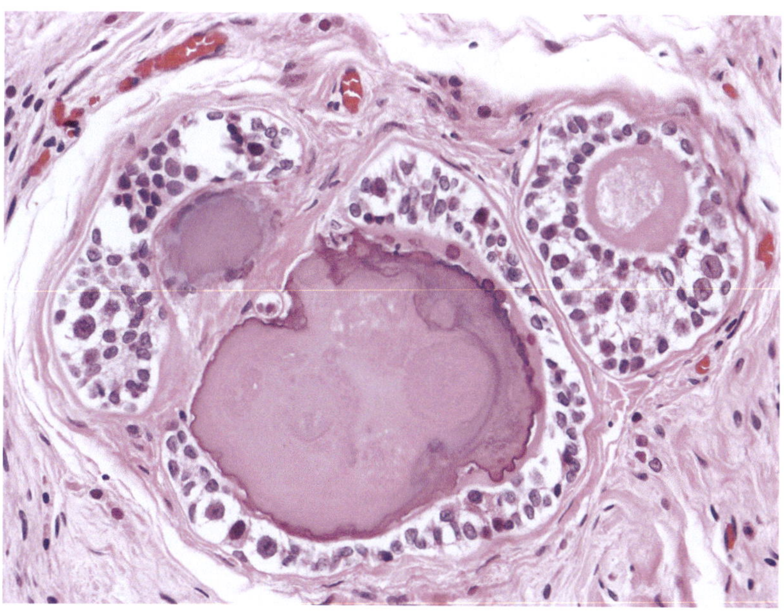

Fig. 3.2 Gonadoblastoma in a 46,XY pure gonadal dysgenesis patient

in autosomes are four- to tenfold more frequent in infertile patients than in men with normozoospermia. The most common anomalies are Robertsonian translocations (present in 0.1 % of the general population and 1 % of the infertile population [14]) and centric fusions. Patients with reciprocal translocations have a high rate of unbalanced spermatozoa due to errors in meiotic segregation. The most common testicular lesions in men with autosomal anomalies are spermatogonial maturation arrest, primary spermatocyte sloughing, and a Sertoli cell-only pattern. An incidence of testicular tumors higher than in the general population has not been observed in patients with autosomal anomalies, with the exception of Down syndrome.

Microdeletions of Y Chromosome

Microdeletions of the long arm of the Y chromosome are present in 10–15 % of men with nonobstructive azoospermia and in 5–10 % of men with severe oligozoospermia [15]. They are the most frequent molecular genetic cause of severe infertility. Most microdeletions occur in three subregions of the Y chromosome (Yq11) known as AZFa, AZFb, and AZFc. Patients with complete deletion of the AZFa subregion (8.3 % of Y chromosome microdeletions) show a Sertoli cell-only pattern in their testicular biopsies [16]. Those with deletion of the AZFb subregion (50 % of Y chromosome microdeletions) have a Sertoli cell-only pattern or maturation arrest. The most frequent of all microdeletions of the Y chromosome is deletion of the AZFc subregion (41–71 %) [17]. The testicular biopsies of patients with AZFc microdeletions show a variable histologic picture in relation to the number of deleted *DAZ* gene copies. The testicular lesion may vary from primary spermatocyte or spermatid arrest to a Sertoli cell-only pattern (Fig. 3.3). Partial deletions in the AZFc subregion have a minimal effect on fertility. Microdeletions of the Y chromosome are not associated with a higher risk of developing tumors or cryptorchidism.

X-Linked Gene Mutations

The two most frequent syndromes associated with the X chromosome are mutations in the androgen receptor gene and in the X-linked

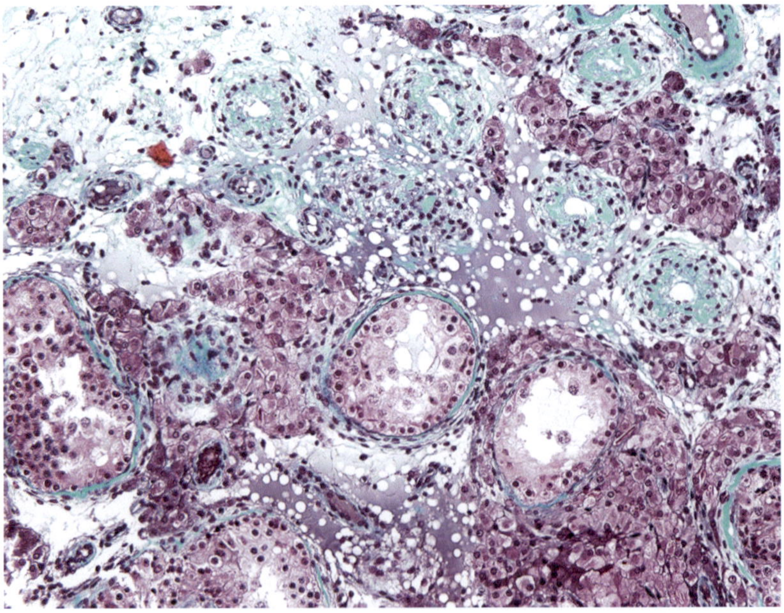

Fig. 3.3 Y chromosome microdeletion. Testicular parenchyma showing hyalinized tubules adjacent to tubules with maturation up to primary spermatocytes and Leydig cell hyperplasia

gene *KAL1*. Androgen receptor gene mutations are the most common cause of sexual differentiation disorders in 46,XY men. The phenotypes can be quite diverse, ranging from a female phenotype known as complete androgen insensitivity syndrome (CAIS), variable grades of undervirilization or partial androgen insensitivity syndrome (PAIS), and men with infertility only or mild androgen insensitivity syndrome (MAIS). The diagnosis in most patients with CAIS is delayed until puberty, when the patient presents with amenorrhea or infertility. The testes in postpubertal CAIS and PAIS men remain in the abdominal cavity or inguinal region. Histologically, the seminiferous tubules are characterized by fetal or infantile development, the absence of androgen receptors, diffuse hyperplasia of Leydig cells, and interstitial fibrosis (Fig. 3.4). The testes may contain one or several Sertoli-Leydig hamartomas. These patients have a higher risk of developing germ cell tumors. The two factors that could be involved are a delay in germ cell maturation with persistence of gonocyte-like cells through infancy and abnormal testicular location.

MAIS patients have a male phenotype, and the most frequent reason for consulting is infertility and underdeveloped external genitalia. Mutations in the androgen receptor gene are observed in 2–3 % of men with azoospermia or severe oligozoospermia [18]. Patients with MAIS typically show complete spermatogenesis (although with a very low sperm count) and diffuse Leydig cell hyperplasia. A higher risk of developing germ cell tumors than in the general population has not been observed.

Mutations in the *KAL1* gene cause the Kallmann syndrome, which is characterized by hypogonadotropic hypogonadism, infertility, and anosmia. The testicular parenchyma of most patients shows prepubertal features in the seminiferous tubules and interstitium. Kallmann syndrome is not associated with germ cell tumors.

Autosomal Gene Mutations

Numerous genes are involved in the regulation of the male reproductive apparatus, but only one of them, the cystic fibrosis transmembrane conductance regulator (*CFTR*) gene, is of clinical importance. The testicular parenchyma usually shows minimal obstructive changes (Fig. 3.5). Other genes, such as insulin-like factor 3 (*INSL3*),

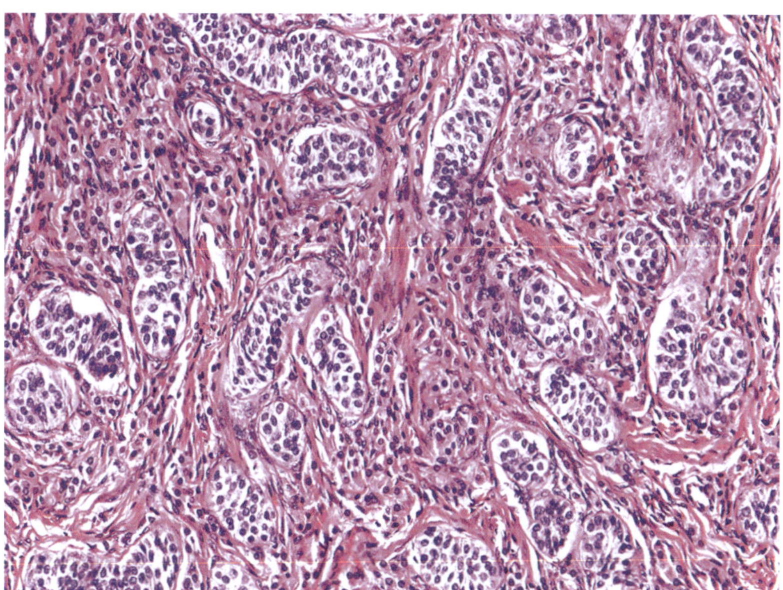

Fig. 3.4 CAIS in an adult patient. Seminiferous tubules showing prepubertal maturation surrounded by Leydig cell hyperplasia and abundantly collagenized and cellular ovarian cortex-like intertubular stroma

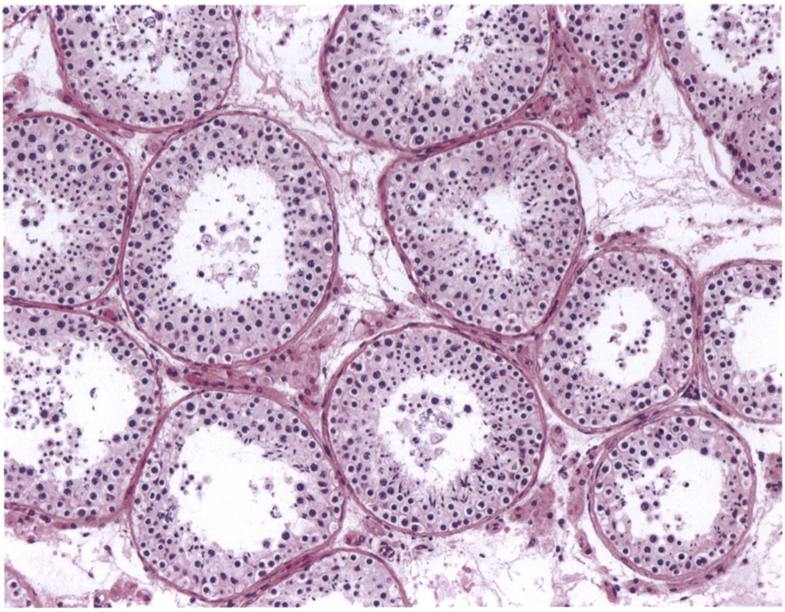

Fig. 3.5 Cystic fibrosis patient with secondary azoospermia showing slight tubular ectasia without interstitial alterations

are involved in the transabdominal stage of testicular descent. Mutations of the *INSL3* gene and its receptor *RHFP2* have been implicated in some cases of cryptorchidism. *INSL3*'s function in infertile patients without cryptorchidism is not known. Mutations in dynein genes are responsible for some cases of male infertility associated with asthenospermias such as primary ciliary dyskinesia. Mutations in a large number of genes such as *GnRH* and *GnRHR*, *FGFR1 (KAL2)*, *FGF8 (KAL6)*, *HS6ST1*, *PROKR2 (KL3)* and *PROK2 (KAL4)*, *KISS1R* and *KISS1*, *TACR3* and *YAC3*, *CHD7*, *NELF*, and *EBF2* [19] are responsible for rare cases of hypogonadotropic hypogonadism (Fig. 3.6). The incidence of bilateral cryptorchidism in patients with hypogonadotropic hypogonadism is very high, whereas testicular germ cell tumors are exceptional.

Defects in DNA Repair

Special interest has centered recently on the study of nuclear damage in sperm. Infertile men have greater sperm DNA fragmentation than the general population or men of proven fertility [20]. Integrity of sperm DNA is of vital importance to the normal functioning of spermatozoa and development of the embryo. Defects in DNA repair will impair both mitosis and meiosis, leading to impaired spermatogenesis and increasing the likelihood of carcinogenesis. The fertilization of an oocyte by a spermatozoon with deranged DNA has a negative impact on the development of the blastocyst. In many cases it is also responsible for failure of implantation, spontaneous abortion, or a negative effect on fetal development or even adulthood [21].

Damage in DNA is manifested by the following alterations: defects in sperm chromatin packaging, DNA fragmentation, oxidative stress, gene mutations, aneuploidy, and apoptosis. Mutations in DNA repair genes can result in deletions or expansions of small repeat DNA sequences, unstable components that have been observed in many forms of cancer. Defects in DNA repair genes have been associated with spermatogenic impairment, infertility, and testicular cancer [22].

Microarray analysis of RNA messenger expression in spermatozoal cytoplasm in the ejaculate of cryptorchid men has shown a significant difference with respect to controls in

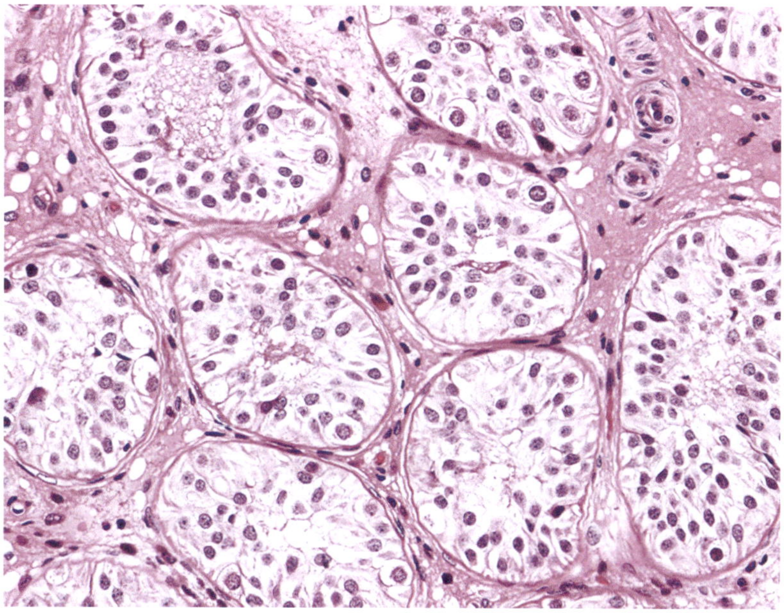

Fig. 3.6 Patient with hypogonadotropic hypogonadism. Note the seminiferous tubules with prepubertal maturation and the absence of Leydig cells in the interstitium

the expression of more than 38 genes [23]. These genes encode transcription factors, anti-apoptotic factors, specific factors of differentiation of germ cells, proteins involved in extracellular transduction signaling, and proteins involved in the S phase of DNA replication [23].

Tumor Suppressor Gene Mutations

Some cases of infertility have been related to deficits in tumor suppressor genes and specifically *TP53* gene defects. Mutations in this gene can give rise to two important events: (1) chromosomal and genomic instability increasing the chances that p53 null cells will become malignant and (2) a high level of reactive oxygen species (ROS) in the semen of infertile patients given the mutation-induced loss of upregulation of some antioxidant agents [24]. Other genes that have been implicated both in sporadic and familial cases of testicular germ cell tumors are *PDE11A*, *KIT* ligand, *SPRY4*, *BAK1* [25], and *CDC27* [26].

Testicular Dysgenesis Syndrome

Sharpe and Skakkebaek proposed in 1993 that male infertility, testicular cancer, cryptorchidism, and hypospadias are different expressions of the same syndrome: the testicular dysgenesis syndrome [27]. This hypothesis was based on a large amount of data observed in several highly industrialized countries. Epidemiologic studies have repeatedly shown an increasing incidence in semen quality alterations, testicular cancer, cryptorchidism, and hypospadias both in certain European countries and countries in other continents [28–32]. The presence of a primary testicular disorder supports the existence of testicular dysgenesis, and this has been confirmed in two groups of patients: patients with cryptorchidism and patients with testicular cancer.

Cryptorchidism is a well-known risk factor for male infertility. It is present in 8–10 % of infertile men and 15–20 % of azoospermic men as opposed to 2.5 % of fertile men [33]. Even in cases where cryptorchidism is apparently unilateral, the contralateral testis frequently shows germ cell diminution. The risk of developing testicular cancer in men with cryptorchidism has been estimated to be five- to tenfold higher than in the general population [34]. The risk of testicular cancer is also increased in the contralateral testis [35].

Fertility is decreased in those patients who will subsequently develop testicular cancer. The incidence of germ cell neoplasia in situ (GCNiS) in infertile men has been estimated to range between 1.1 and 4 %, so infertile men are a risk population for developing testicular cancer [36]. Patients with a testicular germ cell tumor in one testis have a higher risk of developing a tumor in the contralateral testis, a finding which supports the dysgenesis hypothesis.

Testicular Lesions

The most frequent histologic features shared by infertile patients, cryptorchid patients, patients with hypospadias, and patients with testicular germ cell tumors are mixed atrophy, hypoplastic tubules, Sertoli cell nodules, granular changes in Sertoli cells, tubules with germ cell hypoplasia, microlithiasis, focal Leydig cell hyperplasia, and GCNiS.

Mixed Atrophy (Focal Sertoli Cell-Only Tubules)

The testicular area occupied by Sertoli cell-only tubules is variable; it may comprise a group of close tubules that appear to belong to a single lobule, or it may extend through most of the parenchyma. With regard to the morphology of Sertoli cell nuclei, three types of tubules can be distinguished: tubules with dysgenetic Sertoli cells (cells with central spherical or elongated nuclei), tubules with adult Sertoli cells (having triangular nuclei with large central nucleoli), and tubules with involuted Sertoli cells (showing lobulated nuclei and central nucleoli). Sertoli cell-only tubules with dysgenetic Sertoli cells are most frequently found in cases of mixed atrophy associated with other findings of gonadal dysgenesis. These seminiferous tubules do not always show lumina. The number of Sertoli cells is usually increased (Fig. 3.7).

Hypoplastic Tubules

Hypoplastic tubules are small-caliber tubules with Sertoli cells arranged in a pseudostratified pattern. The nuclei are small and hyperchromatic and the nucleoli are also small and eccentric. In

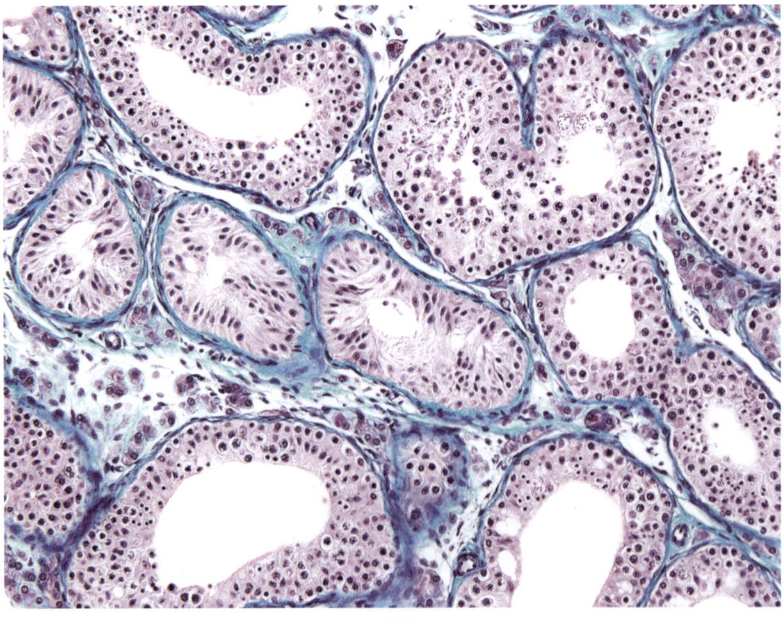

Fig. 3.7 Mixed atrophy in an infertile patient. Sertoli cell-only tubules with incomplete Sertoli cell maturation surrounded by seminiferous tubules with complete spermatogenesis

the apical cytoplasm, small eosinophilic bodies, so-called inhibin bodies, can be observed (Fig. 3.8). Occasionally the hypoplastic tubules contain GCNiS cells and microliths (Fig. 3.9). Immunoexpression of androgen receptor is absent or very weak in hypoplastic tubules (Fig. 3.10).

Sertoli Cell Nodules (Hypoplastic Zones)

These groups of seminiferous tubules are well delimited from the surrounding parenchyma and stand out by their small size (Fig. 3.11). The tubule diameter is markedly reduced and the tubular wall has a variable thickness. The basal lamina frequently has projections that penetrate deeply into the tubules, giving the impression that the component materials (collagen, laminin) are intratubular (Fig. 3.12). The epithelium of the seminiferous tubules is similar to that of hypoplastic tubules. Some tubules may contain microliths. Sertoli cell nodules frequently contain GCNiS cells in patients with germ cell tumors (Fig. 3.13).

Granular Changes in Sertoli Cells

Sertoli cells with granular changes are characterized by cytoplasm filled with eosinophilic granulations that can measure up to 10 μm, the largest of which are surrounded by a clear halo. These granulations are lysosomes, as they express both alpha-1 antitrypsin and CD68; they are ultrastructurally identified as cytolysosomes. These Sertoli cells have an enlarged cytoplasm and a vesicular pyknotic, nucleus with karyorrhexis. Seminiferous tubules containing Sertoli cells with granular changes frequently show a prepubertal development even in adulthood. These types of Sertoli cells can be isolated but are usually the only population in the tubules. As a general rule, seminiferous tubules containing Sertoli cells with granular changes are arranged close together, suggesting they belong to the same lobule (Fig. 3.14). Cytologic changes indicate the evolution of these tubules toward atrophy. Granular changes in Sertoli cells have been observed in decreasing order of frequency in cryptorchidism, CAIS, male infertility with by Sertoli cell-only tubules, and in the peripheral parenchyma of germ cell tumors [37, 38].

Germ Cell Hypoplasia

This form of germ cell hypoplasia is defined by the presence of seminiferous tubules with decreased spermatogenesis associated with

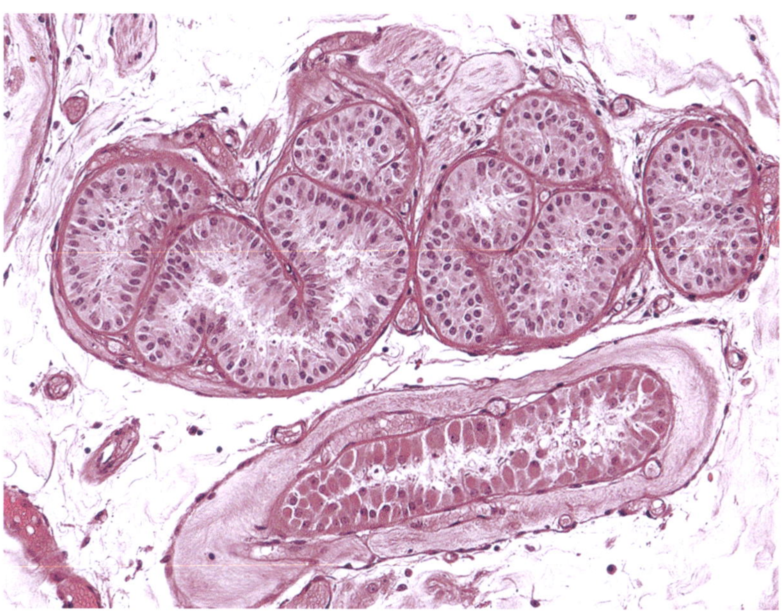

Fig. 3.8 Adult patient with cryptorchidism showing seminiferous tubules with prepubertal maturation. In the apical poles of Sertoli cells, eosinophilic inclusions can be observed which are inhibin bodies

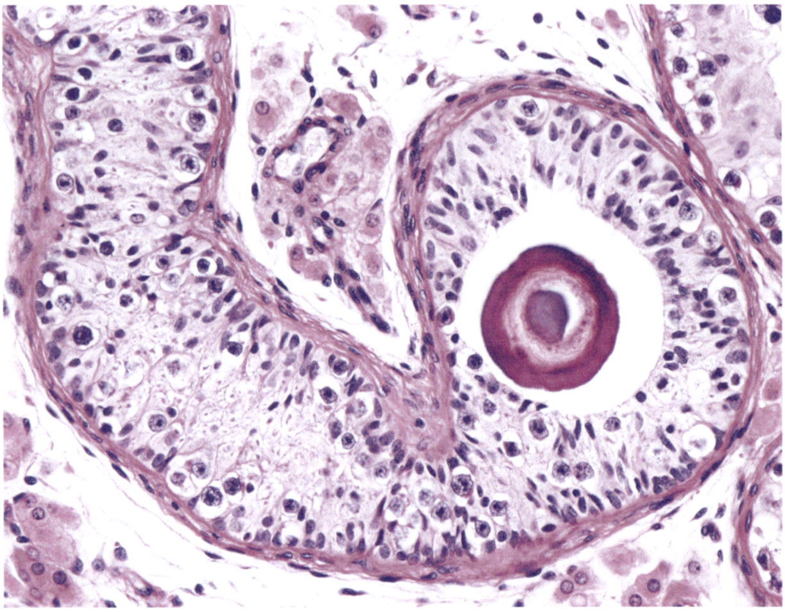

Fig. 3.9 Hypoplastic tubule with Sertoli cells arranged in a pseudostratified pattern intermixed with GCNiS cells both in the center of the tubule and above the basal lamina associated with microlithiasis

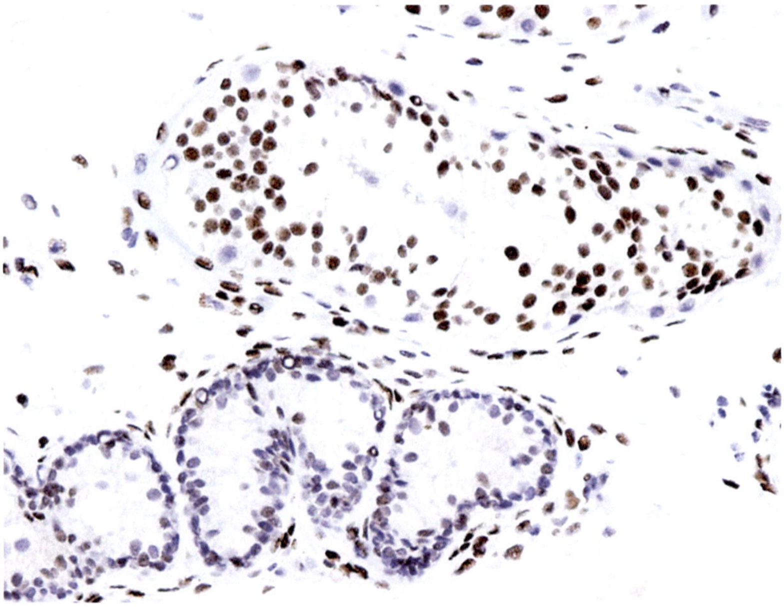

Fig. 3.10 Androgen receptor immunoexpression is observed only in peritubular cells in the hypoplastic tubule while it is positive in all Sertoli cells in the adjacent non-hypoplastic tubule

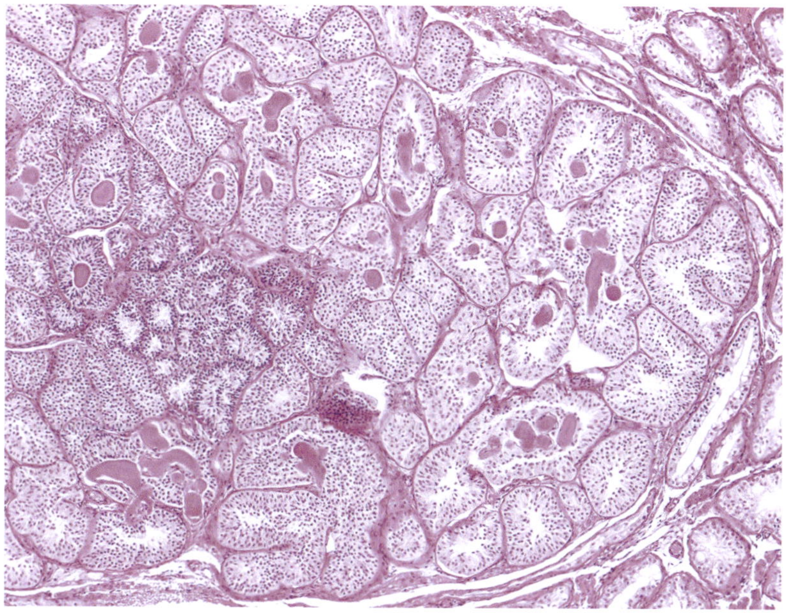

Fig. 3.11 A large Sertoli cell nodule, nonencapsulated but well delimited from the surrounding parenchyma. Note the jumbled arrangement of the tubules with irregularity in shape and size

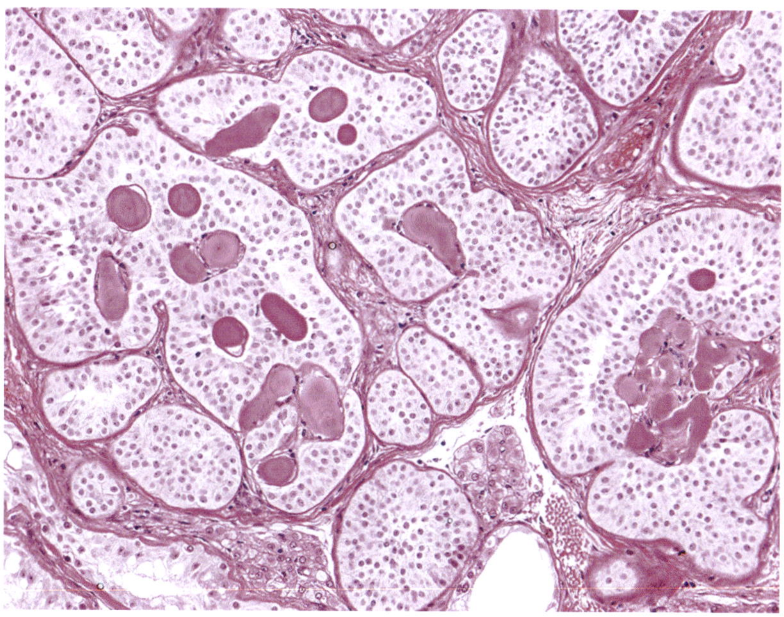

Fig. 3.12 Sertoli cell nodule. PAS stain shows intratubular eosinophilic projections connected to the basal lamina in some tubules. The Sertoli cells have not reached adult maturation and germ cells are absent

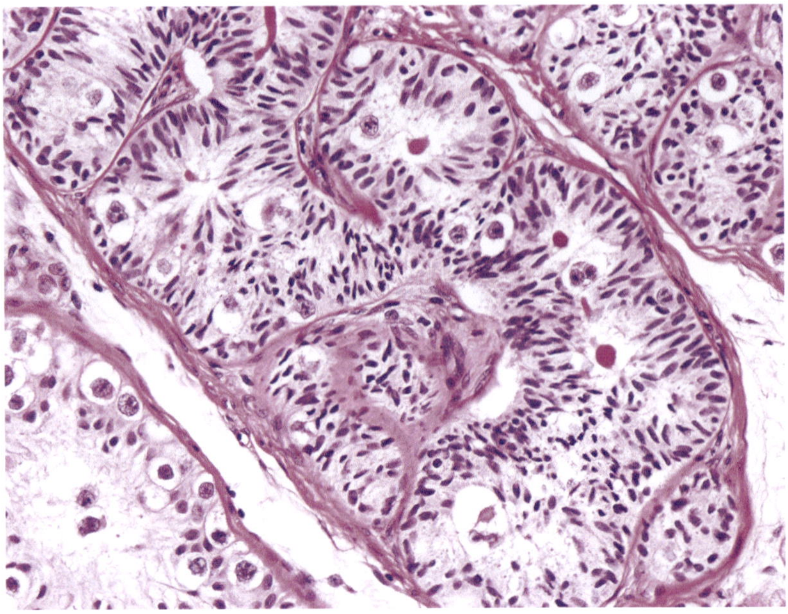

Fig. 3.13 Sertoli cell nodule. Seminiferous tubules with prepubertal features containing GCNiS cells

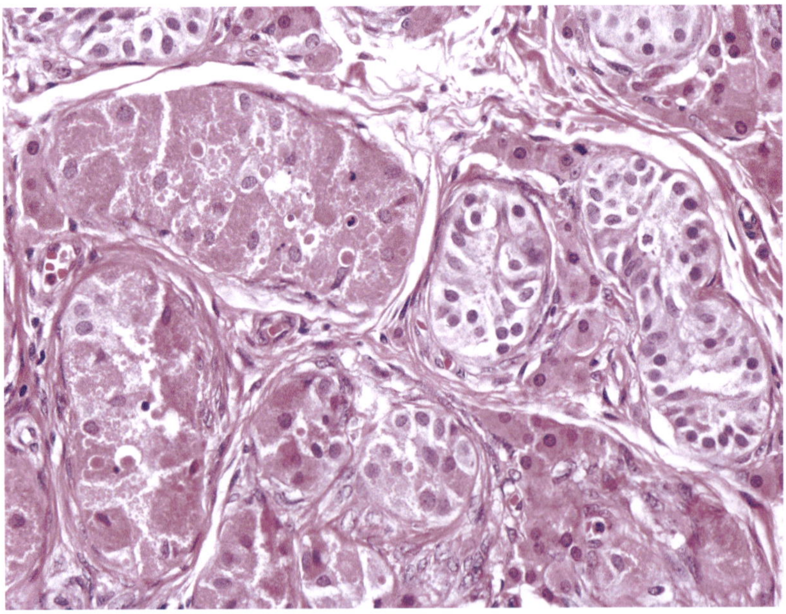

Fig. 3.14 Granular changes in Sertoli cells. Sertoli cell-only seminiferous tubules in a CAIS patient showing hyperchromatic nuclei and numerous variably sized eosinophilic granulations in the cytoplasm

Sertoli cell alterations. Two features are distinctive: the large number of Sertoli cells per tubular cross section and certain marks of immaturity such as the tendency of nuclei to be spherical and the absence of nuclear folds (Fig. 3.15).

Microlithiasis

Microlithiasis is the presence of calcified laminated concentric formations inside seminiferous tubules. These microliths develop in the tubular wall, pass through the basal lamina and seminiferous epithelium, and are eliminated into the lumen of the seminiferous tubule. They probably represent a local anomaly in the cells involved in basal lamina formation (Sertoli cells) and tubular wall formation (myoid cells).

Microlithiasis is present in 2.4–5.6 % of the general population, 4–20 % of subfertile patients (Fig. 3.16), 9.52 % of ex-cryptorchid testes, and half of patients with testicular germ cell tumors [39] (Figs. 3.17 and 3.18). Some patients previously diagnosed with microlithiasis develop testicular germ cell tumors.

Focal Leydig Cell Hyperplasia

Leydig cells are normally arranged in small groups in the interstitium and occasionally inside the tubular wall (peritubular cells). Their number is estimated at 1.2 groups per tubular section [40]. The presence of several groups of more than 14 cells in the interstitium is considered focal Leydig cell hyperplasia, which usually coincides with the absence of Leydig cells in other parts of the testicular parenchyma (Fig. 3.19). Focal Leydig cell hyperplasia is the morphologic expression of loss of the relationship between Leydig cells and seminiferous tubule cells. Functionally, it is associated with a decrease in androgen supply to the seminiferous tubules, and as a result the Sertoli cells cannot maintain effective spermatogenesis.

GCNiS

Germ cell neoplasia in situ or in situ carcinoma is characterized by the presence of cells similar to seminoma cells (i.e., large cells with spherical nuclei, one or two nucleoli, and abundant

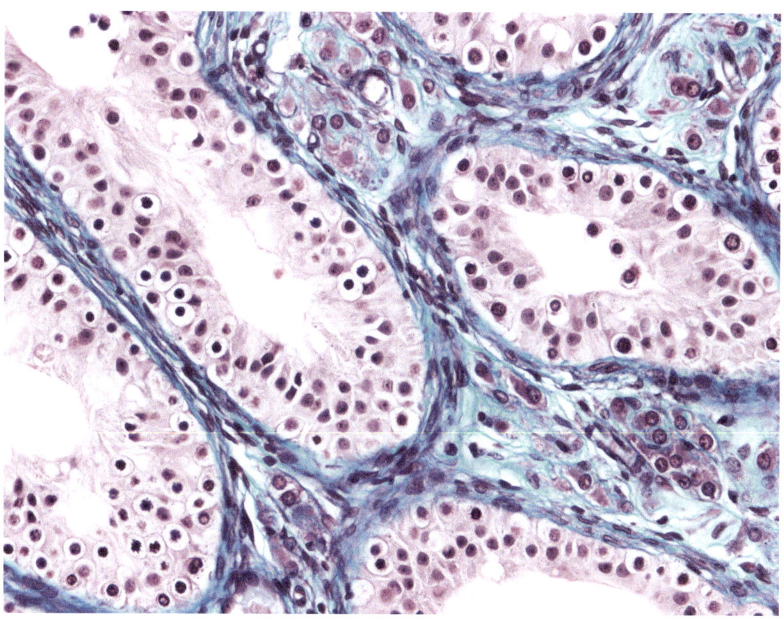

Fig. 3.15 Germ cell hypoplasia. Seminiferous tubules with a large number of incompletely matured Sertoli cells and scanty spermatogenesis (spermatogonia and isolated primary spermatocytes)

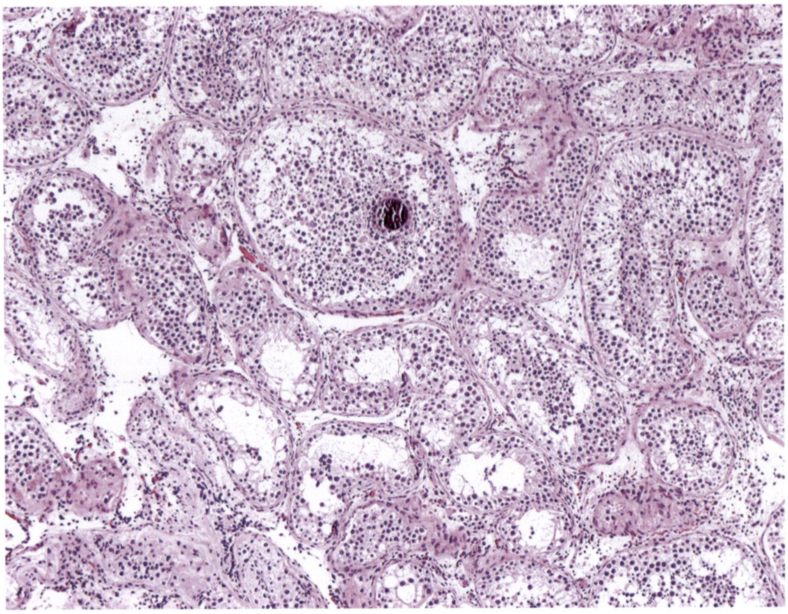

Fig. 3.16 Microlithiasis in an infertile patient. The largest seminiferous tubule has a microlith in its lumen

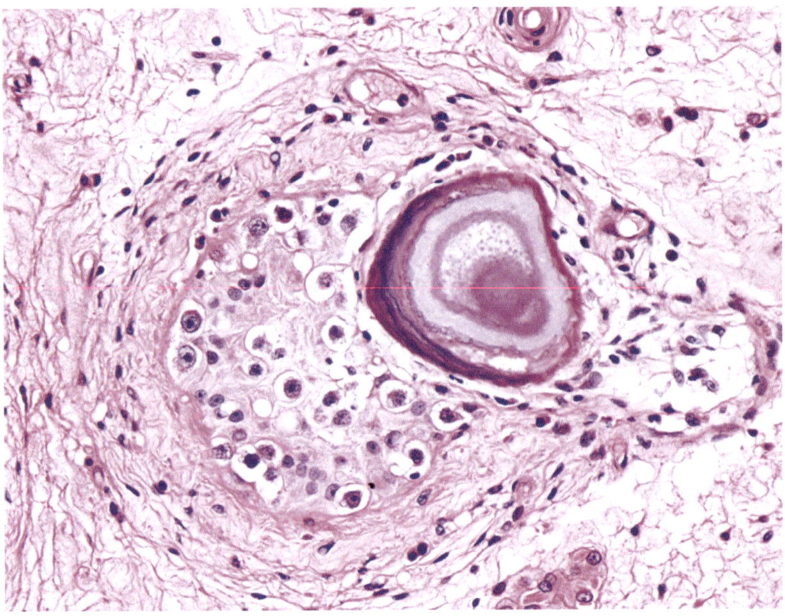

Fig. 3.17 A concentrically laminated microlith inside the wall of a seminiferous tubule that also contains GCNiS cells

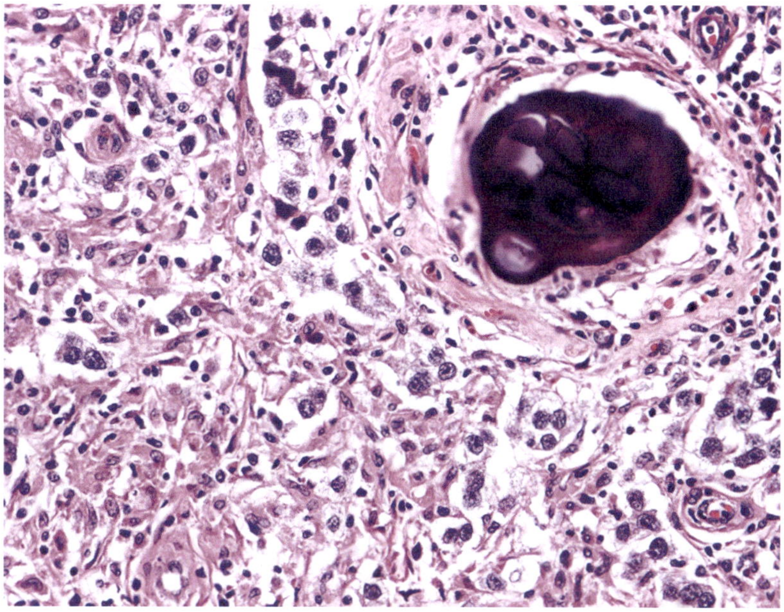

Fig. 3.18 Microlith in a seminoma with abundant lymphoid and granulomatous reaction

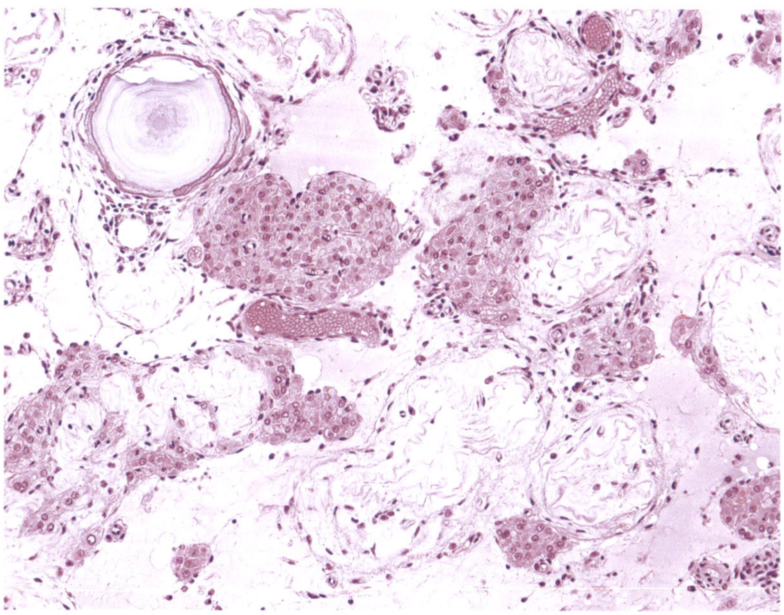

Fig. 3.19 Leydig cell hyperplasia associated with atrophic seminiferous tubules and microlithiasis

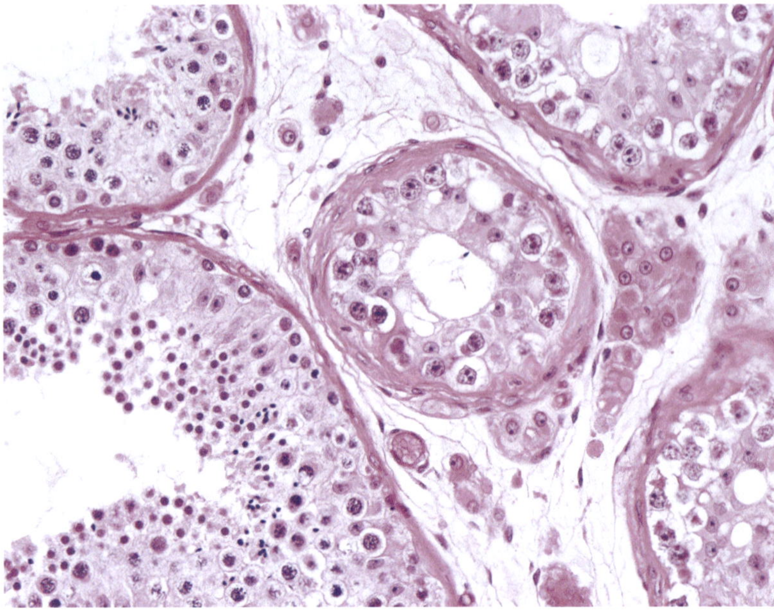

Fig. 3.20 Infertile patient with GCNiS. On the right of the figure, three small seminiferous tubules with uniform cells can be observed that contrast with the cellular variability in the adjacent seminiferous tubule on the left

cytoplasm) located above the basal lamina and displacing the Sertoli cells toward the center of the tubule (Fig. 3.20). In well-fixed specimens these cells are positive to the following antibodies: PLAP, c-kit, D2-40, and OCT3/4 (Fig. 3.21). Sertoli cells in these tubules have small spherical nuclei with small central nucleoli.

The incidence of these lesions in parenchyma peripheral to germ cell tumors is as follows: mixed atrophy 55 %, Sertoli cell nodules 25 %, microlithiasis 47 %, and GCNiS focal (51 %) or diffuse (38 %) [41]. In the testis contralateral to one bearing a germ cell tumor, the incidence of these lesions is mixed atrophy 13.8 %, hypoplastic tubules and Sertoli cell nodules 4.6 %, microlithiasis 6 %, and GCNiS 8.7 %. The cumulative incidence of at least one sign of dysgenesis is 25.2 % [42].

Etiology of the Lesions

The etiology of testicular dysgenesis syndrome is multifactorial. Epidemiologic and experimental studies suggest that environmental factors (endocrine disruptors), alone or combined with a genetic susceptibility, interfere with hormone action during differentiation and development of the reproductive system [43]. Endocrine disruptors are exogenous chemical substances that, once introduced into our organism, modify the function of the endocrine system. The chemical components are not rapidly biodegradable but are bioaccumulative.

Endocrine disruptors may have estrogenic or androgenic activity or both. Among those with estrogenic activity, the actions of bisphenol A and diethylstilbestrol are well known [44, 45]. Exposure to chemical products with antiandrogenic action interferes with hormonal signaling by joining the androgen receptor and blocking its function, thus causing a variety of anomalies in the male reproductive system that include the testicular dysgenesis syndrome [46]. The most studied chemical components with both antiestrogenic and antiandrogenic actions are phthalates, gums, and paints used as plasticizers in PVC products that can be found in children's toys, soaps, shampoos, perfumes, packing materials, agrochemicals, medical devices such as tubing and catheters, and practically any manufactured product that humans are in contact with.

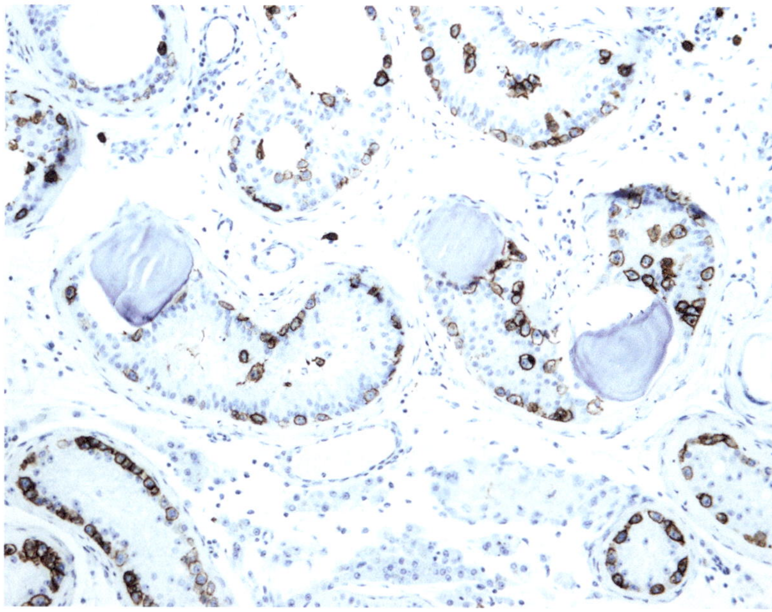

Fig. 3.21 Cryptorchid testis with GCNiS cells showing c-kit immunoexpression

Target Cells of Endocrine Disruptors

Sertoli Cells

Sertoli cells guarantee the viability of the germ cell as soon as primordial germ cells are surrounded by them. Gonocytes, a term that designates germ cells from this moment on, are located in the center of the testicular cords separated from the basal lamina by Sertoli cell cytoplasm. The different stages from a quiescent gonocyte until its complete migration reaching the basal lamina and transforming into a spermatogonium are coordinated by Sertoli cells through several factors, mainly glial cell line-derived neurotrophic factor (GDNF) and platelet-derived growth factor (PDGF).

Estrogens slow down the proliferation of Sertoli cells; as a result, the number of germ cells that depend on those Sertoli cells will be reduced. Estrogens also block the migration of gonocytes from the center of the tubules to their final location above the basal lamina and prevent their transformation into spermatogonia. Those two facts account for a defect in spermatogenesis and the possibility that some persistent gonocytes do not enter apoptosis and keep expressing their pluripotency and self-renewal genes. Clonal proliferation of these cells eventually progresses to GCNiS. Sertoli cells are not essential to maintaining spermatogenesis but to maintaining the phenotype of the peritubular myoid cell and Leydig cell population [47].

Gonocytes

Most germ cell tumors originate from a common cell that is a GCNiS cell. GCNiS cells derive from cells similar to gonocytes that fail in normal intrauterine differentiation into spermatogonia [43]. Gonocyte differentiation starts at about 20 weeks of gestation and continues until the first months of postnatal life. The persistence of gonocytes without transforming into spermatogonia can be due to an imbalance between estrogens and androgens in favor of the former in the quiescent period of gonocytes. This transformation from gonocytes to GCNiS cells is not due to an inherent germ cell abnormality but to inappropriate age signaling from Sertoli and Leydig cells.

Leydig Cells

Alterations in Leydig cell function are revealed by a deficit in testosterone and *INSL3*, as both hormones are involved in testicular descent. Low levels of testosterone lead to defective fusion of the urethral folds and hypospadias.

Summary

The risk of testicular cancer in infertile patients can be categorized into three groups:

Low risk: Klinefelter syndrome 47,XXY, 46,XX males, 47,XYY males, patients with microdeletions in the long arm of the Y chromosome, structural aberrations in the Y chromosome, anomalies in autosomes, gene mutations in autosomes, and ovotesticular disorder of sexual development.

Medium risk (2.2–15 %): Nonobstructive azoospermia, cryptorchidism, contralateral testis, to undescended testis defects in DNA repair genes, family history of testicular cancer, and history of testicular cancer in contralateral testis.

High risk (15–45 %): Androgen insensitivity syndrome (CAIS, PAIS), complete XY gonadal dysgenesis, 45,X0/46XY females, and mutations in *SRY* gene.

References

1. Pizzol D, Bertoldo A, Foresta C. Male infertility: biomolecular aspects. Biomol Concepts. 2014;5:449–56.
2. Walsh TJ, Croughan MS, Schembri M, Chan JM, Turek PJ. Increased risk of testicular germ cell cancer among infertile men. Arch Intern Med. 2009;169:351–6.
3. Jacobsen R, Bostofte E, Engholm G, Hansen J, Olsen JH, Skakkebaek NE, Moller H. Risk of testicular cancer in men with abnormal semen characteristics: cohort study. BMJ. 2000;321:789–92.
4. Practice Committee of the American Society for Reproductive Medicine. Electronic address: ASRM@asrm.org. Diagnostic evaluation of the infertile male: a committee opinion. Fertil Steril. 2015;103:e18–25.
5. Shi Q, Martin RH. Aneuploidy in human sperm: a review of the frequency and distribution of aneuploidy, effects of donor age and lifestyle factors. Cytogenet Cell Genet. 2000;90:219–26.
6. Glander HJ. Infertility in the Klinefelter syndrome. MMW Fortschr Med. 2005;147:39–41.
7. Rives N, Siméon N, Milazzo JP, Barthélémy C, Macé B. Meiotic segregation of sex chromosomes in mosaic and non-mosaic XYY males: case reports and review of the literature. Int J Androl. 2003;26:242–9.
8. Kim JW, Bak CW, Chin MU, Cha DH, Yoon TK, Shim SH. SRY-negative 46,XX infertile male with Leydig cell hyperplasia: clinical, cytogenetic, and molecular analysis and review of the literature. Fertil Steril. 2010;94:753.e5–9.
9. Pacenza N, Pasqualini T, Gottlieb S, Knoblovits P, Costanzo PR, Stewart Usher J, Rey RA, Martínez MP, Aszpis S. Clinical presentation of Klinefelter's syndrome: differences according to age. Int J Endocrinol. 2012;2012:324835.
10. Kriplani A, Agarwal N, Parul, Sharma MC, Manchanda R. Bilateral seminomas in a 45X/46XY mosaic with Turner's phenotype: an unusual case of mixed gonadal dysgenesis. J Obstet Gynaecol Res. 2003;29:63–6.
11. Cools M, Looijenga LH, Wolffenbuttel KP, T'Sjoen G. Managing the risk of germ cell tumourigenesis in disorders of sex development patients. Endocr Dev. 2014;27:185–96.
12. Bianco B, Lipay M, Guedes A, Oliveira K, Verreschi IT. SRY gene increases the risk of developing gonadoblastoma and/or nontumoral gonadal lesions in turner syndrome. Int J Gynecol Pathol. 2009;28:197–202.
13. Hersmus R, van der Zwan YG, Stoop H, Bernard P, Sreenivasan R, Oosterhuis JW, Brüggenwirth HT, de Boer S, White S, Wolffenbuttel KP, Alders M, McElreavy K, Drop SL, Harley VR, Looijenga LH. A 46, XY female DSD patient with bilateral gonadoblastoma, a novel SRY missense mutation combined with a WT1 KTS splice-site mutation. PLoS One. 2012;7:e40858.
14. Nielsen J, Wohlert M. Chromosome abnormalities found among 34,910 newborn children: results from a 13-year incidence study in Arhus. Denmark Hum Genet. 1991;87:81–3.
15. Foresta C, Moro E, Ferlin A. Y chromosome microdeletions and alterations of spermatogenesis. Endocr Rev. 2001;22:226–39.
16. Krausz C, McElreavey K. Y chromosome and male infertility. Front Biosci. 1999;4:E1–8.
17. Vogt PH, Edelmann A, Kirsch S, Henegariu O, Hirschmann P, Kiesewetter F, Köhn FM, Schill WB, Farah S, Ramos C, Hartmann M, Hartschuh W, Meschede D, Behre HM, Castel A, Nieschlag E, Weidner W, Gröne HJ, Jung A, Engel W, Haidl G. Human Y chromosome azoospermia factors (AZF) mapped to different subregions in Yq11. Hum Mol Genet. 1996;5:933–43.
18. Massin N, Bry H, Vija L, Maione L, Constancis E, Haddad B, Morel Y, Claessens F, Young J. Healthy birth after testicular extraction of sperm and ICSI from an azoospermic man with mild androgen insensitivity syndrome caused by an androgen receptor partial loss-of-function mutation. Clin Endocrinol (Oxf). 2012;77:593–8.
19. Bonomi M, Libri DV, Guizzardi F, Guarducci E, Maiolo E, Pignatti E, Asci R, Persani L, Idiopathic Central Hypogonadism Study Group of the Italian Societies of Endocrinology and Pediatric Endocrinology and Diabetes. New understandings of the genetic basis of isolated idiopathic central hypogonadism Asian. J Androl. 2012;14:49–56.

20. Schulte RT, Ohl DA, Sigman M, Smith GD. Sperm DNA damage in male infertility: etiologies, assays, and outcomes. J Assist Reprod Genet. 2010;27:3–12.
21. Aitken RJ, Bronson R, Smith TB, De Iuliis GN. The source and significance of DNA damage in human spermatozoa; a commentary on diagnostic strategies and straw man fallacies. Mol Hum Reprod. 2013;19:475–85.
22. Hughes CM, Lewis SE, McKelvey-Martin VJ, Thompson W. A comparison of baseline and induced DNA damage in human spermatozoa from fertile and infertile men, using a modified comet assay. Mol Hum Reprod. 1996;2:613–9.
23. Nguyen MT, Delaney DP, Kolon TF. Gene expression alterations in cryptorchid males using spermatozoal microarray analysis. Fertil Steril. 2009;92:182–7.
24. Tourtellotte WG, Nagarajan R, Auyeung A, Mueller C, Milbrandt J. Infertility associated with incomplete spermatogenic arrest and oligozoospermia in Egr4-deficient mice. Development. 1999;126:5061–71.
25. Greene MH, Kratz CP, Mai PL, Mueller C, Peters JA, Bratslavsky G, Ling A, Choyke PM, Premkumar A, Bracci J, Watkins RJ, McMaster ML, Korde LA. Familial testicular germ cell tumors in adults: 2010 summary of genetic risk factors and clinical phenotype. Endocr Relat Cancer. 2010;17:R109–21.
26. Litchfield K, Summersgill B, Yost S, Sultana R, Labreche K, Dudakia D, Renwick A, Seal S, Al-Saadi R, Broderick P, Turner NC, Houlston RS, Huddart R, Shipley J, Turnbull C. Whole-exome sequencing reveals the mutational spectrum of testicular germ cell tumours. Nat Commun. 2015;6:5973.
27. Sharpe RM, Skakkebaek NE. Are oestrogens involved in falling sperm counts and disorders of the male reproductive tract? Lancet. 1993;341:1392–5.
28. Toppari J, Larsen JC, Christiansen P, Giwercman A, Grandjean P, Guillette Jr LJ, Jégou B, Jensen TK, Jouannet P, Keiding N, Leffers H, McLachlan JA, Meyer O, Müller J, Rajpert-De Meyts E, Scheike T, Sharpe R, Sumpter J, Skakkebaek NE. Male reproductive health and environmental xenoestrogens. Environ Health Perspect. 1996;104 Suppl 4:741–803.
29. Sharpe RM, Irvine DS. How strong is the evidence of a link between environmental chemicals and adverse effects on human reproductive health? BMJ. 2004; 328:447–51.
30. Burns WR, Sabanegh E, Dada R, Rein B, Agarwal A. Is male infertility a forerunner to cancer? Int Braz J Urol. 2010;36:527–36.
31. Eisenberg ML, Betts P, Herder D, Lamb DJ, Lipshultz LI. Increased risk of cancer among azoospermic men. Fertil Steril. 2013;100:681–5.
32. Serrano T, Chevrier C, Multigner L, Cordier S, Jégou B. International geographic correlation study of the prevalence of disorders of male reproductive health. Hum Reprod. 2013;28:1974–86.
33. Lee PA, Coughlin MT. Fertility after bilateral cryptorchidism. Evaluation by paternity, hormone, and semen data. Horm Res. 2001;55:28–32.
34. Pettersson A, Richiardi L, Nordenskjold A, Kaijser M, Akre O. Age at surgery for undescended testis and risk of testicular cancer. N Engl J Med. 2007;356:1835–41.
35. Dieckmann KP, Pichlmeier U. Clinical epidemiology of testicular germ cell tumors. World J Urol. 2004; 22:2–14.
36. Skakkebaek NE, Rajpert-De Meyts E, Main KM. Testicular dysgenesis syndrome: an increasingly common developmental disorder with environmental aspects. Hum Reprod. 2001;16:972–8.
37. Nistal M, Garcia-Rodeja E, Paniagua R. Granular transformation of Sertoli cells in testicular disorders. Hum Pathol. 1991;22:131–7.
38. Nistal M, Regadera J, Winitzky P, Tejerina E, Chemes H. Granular changes in Sertoli cells in children and pubertal patients. Fertil Steril. 2005;83:1489–99.
39. Nistal M, Paniagua R, Gonzalez-Peramato P, Reyes-Múgica M. Calcifications in the testis and paratesticular structures. Pediatr Dev Pathol. 2014 Aug 8; Epub ahead of print.
40. Nistal M, Paniagua R, González-Peramato P. Nonneoplastic diseases of the testis. In: Bostwick DG, Cheng L, editors. Urologic surgical pathology. 3rd ed. Philadelphia: Elsevier Saunders Ed; 2014. p. 560–735. ISBN 978-1-4557-4327-8.
41. Nistal M, Gonzalez-Peramato P, Regadera J, Serrano A, Tarin V, De Miguel MP. Primary testicular lesions are associated with testicular germ cell tumors of adult men. Am J Surg Pathol. 2006;30:1260–8.
42. Hoei-Hansen CE, Holm M, Rajpert-De Meyts E, Skakkebaek NE. Histological evidence of testicular dysgenesis in contralateral biopsies from 218 patients with testicular germ cell cancer. J Pathol. 2003;200:370–4.
43. Rajpert-De Meyts E. Developmental model for the pathogenesis of testicular carcinoma in situ: genetic and environmental aspects. Hum Reprod Update. 2006;12:303–23.
44. Talsness CE, Andrade AJ, Kuriyama SN, Taylor JA, vom Saal FS. Components of plastic: experimental studies in animals and relevance for human health. Philos Trans R Soc Lond B Biol Sci. 2009;364:2079–96.
45. Palmer JR, Herbst AL, Noller KL, Boggs DA, Troisi R, Titus-Ernstoff L, Hatch EE, Wise LA, Strohsnitter WC, Hoover RN. Urogenital abnormalities in men exposed to diethylstilbestrol in utero: a cohort study. Environ Health. 2009;8:37.
46. Diamanti-Kandarakis E, Bourguignon JP, Giudice LC, Hauser R, Prins GS, Soto AM, Zoeller RT, Gore AC. Endocrine-disrupting chemicals: an endocrine society scientific statement. Endocr Rev. 2009;30:293–342.
47. Rebourcet D, O'Shaughnessy PJ, Monteiro A, Milne L, Cruickshanks L, Jeffrey N, Guillou F, Freeman TC, Mitchell RT, Smith LB. Sertoli cells maintain Leydig cell number and peritubular myoid cell activity in the adult mouse testis. PLoS One. 2014;9:e105687.

Germ Cell Tumors of Infancy and Childhood

4

Manuel Nistal and Pilar González-Peramato

Introduction

Testicular tumors in the prepubertal period are rare. The annual incidence is estimated to range from 0.5 to 2.0 per 100,000 boys, accounting for 1–2 % of all solid pediatric tumors although it is increasing [1, 2]. The age distribution of prepubertal testicular tumors is bimodal, with one peak occurring in the first 2 years of life and a second occurring in young adulthood. The frequency of the distinct testicular tumors in pediatric age varies among series, depending on whether the adolescence period is included or not. Germ cell tumors account for 71 % (yolk sac tumors [YSTs], 49 %; teratomas, 13 %; seminoma and mixed germ cell tumors, 9 %), and gonadal stromal tumors account for 29 % of prepubertal testicular tumors [3]. About 70–75 % of prepubertal tumors are benign [4].

M. Nistal (✉)
Department of Anatomy, Histology and Neuroscience, Autonoma University of Madrid, Madrid, Spain
e-mail: manuel.nistal@salud.madrid.org

P. González-Peramato
Department of Pathology, Autonoma University of Madrid, Hospital University La Paz, Madrid, Spain
e-mail: mpilar.gonzalezperamato@salud.madrid.org

Germ Cell Tumors (GCTs)

There are several differences between GCTs occurring in children and those of adults from the histopathologic, molecular biology and biologic behavior points of view. Most are pure YSTs or teratomas [5, 6]. GCTs account for 71 % of testicular tumors in childhood versus 96 % in adulthood. Cryptorchidism does not play an important role as an underlying factor, as fewer than 40 cases have been reported in undescended testes [7]. By contrast, ethnicity is important: prepubertal tumors are more frequent in Asian-Pacific Islanders than in white men, while the incidence is lowest among blacks [8]. The peritumoral parenchyma rarely shows germ cell neoplasia in situ (GCNiS) also known as carcinoma in situ (CIS), which suggests that GCTs in prepubertal boys have a different origin from those in adolescents and adults [9].

Moreover, it should be emphasized that the cytokinetic profile for the same histologic tumor type is different. YSTs in prepubertal children show chromosome 1 imbalances, loss of 6q, and chromosome 20 anomalies [10–13], while isochromosome 12p is present in 80 % of adult cases and enlargement of 12p segments is found in the remaining adult cases. Both YSTs and teratomas in childhood are diploid [14].

GCTs appearing in pubertal age or immediately afterward do not have any morphologic,

M. Colecchia (ed.), *Pathology of Testicular and Penile Neoplasms*,
DOI 10.1007/978-3-319-27617-5_4

immunohistochemical, or cytogenetic differences with respect to adult GCTs [15–18].

Yolk Sac Tumors, Prepubertal Type

This is the most common testicular tumor in infancy and childhood, accounting for about 70 % of pediatric GCTs [19]. The age of onset varies from birth to 9 years of age, with a peak incidence at 18 months. Most YSTs in children are pure, unlike those in adults [20]. One case associated to microlithiasis has been reported [21].

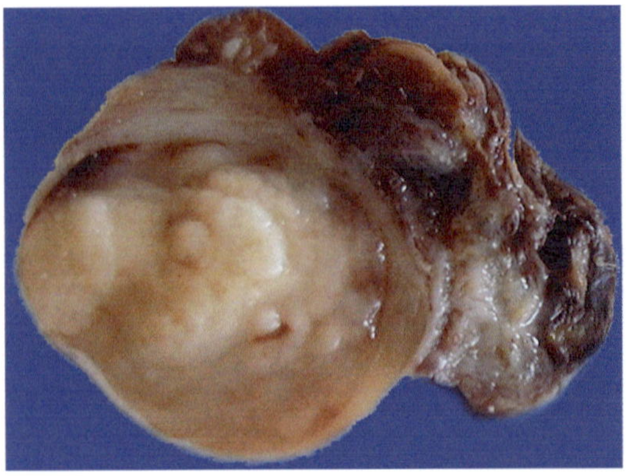

Fig. 4.1 Yolk sac tumor. The whitish multinodular tumor replaces two-thirds of the testicular parenchyma

Clinical Features

The most common presentation (>90 %) is of a painless scrotal mass. A hydrocele is associated with a testicular tumor in 15–50 % of cases [22], and in 6 % of patients, metastasis has been reported as the first finding [23]. One percent of YSTs are bilateral, while in unilateral cases, there is a slight predilection for the right testis. The diameter ranges between 2 and 4 cm. Ninety percent of patients have significant elevation of serum alpha-fetoprotein (AFP) [24]; this should, however, be interpreted with caution as such elevation can overlap with normal levels. Regarding AFP levels in infants, it should be taken into account that 50,000 ng/mL is considered normal at birth; the level then decreases progressively to 10,000 ng/mL at 2 weeks, 300 ng/mL at 2 months, and 12 ng/mL at 6 months [25].

Pathologic Features

The macroscopic appearance of YST in children is a solid, white to gray mass replacing most of the testicular parenchyma. The cut surface is microcystic, myxoid, or gelatinous. Small foci of necrosis and hemorrhage can be observed (Fig. 4.1).

Numerous microscopic patterns including microcystic, endodermal sinus, papillary, solid, glandular, myxomatous, sarcomatoid, macrocystic, polyvesicular vitelline, hepatoid, enteric, and parietal patterns can be found in YSTs [20, 26–28].

The *microcystic pattern* is the most common and is characterized by a reticular pattern that recalls a disorganized spider web of cells with large intracellular vacuoles (Fig. 4.2). The cytoplasm is reduced to a thin peripheral ring resembling false lipoblasts, as the vacuoles do not contain lipid. Cells can also be arranged around variably sized small cysts. In this case the cells are small, benign in appearance, and with numerous hyaline globules.

The *glandular pattern* is defined by the presence of glandular or tubular structures, simple or complex, and contiguous to other patterns such as microcystic, myxomatous, solid, or polyvesicular vitelline. Glands may present intestinal differentiation (enteric pattern). In other cases the glands show subnuclear vacuoles resembling secretory endometrium. These glands can be distinguished from teratomatous glands by the lack of a smooth muscle component and the absence of other teratomatous elements.

The *myxomatous pattern* consists of a proliferation of spindle or stellate cells dispersed in a mucopolysaccharide-rich stroma. This pattern usually has a prominent vascular network described as "angioblastic mesenchyme" [27]. The cells resembling extraembryonic mesenchyme are pluripotential, with the capacity to form differentiated tissues such as the skeletal muscle, cartilage, or bone. The differential diagnosis with teratoma is established by the absence of other surrounding teratomatous elements.

The *endodermal sinus pattern* consists of a central vessel surrounded by tumor cells, contained within a cystic space lined with flattened tumor cells. The papillary structures are termed glomeruloid or Schiller-Duval bodies

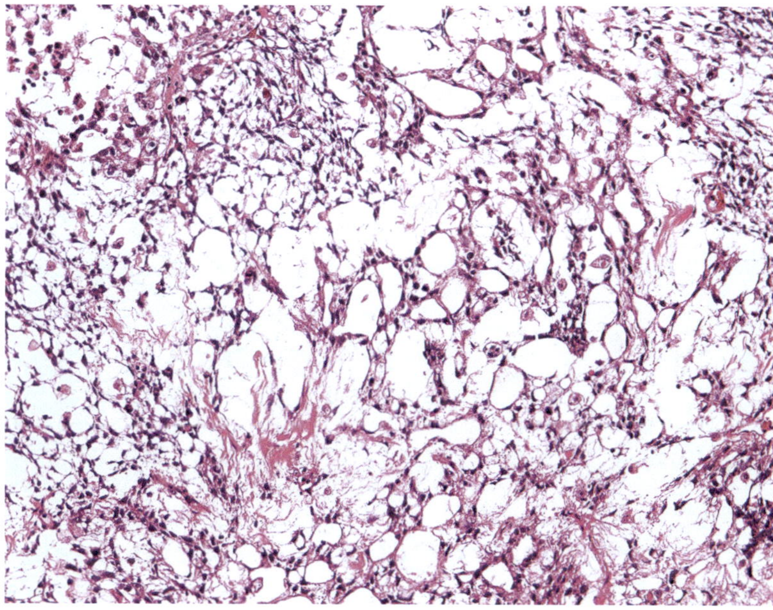

Fig. 4.2 Microcystic pattern of yolk sac tumor showing cells with a large vacuole in the cytoplasm and microcysts created by cords of cells surrounding the extracellular space

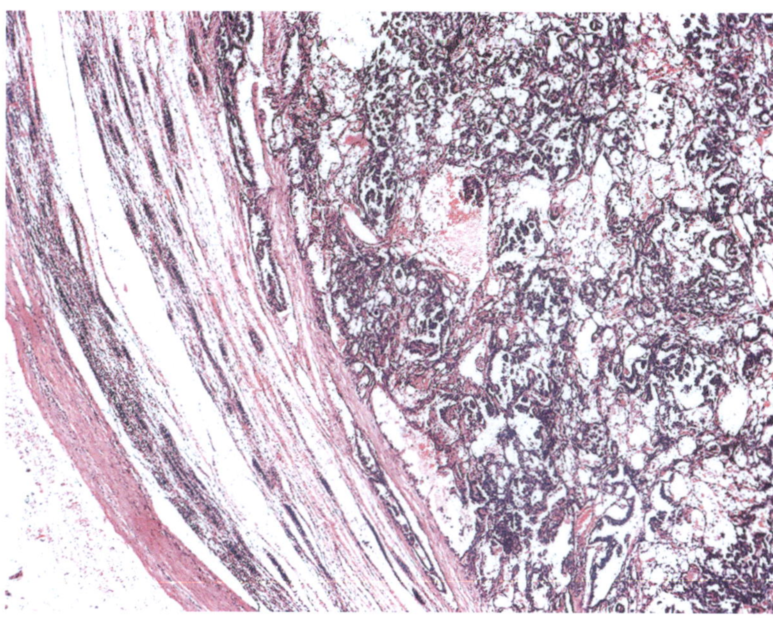

Fig. 4.3 Endodermal sinus pattern of yolk sac tumor showing numerous cystic spaces with glomeruloid structures inside that are formed by tumor cells

because they resemble the endodermal sinus of the placenta of the rat and are responsible for the name by which this tumor was previously known, endodermal sinus tumor. These bodies, although not very numerous, are characteristic of YST (Figs. 4.3 and 4.4).

The *papillary pattern* is recognized by the presence of numerous small papillae, with or without a fibrovascular core, that project into cystic spaces. The cells are cubical or low columnar with hobnail nuclei, resulting in a jigsaw configuration.

The *solid pattern* consists of sheets of uniform cells with clear cytoplasm and well-defined borders. Cells show marked pleomorphism and atypia (Fig. 4.5). The solid pattern of YST is almost always

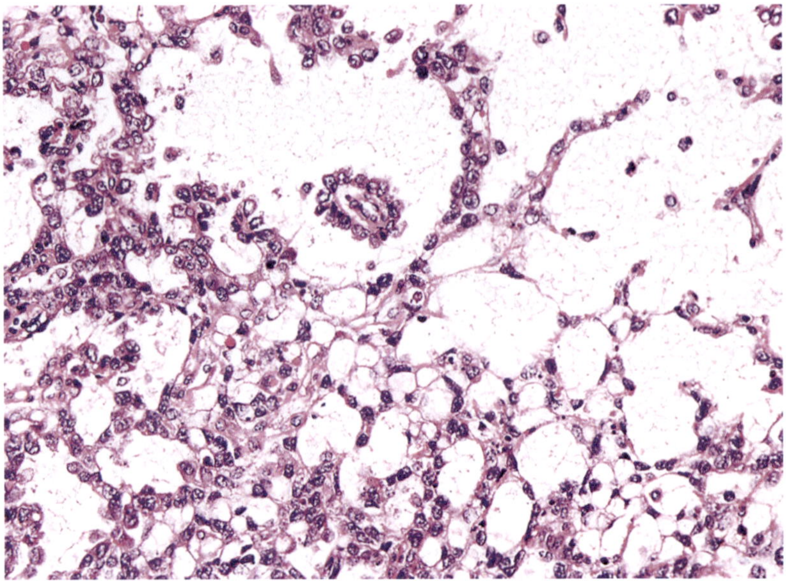

Fig. 4.4 Schiller-Duval body in a yolk sac tumor with microcystic pattern

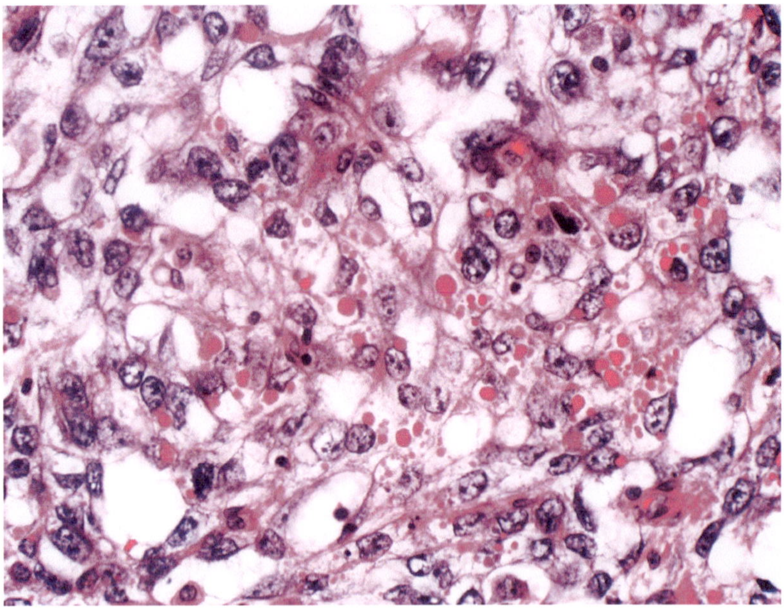

Fig. 4.5 Solid and microcystic patterns of a yolk sac tumor. Numerous eosinophilic bodies can be observed in the cytoplasm of tumor cells

associated with other patterns, most commonly microcystic/reticular (75 %), glandular (35 %), and myxoid (25 %). This tumor may resemble a seminoma that, although rarely, can present in late childhood and puberty, but fibrous septa and a lymphoid component are absent in YST. Moreover, the immunophenotype is different [29].

The *sarcomatoid pattern* consists of a spindle cell proliferation commonly inside a microcystic pattern.

The *macrocystic pattern* usually arises from the coalescence of microcystic spaces to form a large cyst. The cells lining the cysts are flattened and show mild atypia.

The *polyvesicular vitelline pattern* is characterized by the presence of cysts with a central constriction producing two vesicles that remain connected, dispersed in a myxoid stroma (Fig. 4.6). The name refers to the image observed when the secondary yolk sac is formed in a

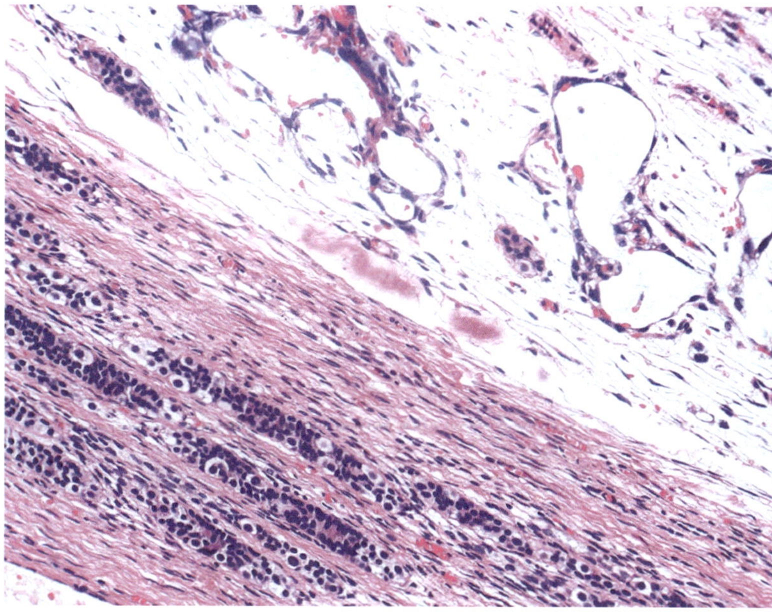

Fig. 4.6 Polyvesicular vitelline pattern of yolk sac tumor. Vesicle-like structures with a partial constriction lined with flattened epithelium in a myxoid stroma

normal embryo. The epithelium lining the second vesicle is commonly columnar, which contrasts with the flattened epithelium of the original cavity. The cells frequently show hyaline globules. The occasional presence of glands with mucous cells or cells with brush borders is interpreted as a differentiation of this second cavity. There is an established parallelism with gastrointestinal differentiation from the secondary yolk sac in the normal embryo.

The *hepatoid pattern* is also interpreted as a differentiation from yolk sac. It is characterized by clusters of polygonal cells arranged in sheets, nests, or cords. The cells have large, round, vesicular nuclei with prominent nucleoli. Atypia and mitosis are common. The cytoplasm may be clear, slightly amphophilic or basophilic, and may contain hyaline globules. This pattern is more common in adult tumors than in children and is almost always focal.

The *parietal pattern* has extensive and irregular deposits of extracellular basement membrane. Tumor cells are arranged surrounding or inside these masses. This pattern is named after the resemblance of the thick basement membrane (Reichert's membrane) of the parietal layer of the vitelline sac of rodents.

Most times YST is formed by different patterns in a myxoid or fibrous stroma or a highly cellular mesenchyme. The most common patterns are microcystic, solid, and myxomatous. The polyvesicular vitelline, sarcomatoid, and parietal patterns are rare. The glandular and parietal patterns are most often seen after chemotherapy.

Immunohistochemistry

Most tumor cells show positivity for cytokeratins and glypican-3 by immunohistochemistry, while staining for OCT3/4 is uniformly negative. Placental-like alkaline phosphatase (PLAP) positivity is found in 39–85 % of tumors [26]. AFP is focally observed in most tumors except for those with a hepatoid pattern that is diffuse, with or without a relationship with hyaline globules. Fifty percent of tumors show positivity for alpha-1 antitrypsin, while vimentin is positive in YSTs with myxomatous and sarcomatoid patterns. Laminin is characteristically positive in the parietal pattern. The enteric glands express carcinoembryonic antigen [28].

Biologic Behavior

YSTs in children have a much better prognosis than those in adults [30]. The prognosis of pediatric YST is correlated with age, with slower growth rates and lower grades of malignancy observed in younger children. In children younger than 5 years, the incidence of metastasis is no higher than 5 %, which increases to 20 % in adults [31]. The most common route of dissemination is hematogenous and the lung is the most common metastatic location [22]. In stage I YSTs, orchiectomy is sufficient, or even testis-sparing tumor excision and follow-up with chest and abdominal imaging and serum AFP measurement, as these tumors are not associated with GCNiS in the peritumoral parenchyma. Survival rates in stage I are higher than 80 % [32, 33]. In case of recurrence or metastasis, patients can be successfully treated with platinum-based chemotherapy (etoposide, carboplatin, and bleomycin) [34–36].

Teratoma, Prepubertal Type

Teratoma is the second most common testicular GCT in pediatric age according to the Prepubertal Testicular Tumor Registry of the American Academy of Pediatrics [37]. However, there is reason to believe that its incidence has been underestimated and that the real number is not accounted for in large series as not all cases are included because of their benign behavior. The incidence of teratomas may actually be higher than that of YSTs [38–40]. The median age at presentation is 13 months. Some cases have been reported in the neonatal period [41], and teratomas are unusual in children older than 4 years of age. Testicular teratomas in children are different from teratomas in adults in many aspects. Teratoma is not associated with other forms of GCT and bilateralism is exceptional in children [42]. A wide variety of congenital malformations such as spina bifida, retrocaval ureter, hemihypertrophy, and hernia can be associated with testicular teratomas. A total of 30 cases have been reported of teratomas originating in intra-abdominal undescended testes [43].

Clinical Features

Most patients with testicular teratomas present with a testicular mass detected during clinical exploration. Some teratomas contain large cysts filled with mucus or fluid that can be misdiagnosed as hydrocele [44] or may contain simple cysts [45], delaying the diagnosis by 6 months on average [46]. Ultrasonography is a useful method to identify a well-delimited, partially cystic intratesticular lesion. In teratomas occurring at prepubertal age, serum markers such as beta-HCG and AFP show normal levels except for teratomas with intestinal glands, which show moderate elevation of AFP.

Pathologic Features

Macroscopically, teratomas are cystic tumors with solid areas. The cysts may measure up to 1 cm in diameter and contain mucous, watery fluid or keratin. Solid areas may contain cartilage or bone.

Microscopically, teratomas are neoplasms that can show endoderm-, mesoderm-, or ectoderm-derived tissues in a disorganized or organoid arrangement. Like teratomas, postpubertal type childhood teratomas can contain mature and immature tissues. Mature teratomas contain cysts lined with squamous, ciliated respiratory-type or intestinal-type epithelium next to smooth muscle, cartilage, bone trabeculae, neuroglia, choroid plexus, and occasionally pigmented epithelium and pancreatic tissue (Figs. 4.7 and 4.8). Immature teratomas contain different types of immature tissues such as neuroepithelium (small cells in tubular or rosette arrangement) and blastema (nodular collections of cells with hyperchromatic nuclei and scant cytoplasm with or without tubular structures inside). The seminiferous tubules in the peripheral parenchyma show hypertrophic or multinucleated germ cells.

Dermoid cyst is a variant of prepubertal, type teratoma, uncommonly present in childhood [47, 48]. Macroscopically, it consists of one large cavity filled with cellular detritus and hair. Microscopically, all epidermal and dermal components are represented. Sebaceous glands are usually numerous (Figs. 4.9 and 4.10). Some authors accept as dermoid cysts tumors containing in their walls other tissues such as smooth muscle, adipose tissue, cartilage, bone, thyroid, salivary gland, gastrointestinal tissue, respiratory-type epithelium, and mature neural tissue [49].

Epidermoid cyst is defined as an encapsulated cyst lined with keratinized stratified flat

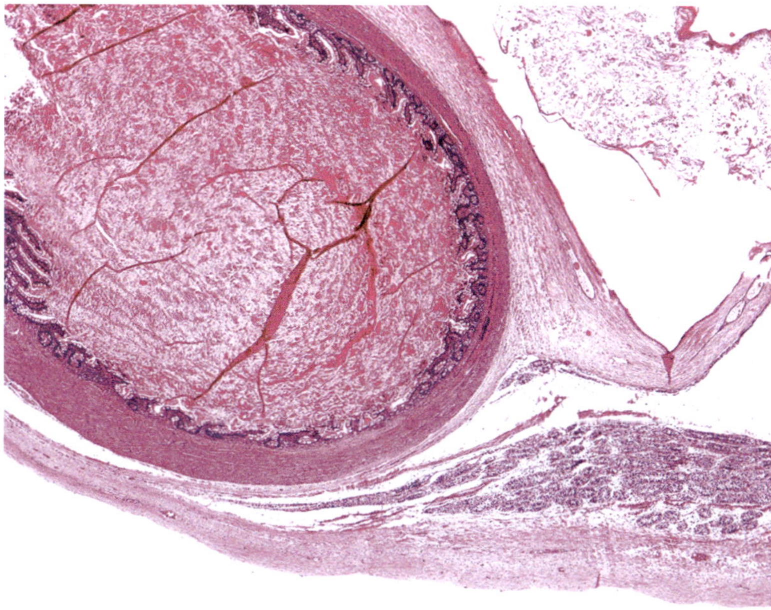

Fig. 4.7 Cystic organoid teratoma in a 10-year-old boy. The spherical formation resembles a complete intestinal wall. The remaining content of the cyst is made up of abundant keratin material

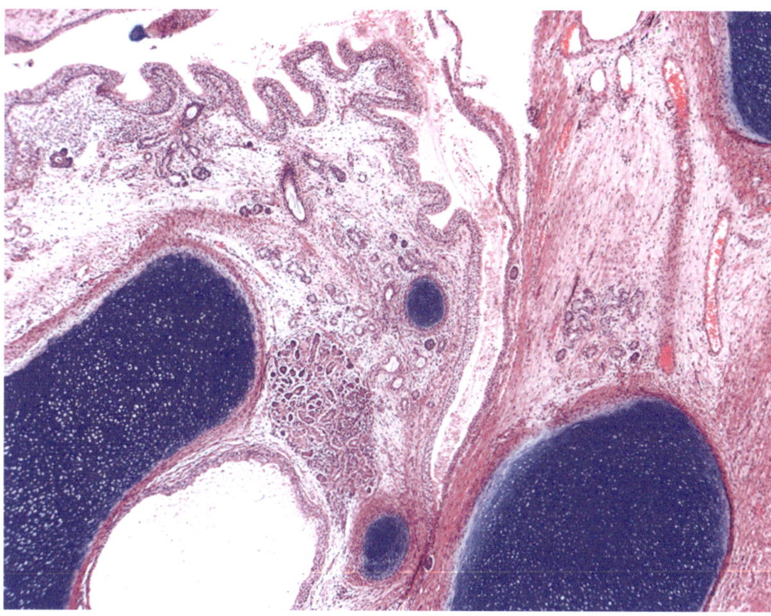

Fig. 4.8 Mature teratoma with islands of hyaline cartilage and cysts lined with nonkeratinized epithelium and glandular structures

epithelium without skin adnexal structures [50]. The keratin masses that fill the cyst produce a characteristic ultrasonographic image resembling onion layers or a dartboard. Most authors consider this lesion as nontumoral and some consider it a as monodermal teratoma. Epidermoid cysts are rare in the pediatric age [51].

Testicular primary carcinoid tumors have been reported as monodermal teratomas [52].

Biologic Behavior

The biologic behavior of teratomas in prepubertal age is benign, independent of their maturity or immaturity (unlike teratomas in adulthood). The nonmalignant behavior justifies enucleating or testis-sparing surgery in cases of bilateral tumors or unique testis [53]. This biologic behavior is related to the absence in childhood (except in 1 reported case [54]) of GCNiS in the

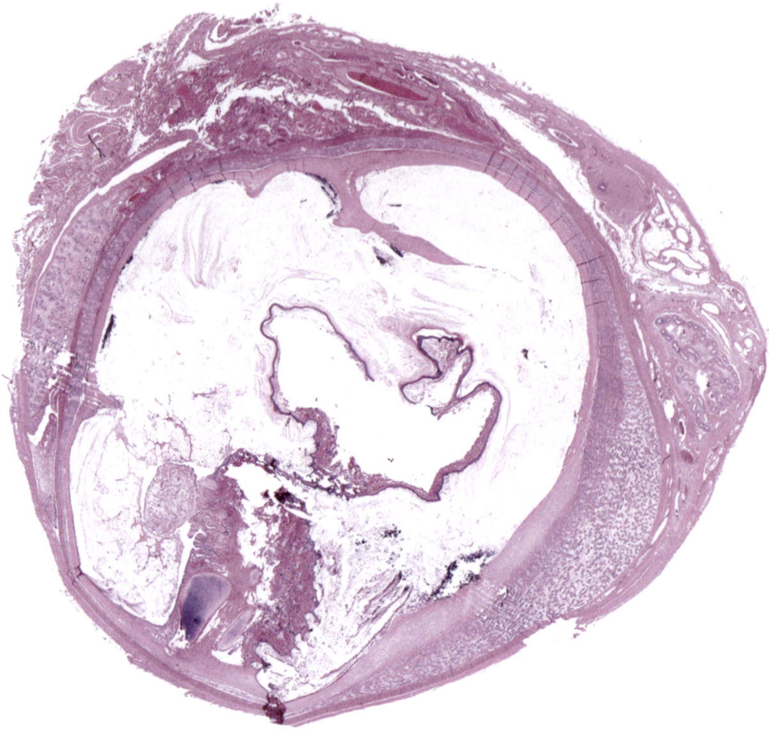

Fig. 4.9 Dermoid cyst. The encapsulated cyst comprises the testicular parenchyma

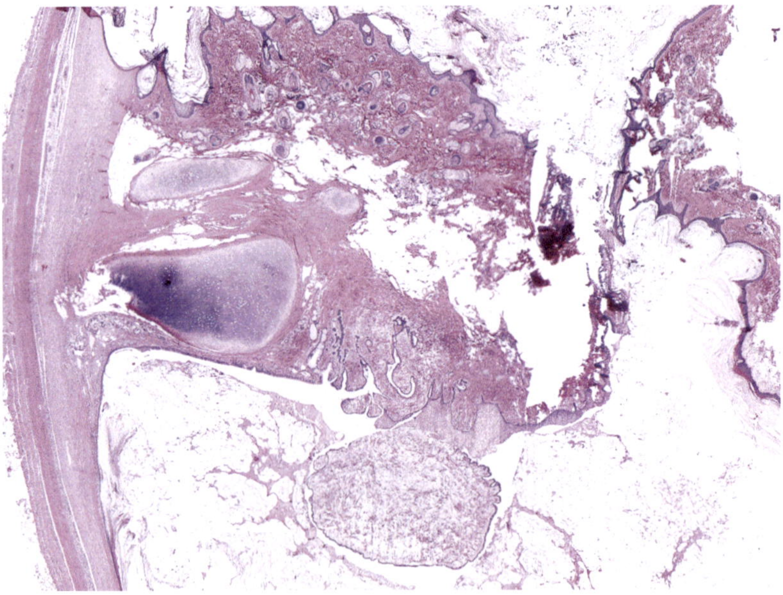

Fig. 4.10 Dermoid cyst partially lined with skin and adnexal pilosebaceous structures as well as respiratory-type epithelium in the septa. Note several islands of cartilage as another component

residual parenchyma, as previously mentioned [55]. In adolescents, orchiectomy and evaluation with the same protocols as used in adult GCTs are recommended. A small percentage of pediatric teratomas have a malignant somatic component, as is frequently observed in adult testis. In these unusual cases, treatment should be completed with chemotherapy or surgery depending on the nature of the malignant component [56].

Other Germ Cell Tumors

Some cases of embryonal carcinoma [34], seminoma [57], and mixed GCT [58] have been reported in childhood and more frequently adolescence. These tumors have a very aggressive behavior, presenting as metastatic disease at diagnosis [59, 60]. After puberty, these tumors are similar to those in adults [61].

Gonadoblastoma

Gonadoblastoma is a mixed tumor composed of a mixture of germ cells and cells resembling Sertoli/granulosa cells arranged in a preferably nodular pattern in an ovarian-type stroma [62]. It characteristically arises in dysgenetic gonads in patients with disorders in sexual differentiation who have either the whole or a part of the Y chromosome in their genome. The most common clinical entities where gonadoblastoma develops are 46XY pure gonadal dysgenesis (patients with bilateral streak gonads) [63–65], mixed gonadal dysgenesis (streak gonad on one side and testicular dysgenesis in the contralateral testis), dysgenetic male pseudohermaphroditism (both gonads with testicular dysgenesis features), ovotesticular disorder [66], patients with Turner syndrome and Y chromosome residual material [67, 68], and androgen receptor insensitivity. Exceptionally, gonadoblastoma has been observed in a normal testis [69].

Eighty percent of patients with gonadoblastomas are phenotypically female, and 20 % are phenotypically male [70]. The *TSPY1* gene (which encodes a testis-specific protein) located at the GBY locus in the centromeric portion of the short arm of the Y chromosome is involved in the genesis of most gonadoblastomas [71, 72]. Gonadoblastoma is assumed to arise from OCT3/4-positive surviving germ cells in undifferentiated gonadal tissue of dysgenetic gonads [73].

The size varies from microscopic to 8 cm in diameter [74]. The tumors are solid and gray or yellow in color. Most gonadoblastomas arise from streak gonads. The remainder arise from testes with a thin and poorly collagenized tunica albuginea resembling the ovarian cortex, with irregular cellular cords or tubules that go through the albuginea to reach the testicular surface [75]. One-third of patients have bilateral gonadoblastomas.

Gonadoblastoma cells are arranged in nests or cords and less frequently in a diffuse pattern; the same tumor can show different patterns. Gonadoblastoma is composed of two types of cells. The first type is germ cells appearing like gonocytes or with seminoma-like morphology because of their large size, voluminous nuclei with one or two nucleoli, and pale cytoplasm. Mitosis can also be seen. The second type of cells is smaller cells with ovoid hyperchromatic nuclei and Charcot-Böttcher filaments in their cytoplasm like Sertoli cells that are admixed with germ cells. Cells with Sertoli features are arranged as an outer palisade in the nodules and around eosinophilic bodies or hyaline nodules that are dispersed by the tumor and formed by basement membrane material (Fig. 4.11). These tumors show prominent calcifications that arise from hyaline bodies. Leydig cells can be observed in the stroma among cords or nests.

Immunohistochemistry

Gonocyte-like cells express OCT3/4, PLAP (Fig. 4.12), c-kit, TSPY, and D2-40 [76], while Sertoli/granulosa cells show inhibin in their cytoplasm and SOX9 and more commonly FOXL2 in the nuclei [77]. Leydig cells are inhibin and calretinin positive.

Gonadoblastoma is considered to be an in situ neoplasia precursor of infiltrating tumors like germ cell neoplasia, in situ. The level of testicularization of the gonad will determine the histologic composition of the precursor lesion, either gonadoblastoma or GCNiS [78]. When germ cells proliferate, they actively destroy the nodular arrangement of the tumor and infiltrate the gonad, giving rise to any type of GCT, although the most common are seminoma and dysgerminoma [79] (Fig. 4.13). Gonadectomy is recommended in all cases because of the infiltrating ability of the tumor.

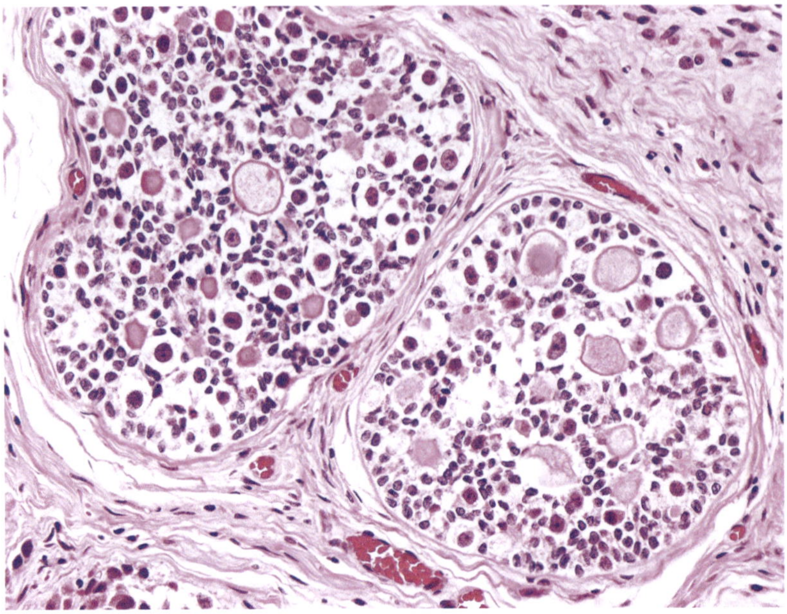

Fig. 4.11 Gonadoblastoma. Nests made up of two cell types. The smaller cells have hyperchromatic nuclei and are arranged above the basement membrane and surrounding the abundant eosinophilic matrix. The larger cells have clear cytoplasm and prominent nucleoli

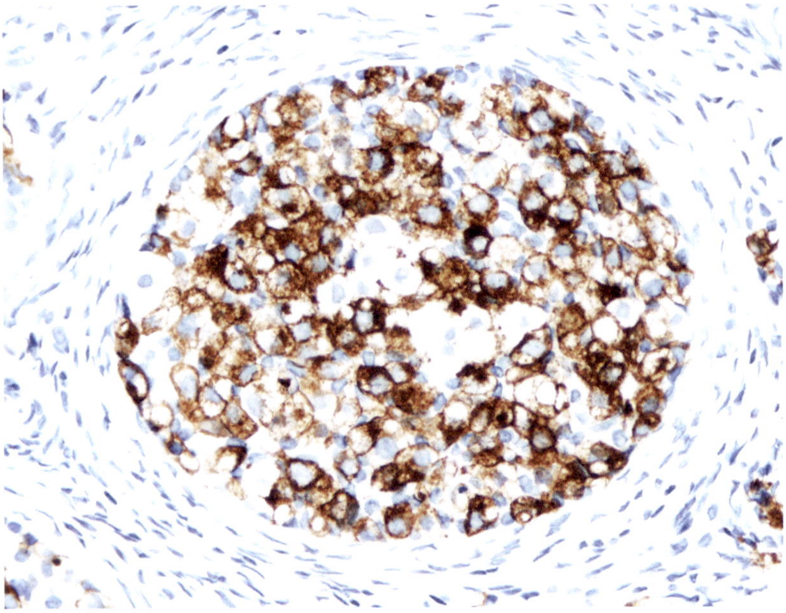

Fig. 4.12 Gonocyte-like cells of a gonadoblastoma show PLAP membranous immunostaining

The differential diagnosis of gonadoblastoma in childhood includes fetal gonadoblastoid testicular dysplasia (abnormally differentiated testicular parenchyma that is associated with Walker-Warburg syndrome) as well as ureter malformations and renal cystic dysplasia. The peripheral testicular parenchyma shows a crescent-like zone with spherical or irregular solid nests, cords, and malformed tubules that are embedded in an undifferentiated stroma. Each structure is composed of three cell types: cells with vesicular nuclei and vacuolated cytoplasm, cells with hyperchromatic nuclei, and germ cell-like cells. However, gonocyte or dysgerminoma-like cells are absent unlike gonadoblastomas.

In postpubertal patients, Sertoli cell nodules colonized by GCNiS cells may be misinterpreted

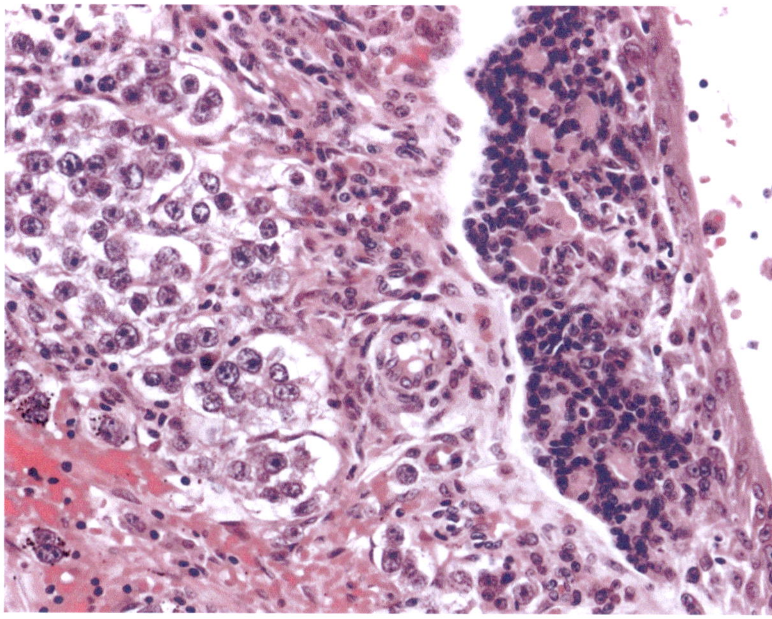

Fig. 4.13 Dysgerminoma originated from gonadoblastoma. Remnants of gonadoblastoma can be recognized with Sertoli/granulosa cells and Call-Exner bodies

as gonadoblastoma. Sertoli cell nodules are common in cryptorchid testes of postpubertal patients without any intersexual condition. Sertoli cell nodules colonized by GCNiS cells are usually in the vicinity of seminoma or seminiferous tubules with GCNiS. Sertoli/granulosa cells express both SOX9 and FOXL2, and this is evidence of their incomplete differentiation. In contrast, Sertoli cell nodules with GCNiS show diffuse and intense positivity for SOX9 and SF-1 and absence of immunoexpression for FOXL2 as evidence of their complete differentiation [80].

Pediatric-Type GCTs (Type I) in Adults

Several types of GCNiS, varying from mature teratomas to monophyletic immature teratomas to YSTs, have been reported in adults that, except for the patient's age, have all the characteristics of pediatric GCTs (type I). These tumors differ from adult GCTs in the following features [81]:

- Absence of GCNiS in the peripheral parenchyma confirmed by OCT3/4 and PLAP.
- Absence of testicular scar or burned-out tumor.
- Absence of inflammatory infiltrates; minimal infiltrates or plasma cell inflammatory infiltrates are accepted.
- Demonstration by FISH of two centromeres in chromosome 12 and absence of 12p excess.
- Complete spermatogenesis.

The behavior of this group of tumors is benign, and the recommended treatment should be orchiectomy or even testis-sparing surgery.

The origin of type I GCT in adults is probably a germ cell that is directly reprogrammed to pluripotentiality without going through a GCNiS stage. Like their pediatric counterparts, these tumors probably originate in the neonatal period or some years later, presenting clinical symptoms in puberty or adulthood [82].

Germ Cell Neoplasia In Situ (GCNiS)

Germ cell neoplasia in situ presumably originates during fetal life from gonocytes that do not differentiate properly and maintain their original immature and multipotent features. Morphologic, immunohistochemistry, and genetic profile similarities support this hypothesis [83–85]. The microscopic morphology of GCNiS in childhood

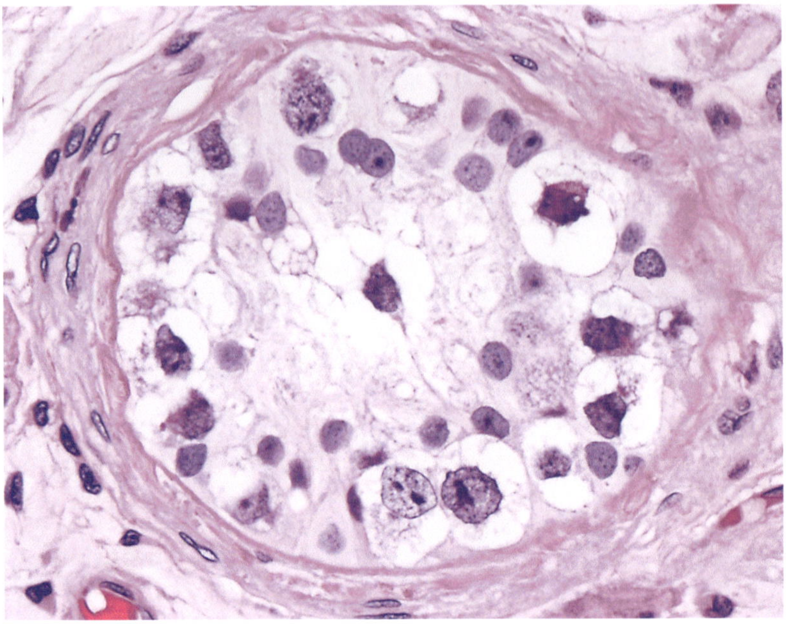

Fig. 4.14 GCNiS cells above the basement membrane displacing Sertoli cells toward the lumen of the tubule. The cells are large and show one or two prominent nucleoli

is different from GCNiS in adults. Before making a diagnosis of GCNiS in infancy or childhood, it is important that one is familiar with the following features: (a) GCNiS features in adult testis, (b) proliferation and differentiation of fetal germ cells, (c) the most useful criteria in the differential diagnosis between a delay in gonocyte maturation and GCNiS in postnatal life, and (d) knowledge of situations with atypical-looking germ cells but without enough criteria to establish a diagnosis of GCNiS.

GCNiS Features in Adult Testis

Germ cell neoplasia in situ is the preinvasive phase of all types of GCTs except for pediatric GCTs and spermatocytic tumor. It is usually found in groups of small seminiferous tubules devoid of spermatogenesis that probably belong to the same lobule. These small tubules are often separated by larger tubules with complete spermatogenesis. The tumor cells are typically confined to the basal compartment of the seminiferous tubule, displacing Sertoli cells luminally. GCNiS cells are large cells with clear cytoplasm because of the high glycogen content and a sharply defined plasma membrane. The nuclei are large, spherical, and hyperchromatic, often with one or two prominent nucleoli and coarse chromatin (Fig. 4.14). Mitosis can be observed. Sertoli cells commonly show spherical instead of the normal triangular nuclei. The nucleoli are central but small, suggesting incomplete maturation [83]. Sertoli cell dysfunction is probably established in fetal life, leading to a defect in the mechanisms of interaction between Sertoli and germ cells and a consequent defect in gonocyte maturation. In 50 % of cases, GCNiS cells acquire infiltrating capacity after 5 years, and a GCT develops [86]. GCNiS cell transformation into seminoma is slower than transformation into a nonseminomatous tumor, which is related to the more aggressive behavior of the latter.

The classical immunohistochemical markers of GCNiS are the transcription factor OCT3/4 [87, 88] and PLAP [89] (Fig. 4.15). GCNiS cells are also positive for the AP2 transcription factor AP2γ [90], podoplanin [91, 92], and c-kit [93]. OCT3/4 is expressed in the nuclei, whereas PLAP shows membranous expression. Most cells that express OCT3/4 also express PLAP. The average nuclear DNA content of CIS cells is about 4C.

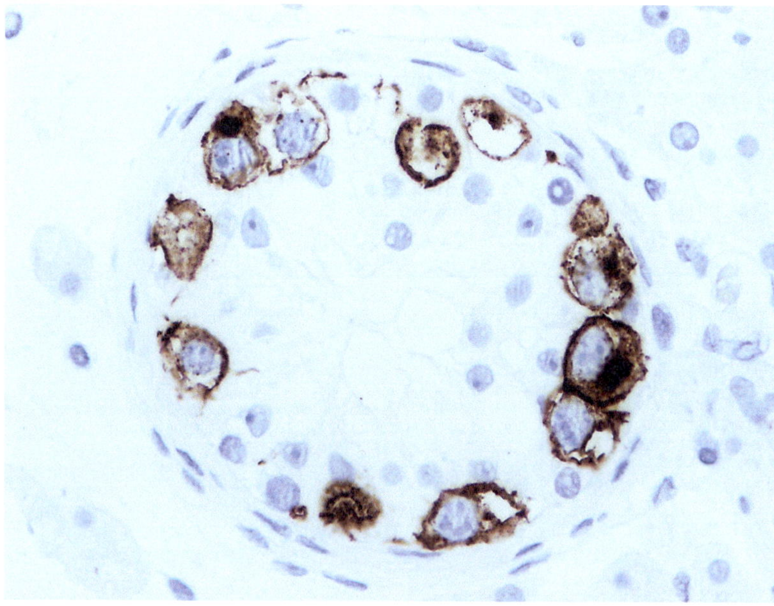

Fig. 4.15 PLAP immunoexpression in the membrane of GCNiS cells

Proliferation and Differentiation of Fetal Germ Cells

Three different morphologic and immunohistochemical types of germ cells have been identified in the testis during the fetal period; these types represent three different stages in the differentiation from primordial germ cell to spermatogonium. One characteristic feature of human fetal testis is the concurrence during several months of the three cell types as opposed to the homogeneous population of gonocytes in other mammalian species.

Gonocytes

Once the primordial germ cells in the genital ridge are surrounded by cells deriving from the coelomic epithelium (pre-Sertoli cells), they transform into gonocytes: gonocytes are identified in the center of the seminiferous cords separated from the basement membrane by Sertoli cells. Gonocytes are large cells that have spherical euchromatic nuclei with one or two nucleoli [94, 95]. The gonocyte immunophenotype is OCT3/4, c-kit, and PLAP positive and melanoma-associated antigen 4 (MAGEA4) negative [96–98].

Intermediate Cells

Intermediate cells (transitional gonocytes) are morphologically similar to gonocytes, although they differ in their distribution in the seminiferous cords and in their immunophenotype. Intermediate cells are located in the periphery of the seminiferous cords in contact with the basement membrane. Their immunophenotype is negative for both c-kit and MAGEA4, whereas they show weak or negative staining for OCT4 and positive staining for proliferating cell nuclear antigen (PCNA), indicating active proliferation. It has been suggested that when these cells get in contact with the basement membrane, they lose their pluripotency and start to differentiate.

Fetal Spermatogonia

Fetal spermatogonia (or pre-spermatogonia) are grouped at the periphery of the seminiferous cords above the basement membrane. They are the germ stem cells of the adult testis. Immunohistochemistry shows MAGEA4 staining, and the cells are negative for c-kit and PCNA.

At the tenth week of gestation, most germ cells are gonocytes; at approximately the 15th week, many intermediate cells are present together with gonocytes, and fetal spermatogonia

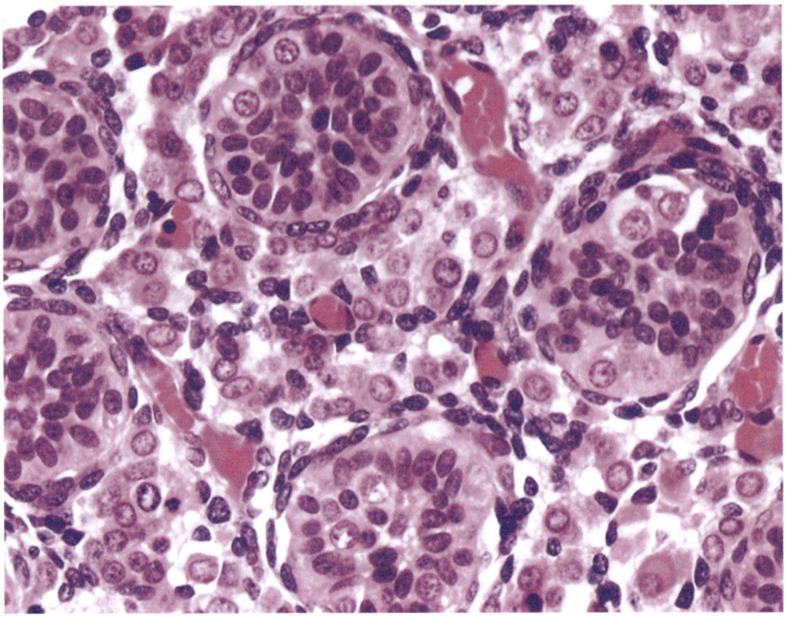

Fig. 4.16 Fetal testis (30 weeks of gestation). Most germ cells are pre-spermatogonia located above the basement membrane

can be observed for the first time. From the 22nd week onward, most germ cells are fetal spermatogonia. Some gonocytes persist even after birth. Most of them differentiate into spermatogonia between 30 and 90 days after birth at the stage known as mini-puberty; the remainder undergo apoptosis. The lack of synchronization of these stages in the human fetal testis may serve to protect the number of spermatogonial stem cells (and thus future fertility) from various insults that may occur throughout fetal life.

In summary, in parallel with germ cell differentiation, a change in the expression of several proteins takes place. PLAP is positive mainly in young gonocytes and less in pre-spermatogonia. The largest number of positive cells is observed in the first trimester of gestation, decreasing as gestation progresses (Fig. 4.16). At birth PLAP is positive only in isolated cells (less than 1 per tubule) and located in the center of the tubule. C-kit is expressed in the second and third trimesters of gestation in a similar proportion in gonocytes and pre-spermatogonia. OCT3/4 is most expressed in the first trimester and the first half of the second trimester (4–6 cells per tubule), mainly in gonocytes. Its expression decreases to three cells per tubule in the second half of the second trimester. At the end of gestation, positivity is only observed in isolated gonocytes in the center of the tubule. TSPY is positive throughout gestation exclusively in spermatogonia. Ki67 is predominantly expressed in gonocytes up to the 24th week. From that week onward, the number of positive gonocytes and pre-spermatogonia is similar. The number of positive cells decreases as gestation progresses. At birth positivity persists only in isolated gonocytes in the center of the tubule, and pre-spermatogonia seem to have entered a quiescent period [97, 99] (Table 4.1).

GCNiS Cell Features in Childhood (Pre-GCNiS)

In childhood, seminiferous tubules with GCNiS have no lumen, and their size is similar to that of normal tubules. Gonocyte-like cells are located both in the center of the tubule and above the basement membrane. These cells show similar nuclear and cytoplasmic features to GCNiS cells in adults [100]. They occasionally show mitosis (Fig. 4.17). Like GCNiS cells, these pre-GCNiS cells are strongly positive for OCT3/4, TSPY, and PLAP and focally for SCF [101]. OCT3/4 suppresses apoptosis of gonocytes, TSPY enhances the proliferation of these cells, and SCF is a survival and growth factor for these cells [102].

Table 4.1 Evolution through fetal life of the immunoexpression of different markers in germ cells

Marker	Germ cell type	First trimester	Second trimester	Third trimester	First year of life
PLAP	Gonocyte	+++	++	+	+
	Pre-spermatogonia	++	+	–	–
c-KIT	Gonocyte	+++	+++	++	+
	Pre-spermatogonia	+++	+++	++	+
OCT 3/4	Gonocyte	+++	+++	+	+
	Pre-spermatogonia	–	–	–	–
TSPY	Gonocyte	–	–	–	–
	Pre-spermatogonia	++	++	++	++
Ki67	Gonocyte	+++	+++	+	+
	Pre-spermatogonia	++	++	+	–

+ Less than one positive cell per tubule (isolated), ++ 1–3 positive cells per tubule, +++ 4–6 positive cells per tubule

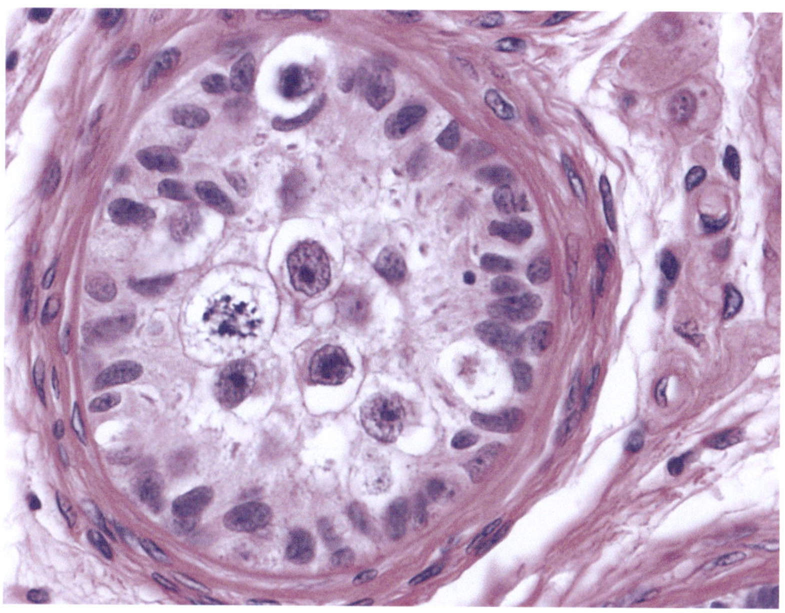

Fig. 4.17 Cross section of seminiferous tubule of a 9-year-old patient showing Sertoli cells in a pseudostratified arrangement and several large cells in the center, one of them in mitosis

GCNiS cells in children have DNA contents in a hypertriploid or hypertetraploid range [103, 104]. Seminiferous tubules with germ cells are arranged in small groups preferably beneath the tunica albuginea. Gonocytes in the center of the tubule retain an embryonic phenotype that persists beyond fetal development and childhood (OCT3/4 positive). These arrested gonocytes fail to differentiate due to impaired functioning of Sertoli cells in fetal development that prevents the movement of gonocytes from the center of the tubule to the periphery to get in contact with the basement membrane [105, 106]. This pattern is maintained until puberty, when the increase in hormone production produces changes in the spermatogonial niche to induce meiosis and haploid spermatozoa. At the same time that these changes take place, GCNiS cells start to proliferate. The result is a progressive transformation of a GCNiS cell phenotype from infantile to adult.

Delayed Maturation of Gonocytes Versus Infantile GCNiS

The finding of gonocyte-like cells in an infantile testis after the third month of postnatal life, when

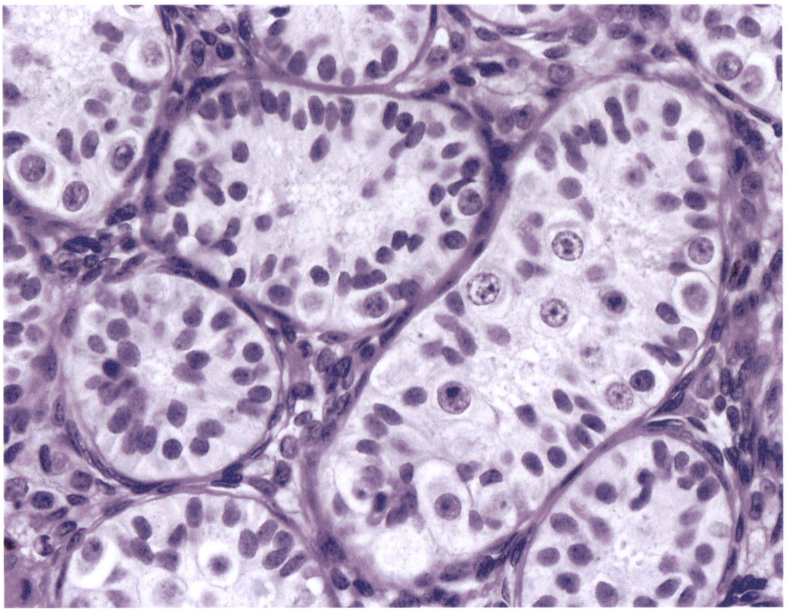

Fig. 4.18 Infantile testis of a patient with 46XY disorder of sex development with Müllerian remnants showing seminiferous tubules with intratubular gonocytes both above the basement membrane and at the center of the tubule

mini-puberty finishes, raises the possibility of a delay in the maturation of gonocytes instead of an infantile GCNiS. This differential diagnosis is of great prognostic importance since the malignant potential of delayed maturation of gonocytes is practically nonexistent, while infantile GCNiS has a high risk of malignant evolution [101, 107, 108]. The problem becomes more difficult when these cells appear in populations with a high risk of GCTs, such as individuals with gonadal dysgenesis, Down syndrome, and undervirilization syndromes [109]. The differential diagnosis should be supported by the age of the patient together with cytologic, histologic, immunohistochemical, and ploidy marker data. Gonocytes with delayed maturation are uniformly dispersed in the entire testis and more or less randomly placed in the seminiferous tubules instead of in groups of seminiferous tubules (Fig. 4.18). These cells have cytologic features of gonocytes located both in the center of the tubule and above the basement membrane. In spite of their similar morphology to pre-GCNiS cells, the immunophenotype is different. OCT3/4 is expressed only in germ cells with delayed maturation that are in the center of the tubule and occasionally in the cells above the basement membrane. They are also PLAP positive (Fig. 4.19). The cells in the periphery of the tubule are TSPY positive as well. SCF is negative in delayed maturation. Inconsistent OCT3/4 expression in TSPY-positive cells in the absence of SCF expression indicates a delay in maturation.

Atypical Germ Cells that May Simulate GCNiS

Two types of germ cells can be misinterpreted as GCNiS cells because of their morphology, especially if the specimen has not been properly fixed. These cell types are hypertrophic and multinucleated spermatogonia. Both can be seen in the testicular parenchyma peripheral to GCTs in childhood.

Hypertrophic spermatogonia characteristically have large hyperchromatic nuclei without nucleoli and clear, abundant cytoplasm. They are polyploid cells that were probably arrested in the S phase of the cell cycle [110]. They are observed in cryptorchid testes and exceptionally in normal testes. Hyperchromatic spermatogonia are numerous in seminiferous tubules surrounding teratomas and have been observed around YSTs. These cells are negative for OCT3/4 and PLAP and positive for PCNA and p53, which is a sign of their non-tumor-proliferative nature [9, 111].

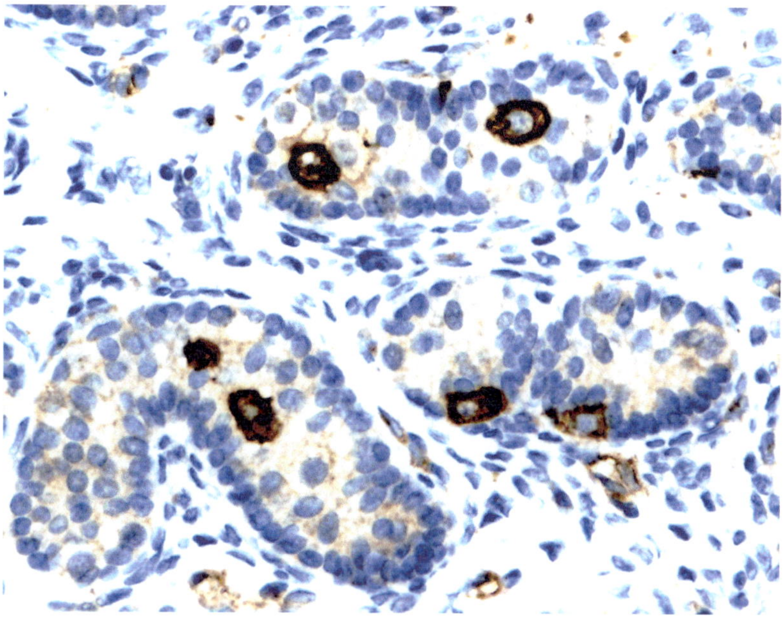

Fig. 4.19 PLAP-positive cells inside a seminiferous tubule

Multinucleated spermatogonia commonly show three or four nuclei, but the number can be higher. The nuclei can show features of spermatogonia type A dark, A pale, or a mixture of both. Multinucleated spermatogonia have been observed in cryptorchid testis with or without GCNiS. They have not been reported in normal testes. Multinucleated spermatogonia are produced by amitotic cell division [112].

References

1. Kay R. Prepubertal testicular tumor registry. J Urol. 1993;150:671–4.
2. Coppes MJ, Rackley R, Kay R. Primary testicular and paratesticular tumors of childhood. Med Pediatr Oncol. 1994;22:329–40.
3. Ross JH, Kay R. Prepubertal testis tumors. Rev Urol. 2004;6:11–8.
4. Pohl HG, Shukla AR, Metcalf PD, Cilento BG, Retik AB, Bagli DJ, Huff DS, Rushton H. Prepubertal testis tumors: actual prevalence rate of histological types. J Urol. 2004;172:2370–2.
5. Schneider DT, Calaminus G, Koch S, Teske C, Schmidt P, Haas RJ, Harms D, Göbel U. Epidemiologic analysis of 1,442 children and adolescents registered in the German germ cell tumor protocols. Pediatr Blood Cancer. 2004;42:169–75.
6. Murphy FL, Law H, Mushtaq I, Sebire NJ. Testicular and paratesticular pathology in infants and children: the histopathological experience of a tertiary paediatric unit over a 17 year period. Pediatr Surg Int. 2007;23:867–72.
7. Mittal D, Agarwala S, Yadav DK, Pramanik DD, Sharma MC, Bagga D. Testicular tumors in undescended testes in children below 5 y of age. Indian J Pediatr. 2015;82:549–52.
8. Walsh TJ, Davies BJ, Croughan MS, Carroll PR, Turek PJ. Racial differences among boys with testicular germ cell tumors in the United States. J Urol. 2008;179:1961–5.
9. Hawkins E, Heifetz SA, Giller R, Cushing B. The prepubertal testis (prenatal and postnatal): its relationship to intratubular germ cell neoplasia: a combined Pediatric Oncology Group and Children's Cancer Study Group. Hum Pathol. 1997;28:404–10.
10. Perlman EJ, Cushing B, Hawkins E, Griffin CA. Cytogenetic analysis of childhood endodermal sinus tumors: a Pediatric Oncology Group study. Pediatr Pathol. 1994;14:695–708.
11. Mostert M, Rosenberg C, Stoop H, Schuyer M, Timmer A, Oosterhuis W, Looijenga L. Comparative genomic and in situ hybridization of germ cell tumors of the infantile testis. Lab Invest. 2000;80: 1055–64.
12. van Echten J, Timmer A, van der Veen AY, Molenaar WM, de Jong B. Infantile and adult testicular germ cell tumors. a different pathogenesis? Cancer Genet Cytogenet. 2002;135:57–62.
13. Harms D, Zahn S, Göbel U, Schneider DT. Pathology and molecular biology of teratomas in childhood and adolescence. Klin Padiatr. 2006;218:296–302.
14. Silver SA, Wiley JM, Perlman EJ. DNA ploidy analysis of pediatric germ cell tumors. Mod Pathol. 1994;7:951–6.

15. Visfeldt J, Jørgensen N, Müller J, Møller H, Skakkebaek NE. Testicular germ cell tumours of childhood in Denmark, 1943–1989: incidence and evaluation of histology using immunohistochemical techniques. J Pathol. 1994;174:39–47.
16. Chaganti RS, Houldsworth J. Genetics and biology of adult human male germ cell tumors. Cancer Res. 2000;60:1475–82.
17. Ulbright TM. Germ cell tumors of the gonads: a selective review emphasizing problems in differential diagnosis, newly appreciated, and controversial issues. Mod Pathol. 2005;18:S61–79.
18. Ulbright TM, Young RH. Testicular and paratesticular tumors and tumor-like lesions in the first 2 decades. Semin Diagn Pathol. 2014;31:323–81.
19. Mostofi FK. Pathology of germ cell tumors of testis: a progress report. Cancer. 1980;45:1735–54.
20. Teilum G. Endodermal sinus tumors of the ovary and testis: comparative morphogenesis of the so-called mesonephroma ovarii (Schiller) and extraembryonic (yolk sac-allantoic) structures of the rat's placenta. Cancer. 1959;12:1092–105.
21. Drut R. Yolk sac tumor and testicular microlithiasis. Pediatr Pathol Mol Med. 2003;22:343–7.
22. Ahmed HU, Arya M, Muneer A, Mushtaq I, Sebire NJ. Testicular and paratesticular tumours in the prepubertal population. Lancet Oncol. 2010;11:476–83.
23. Kaplan GW, Cromie WC, Kelalis PP, Silber I, Tank Jr ES. Prepubertal yolk sac testicular tumors – report of the testicular tumor registry. J Urol. 1988;140:1109–12.
24. Tsuchida Y, Saito S, Ishida M, Omi K, Urano Y. Yolk sac tumor (endodermal sinus tumor) and alpha-fetoprotein. A report of three cases. Cancer. 1973;32: 917–21.
25. Wu JT, Book L, Sudar K. Serum alpha fetoprotein (AFP) levels in normal infants. Pediatr Res. 1981;15: 50–2.
26. Teilum G. Classification of endodermal sinus tumour (mesoblatoma vitellinum) and so-called "embryonal carcinoma" of the ovary. Acta Pathol Microbiol Scand. 1965;64:407–29.
27. Talerman A. Germ cell tumours. Ann Pathol. 1985; 5:145–57.
28. Emerson RE, Ulbright TM. The use of immunohistochemistry in the differential diagnosis of tumors of the testis and paratestis. Semin Diagn Pathol. 2005;22:33–50.
29. Kao CS, Idrees MT, Young RH, Ulbright TM. Solid pattern yolk sac tumor: a morphologic and immunohistochemical study of 52 cases. Am J Surg Pathol. 2012;36:360–7.
30. Lin JN, Wang KL, Hung IJ, Yang CP. Management of yolk sac tumor of the testis in children. J Formos Med Assoc. 1994;93:393–6.
31. Grady RW, Ross JH, Kay R. Patterns of metastatic spread in prepubertal yolk sac tumor of the testis. J Urol. 1995;153:1259–61.
32. Schmidt P, Haas RJ, Göbel U, Calaminus G. Results of the German studies (MAHO) for treatment of testicular germ cell tumors in children – an update. Klin Padiatr. 2002;214:167–72.
33. Zhou XJ, Zhou RS, Fan T, Han CH. Experience with the treatment of testicular yolk sac tumor in children: a report of 14 cases. Eur Rev Med Pharmacol Sci. 2014;18:3831–3.
34. Taskinen S, Fagerholm R, Aronniemi J, Rintala R, Taskinen M. Testicular tumors in children and adolescents. J Pediatr Urol. 2008;4:134–7.
35. Steffens J, Treiyer A, Calaminus G. Management of pediatric testicular tumors: diagnosis, therapy, and follow-up. Urologe A. 2009;48:359–63.
36. Shin YS, Kim HJ. Current management of testicular cancer. Korean J Urol. 2013;54:2–10.
37. Ross JH, Rybicki L, Kay R. Clinical behavior and a contemporary management algorithm for prepubertal testis tumors: a summary of the Prepubertal Testis Tumor Registry. J Urol. 2002;168:1675–8.
38. Walsh C, Rushton HG. Diagnosis and management of teratomas and epidermoid cysts. Urol Clin North Am. 2000;27:509–18.
39. Shukla AR, Woodard C, Carr MC, Huff DS, Canning DA, Zderic SA, Kolon TF, Snyder 3rd HM. Experience with testis sparing surgery for testicular teratoma. J Urol. 2004;171:161–3.
40. Metcalfe PD, Farivar-Mohseni H, Farhat W, McLorie G, Khoury A, Bägli DJ. Pediatric testicular tumors: contemporary incidence and efficacy of testicular preserving surgery. J Urol. 2003;170:2412–5.
41. Levy DA, Kay R, Elder JS. Neonatal testis tumors: a review of the Prepubertal Testis Tumor Registry. J Urol. 1994;151:715–7.
42. Herek O, Ulman I, Ozcan C, Avanoğlu A. Bilateral testicular teratoma in infancy: report of a rare case treated by testis-sparing surgery. Eur J Pediatr Surg. 2004;14:209–11.
43. Yam B, Georgiou NA, Khullar P, Coren CV, Katz DS. Radiology-pathology conference: mature teratoma arising from an intra-abdominal undescended testis in a 7-month-old infant. Clin Imaging. 2010; 34:466–71.
44. Lin HC, Clark JY. Testicular teratoma presenting as a transilluminating scrotal mass. Urology. 2006;67: 1290.e3–5.
45. Di Renzo D, Persico A, Sindici G, Lelli Chiesa P. Testicular teratoma, mimicking a simple testicular cyst, in an infant. Urology. 2013;82:701–3.
46. Brosman SA. Testicular tumors in prepubertal children. Urology. 1979;13:581–8.
47. Assaf G, Mosbah A, Homsy Y, Michaud J. Dermoid cyst of testis in five-year-old-child. Urology. 1983; 22:432–4.
48. Jesus LE, Pena CR, Leao AP. Pre-pubertal testicular dermoid cyst treated with conservative surgery. Int Braz J Urol. 2005;31:359–61.
49. Ulbright TM, Srigley JR. Dermoid cyst of the testis: a study of five postpubertal cases, including a pilomatrixoma-like variant, with evidence supporting its separate classification from mature

testicular teratoma. Am J Surg Pathol. 2001;25: 788–93.
50. Price Jr EB. Epidermoid cysts of the testis: a clinical and pathologic analysis of 69 cases from the testicular tumor registry. J Urol. 1969;102:708–13.
51. Aneiros-Fernandez J, Arias-Santiago S, Cancela-Diez B, O'Valle F, Cachaza JA. Intratesticular epidermoid cyst: a rare tumor. J Clin Med Res. 2010;2:281–3.
52. Leake J, Levitt G, Ramani P. Primary carcinoid of the testis in a 10-year-old boy. Histopathology. 1991;19:373–5.
53. Rushton HG, Belman AB, Sesterhenn I, Patterson K, Mostofi FK. Testicular sparing surgery for prepubertal teratoma of the testis: a clinical and pathological study. J Urol. 1990;144:726–30.
54. Stamp IM, Jacobsen GK. Infant intratubular germ cell neoplasia. Am J Surg Pathol. 1995;19:489.
55. Renedo DE, Trainer TD. Intratubular germ cell neoplasia (ITGCN) with p53 and PCNA expression and adjacent mature teratoma in an infant testis. An immunohistochemical and morphologic study with a review of the literature. Am J Surg Pathol. 1994; 18:947–52.
56. Terenziani M, D'Angelo P, Bisogno G, Boldrini R, Cecchetto G, Collini P, Conte M, De Laurentis T, Ilari I, Indolfi P, Inserra A, Piva L, Siracusa F, Spreafico F, Tamaro P, Lo Curto M. Teratoma with a malignant somatic component in pediatric patients: the Associazione Italiana Ematologia Oncologia Pediatrica (AIEOP) experience. Pediatr Blood Cancer. 2010;54:532–7.
57. Tanini R. On a case of testicular seminoma in infancy. Atti Accad Fisiocrit Siena Med Fis. 1964;13:107–27.
58. Frey P, Fliegel C, Herzog B. Testicular tumours in infancy and childhood – a review of 10 germ cell tumours and 10 non germ cell tumours. Z Kinderchir. 1990;45:229–34.
59. Sokoloff MH, Joyce GF, Wise M, Urologic Diseases in America Project. Testis cancer. J Urol. 2007;177: 2030–41.
60. Cost NG, Lubahn JD, Adibi M, Romman A, Wickiser JE, Raj GV, Sagalowsky AI, Margulis V. A comparison of pediatric, adolescent, and adult testicular germ cell malignancy. Pediatr Blood Cancer. 2014;61:446–51.
61. Marulaiah M, Gilhotra A, Moore L, Boucaut H, Goh DW. Testicular and paratesticular pathology in children: a 12-year histopathological review. World J Surg. 2010;34:969–74.
62. Scully RE. Gonadoblastoma; a gonadal tumor related to the dysgerminoma (seminoma) and capable of sex-hormone production. Cancer. 1953;6: 455–63.
63. Ng SB, Yong MH, Knight LA, Lee VK, Nadarajah S, Stoop H, Looijenga LH. Gonadoblastoma-associated mixed germ cell tumour in 46, XY complete gonadal dysgenesis (Swyer syndrome): analysis of Y chromosomal genotype and OCT3/4 and TSPY expression profile. Histopathology. 2008;52:644–6.
64. Ben Temime R, Chachial A, Attial L, Ghodbanel I, Makhloufl T, Koubaal A, Kourda N, Ben Jilani S, Dammak T, El May A, Rahal K. 46 XY pure gonadal dysgenesis with gonadoblastoma and dysgerminoma. Tunis Med. 2008;86:710–3.
65. Fernandes GC, Sathe PA, Naik LP, Kane SV. Bilateral gonadoblastomas with unilateral dysgerminoma in a case of 46 XY pure gonadal dysgenesis (Swyer syndrome). Indian J Pathol Microbiol. 2010;53: 376–8.
66. Kini U, Bantwal G, Ayyar V, Idiculla J. Bilateral gonadoblastomas with a left sided dysgerminoma in a true hermaphrodite (disorder of sexual differentiation) with 46, XY karyotype. J Assoc Physicians India. 2008;56:549–51.
67. Mazzanti L, Cicognani A, Baldazzi L, Bergamaschi R, Scarano E, Strocchi S, Nicoletti A, Mencarelli F, Pittalis M, Forabosco A, Cacciari E. Gonadoblastoma in Turner syndrome and Y-chromosome-derived material. Am J Med Genet A. 2005;135:150–4.
68. Matsumoto F, Shimada K, Ida S. Tumors of bilateral streak gonads in patients with disorders of sex development containing y chromosome material. Clin Pediatr Endocrinol. 2014;23:93–7.
69. Hatano T, Yoshino Y, Kawashima Y, Shirai H, Iizuka N, Miyazawa Y, Sakata A, Onishi T. Case of gonadoblastoma in a 9-year-old boy without physical abnormalities. Int J Urol. 1999;6:164–6.
70. Verp MS, Simpson JL. Abnormal sexual differentiation and neoplasia. Cancer Genet Cytogenet. 1987; 25:191–218.
71. Li Y, Tabatabai ZL, Lee TL, Hatakeyama S, Ohyama C, Chan WY, Looijenga LH, Lau YF. The Y-encoded TSPY protein: a significant marker potentially plays a role in the pathogenesis of testicular germ cell tumors. Hum Pathol. 2007;38:1470–81.
72. Hertel JD, Huettner PC, Dehner LP, Pfeifer JD. The chromosome Y-linked testis-specific protein locus TSPY1 is characteristically present in gonadoblastoma. Hum Pathol. 2010;41:1544–9.
73. Cools M, Stoop H, Kersemaekers AM, Drop SL, Wolffenbuttel KP, Bourguignon JP, Slowikowska-Hilczer J, Kula K, Faradz SM, Oosterhuis JW, Looijenga LH. Gonadoblastoma arising in undifferentiated gonadal tissue within dysgenetic gonads. J Clin Endocrinol Metab. 2006;91:2404–13.
74. Scully RE. Gonadoblastoma. A review of 74 cases. Cancer. 1970;25:1340–56.
75. Manuel M, Katayama PK, Jones Jr HW. The age of occurrence of gonadal tumors in intersex patients with a Y chromosome. Am J Obstet Gynecol. 1976;124:293–300.
76. Hersmus R, Stoop H, van de Geijn GJ, Eini R, Biermann K, Oosterhuis JW, Dhooge C, Schneider DT, Meijssen IC, Dinjens WN, Dubbink HJ, Drop SL, Looijenga LH. Prevalence of c-KIT mutations in

gonadoblastoma and dysgerminomas of patients with disorders of sex development (DSD) and ovarian dysgerminomas. PLoS One. 2012;7:e43952.
77. Buell-Gutbrod R, Ivanovic M, Montag A, Lengyel E, Fadare O, Gwin K. FOXL2 and SOX9 distinguish the lineage of the sex cord-stromal cells in gonadoblastomas. Pediatr Dev Pathol. 2011;14:391–5.
78. Looijenga LH. Testicular germ cell tumors. Pediatr Endocrinol Rev. 2014;11:251–62.
79. Kersemaekers AM, Honecker F, Stoop H, Cools M, Molier M, Wolffenbuttel K, Bokemeyer C, Li Y, Lau YF, Oosterhuis JW, Looijenga LH. Identification of germ cells at risk for neoplastic transformation in gonadoblastoma: an immunohistochemical study for OCT3/4 and TSPY. Hum Pathol. 2005;36:512–21.
80. Kao CS, Ulbright TM, Idrees MT. Gonadoblastoma: an immunohistochemical study and comparison to sertoli cell nodule with intratubular germ cell neoplasia, with pathogenetic implications. Histopathology. 2014;65:861–7.
81. Zhang C, Berney DM, Hirsch MS, Cheng L, Ulbright TM. Evidence supporting the existence of benign teratomas of the postpubertal testis: a clinical, histopathologic, and molecular genetic analysis of 25 cases. Am J Surg Pathol. 2013;37:827–35.
82. Oosterhuis JW, Stoop JA, Rijlaarsdam MA, Biermann K, Smit VT, Hersmus R, Looijenga LH. Pediatric germ cell tumors presenting beyond childhood? Andrology. 2015;3:70–7.
83. Skakkebaek NE. Possible carcinoma-in-situ of the testis. Lancet. 1972;2:516–7.
84. Rajpert-De Meyts E. Developmental model for the pathogenesis of testicular carcinoma in situ: genetic and environmental aspects. Hum Reprod Update. 2006;12:303–23.
85. Almstrup K, Hoei-Hansen CE, Wirkner U, Blake J, Schwager C, Ansorge W, Nielsen JE, Skakkebaek NE, Rajpert-De Meyts E, Leffers H. Embryonic stem cell-like features of testicular carcinoma in situ revealed by genome-wide gene expression profiling. Cancer Res. 2004;64:4736–43.
86. von der Maase H, Rørth M, Walbom-Jørgensen S, Sørensen BL, Christophersen IS, Hald T, Jacobsen GK, Berthelsen JG, Skakkebaek NE. Carcinoma in situ of contralateral testis in patients with testicular germ cell cancer: study of 27 cases in 500 patients. Br Med J (Clin Res Ed). 1986;293:1398–401.
87. Looijenga LH, Stoop H, de Leeuw HP, de Gouveia Brazao CA, Gillis AJ, van Roozendaal KE, van Zoelen EJ, Weber RF, Wolffenbuttel KP, van Dekken H, Honecker F, Bokemeyer C, Perlman EJ, Schneider DT, Kononen J, Sauter G, Oosterhuis JW. POU5F1 (OCT3/4) identifies cells with pluripotent potential in human germ cell tumors. Cancer Res. 2003;63:2244–50.
88. Jones TD, Ulbright TM, Eble JN, Cheng L. OCT4: a sensitive and specific biomarker for intratubular germ cell neoplasia of the testis. Clin Cancer Res. 2004;10:8544–7.
89. Hustin J, Collette J, Franchimont P. Immunohistochemical demonstration of placental alkaline phosphatase in various states of testicular development and in germ cell tumours. Int J Androl. 1987;10:29–35.
90. Hoei-Hansen CE, Nielsen JE, Almstrup K, Sonne SB, Graem N, Skakkebaek NE, Leffers H, Rajpert-De Meyts E. Transcription factor AP-2gamma is a developmentally regulated marker of testicular carcinoma in situ and germ cell tumors. Clin Cancer Res. 2004;10:8521–30.
91. Yu H, Pinkus GS, Hornick JL. Diffuse membranous immunoreactivity for podoplanin (D2-40) distinguishes primary and metastatic seminomas from other germ cell tumors and metastatic neoplasms. Am J Clin Pathol. 2007;128:767–75.
92. Idrees M, Saxena R, Cheng L, Ulbright TM, Badve S. Podoplanin, a novel marker for seminoma: a comparison study evaluating immunohistochemical expression of podoplanin and OCT3/4. Ann Diagn Pathol. 2010;14:331–6.
93. Biermann K, Stoop H, Looijenga L. c-KIT protein expression does not discriminate neoplastic from non-neoplastic intratubular germ cells. Histopathology. 2012;60:1017–9.
94. Niemi M, Ikonen M. Primordial germ cells in foetal and postnatal human testis. Ann Med Exp Biol Fenn. 1965;43:23–8.
95. Gondos B, Hobel CJ. Ultrastructure of germ cell development in the human fetal testis. Z Zellforsch Mikrosk Anat. 1971;119:1–20.
96. Rajpert-De Meyts E, Bartkova J, Samson M, Hoei-Hansen CE, Frydelund-Larsen L, Bartek J, Skakkebaek NE. The emerging phenotype of the testicular carcinoma in situ germ cell. APMIS. 2003; 111:267–78.
97. Gaskell TL, Esnal A, Robinson LL, Anderson RA, Saunders PT. Immunohistochemical profiling of germ cells within the human fetal testis: identification of three subpopulations. Biol Reprod. 2004;71: 2012–21.
98. Culty M. Gonocytes, the forgotten cells of the germ cell lineage. Birth Defects Res C Embryo Today. 2009;87:1–26.
99. Honecker F, Stoop H, de Krijger RR, Chris Lau YF, Bokemeyer C, Looijenga LH. Pathobiological implications of the expression of markers of testicular carcinoma in situ by fetal germ cells. J Pathol. 2004;203:849–57.
100. Chemes H, Muzulin PM, Venara MC, Mulhmann Mdel C, Martínez M, Gamboni M. Early manifestations of testicular dysgenesis in children: pathological phenotypes, karyotype correlations and precursor stages of tumour development. APMIS. 2003;111: 12–23.
101. Oosterhuis JW, Stoop H, Dohle G, Boellaard W, van Casteren N, Wolffenbuttel K, Looijenga LH. A pathologist's view on the testis biopsy. Int J Androl. 2011;34:e14–9.

102. Stoop H, Honecker F, van de Geijn GJ, Gillis AJ, Cools MC, de Boer M, Bokemeyer C, Wolffenbuttel KP, Drop SL, de Krijger RR, Dennis N, Summersgill B, McIntyre A, Shipley J, Oosterhuis JW, Looijenga LH. Stem cell factor as a novel diagnostic marker for early malignant germ cells. J Pathol. 2008;216:43–54.
103. Müller J, Skakkebaek NE, Nielsen OH, Graem N. Cryptorchidism and testis cancer. Atypical infantile germ cells followed by carcinoma in situ and invasive carcinoma in adulthood. Cancer. 1984;54:629–34.
104. Słowikowska-Hilczer J. Nuclear DNA, content and proliferative potential of human carcinoma in situ cells in testes of intersex children. Folia Histochem Cytobiol. 2001;39:167–8.
105. Rajpert-De Meyts E, Jørgensen N, Brøndum-Nielsen K, Müller J, Skakkebaek NE. Developmental arrest of germ cells in the pathogenesis of germ cell neoplasia. APMIS. 1998;106:198–204.
106. Looijenga LH. Human testicular (non)seminomatous germ cell tumours: the clinical implications of recent pathobiological insights. J Pathol. 2009;218:146–62.
107. Müller J. Abnormal infantile germ cells and development of carcinoma-in-situ in maldeveloped testes: a stereological and densitometric study. Int J Androl. 1987;10:543–67.
108. Cools M, van Aerde K, Kersemaekers AM, Boter M, Drop SL, Wolffenbuttel KP, Steyerberg EW, Oosterhuis JW, Looijenga LH. Morphological and immunohistochemical differences between gonadal maturation delay and early germ cell neoplasia in patients with undervirilization syndromes. J Clin Endocrinol Metab. 2005;90:5295–303.
109. Cools M, Honecker F, Stoop H, Veltman JD, de Krijger RR, Steyerberg E, Wolffenbuttel KP, Bokemeyer C, Lau YF, Drop SL, Looijenga LH. Maturation delay of germ cells in fetuses with trisomy 21 results in increased risk for the development of testicular germ cell tumors. Hum Pathol. 2006;37:101–11.
110. Codesal J, Nistal M, Queizan A, Carretero JL, de Vega RM, Perez A, Paniagua R. Number and DNA content of hypertrophic spermatogonia in normal and cryptorchid human testes. Arch Androl. 1992; 29:157–62.
111. Jørgensen N, Müller J, Giwercman A, Visfeldt J, Møller H, Skakkebaek NE. DNA content and expression of tumour markers in germ cells adjacent to germ cell tumours in childhood: probably a different origin for infantile and adolescent germ cell tumours. J Pathol. 1995;176:269–78.
112. Cortes D, Thorup J, Visfeldt J. Multinucleated spermatogonia in cryptorchid boys: a possible association with an increased risk of testicular malignancy later in life? APMIS. 2003;111:25–30.

The Stem Cell Origin and Pathogenetic Routes of Testicular Germ Cell Tumors

5

Maurizio Colecchia, Alessia Bertolotti, Biagio Paolini, and Gregor Mikuz

Introduction

Different pathogenetic theories have been put forward about the origin of germ cell tumors (GCTs): some of the evidence is strongly supported by widespread consensus among experts, while the oncogenic pathways are still questioned [1]. Most GCTs of the testis evolve from a common neoplastic precursor: germ cell neoplasia in situ (also called carcinoma in situ [CIS], intratubular germ cell neoplasia, and testicular intratubular neoplasia; see Chap. 6). Many experts believe CIS to be at the origin of two different pathways: one leading to seminoma as the end-stage tumor and the other leading to embryonal carcinoma (EC) [2], which is considered a step in the differentiation into yolk sac tumor (YST), teratoma, or choriocarcinoma. The current hypothesis is that CIS cells are the neoplastic counterparts of primordial germ cells or gonocytes [3], with malignant transformation being induced by blocked maturation of the gonocyte in utero, which causes testicular maldevelopment ("dysgenesis") [4, 5]. An alternative hypothesis is that seminomas may evolve into other types of GCT. In 1946 Friedman and Moore [6] reported the existence of seminomas that evolved into ECs; recently, the immunophenotypic switch of tumor cells from seminoma to nonseminomatous features ("reprogramming") with activation of pluripotency was demonstrated [4]. Autopsy findings are consistent with this theory: the presence of nonseminomatous metastases in men with a history of seminoma [7] and the occurrence of retroperitoneal metastases with different histology from the testicular primary are additional evidence supporting it.

Childhood GCTs (YST, teratoma) are believed to arise from primordial germ cells or gonocytes [4]. The most frequent chromosomal aberrations in type I YST are loss of 1p, 4 and 6q and gain of 1q, 12(p13) and 20q, whereas the majority of type I teratomas have a normal chromosomal complement. All cells of intratubular neoplasia are positive for nuclear expression of OCT3/4, like seminomas and ECs, while in the more differentiated tumors (YST, teratoma, choriocarcinoma), OCT3/4 is downregulated [8]. Of the other GCTs, only gonadoblastoma shows OCT3/4-positive cell nuclei, and alteration of the testis-specific protein on

M. Colecchia (✉)
Uropathology Unit, Department of Pathology, Fondazione IRCCS Istituto Nazionale dei Tumori di Milano, Milan, Italy
e-mail: maurizio.colecchia@istitutotumori.mi.it

A. Bertolotti • B. Paolini
Department of Pathology, Fondazione IRCCS Istituto Nazionale dei Tumori di Milano, Milan, Italy
e-mail: alessia.bertolotti@istitutotumori.mi.it; biagio.paolini@istitutotumori.mi.it

G. Mikuz
Institute of Pathology, Medical University of Innsbruck, Innsbruck, Austria
e-mail: Gregor.Mikuz@i-med.ac.at

M. Colecchia (ed.), *Pathology of Testicular and Penile Neoplasms*,
DOI 10.1007/978-3-319-27617-5_5

Y chromosome (*TSPY*) gene seems to play an important role in the development of this cancer [9]. OCT3/4 (also known as POU5F1) is a transcription factor that has a key function in the maintenance of pluripotency in embryonic stem cells and primordial germ cells, resulting in the capacity of giving rise to most somatic and extraembryonic lineages [8]. An open question is whether OCT3/4 expression is a driving force in the pathogenesis of GCT or merely the marker of the origin of this cancer [4, 8, 10]. Many studies have found OCT3/4 to be an extremely useful tool in the diagnosis of testicular CIS, especially in small biopsy specimens from patients with previous contralateral GCT, a history of cryptorchidism, or gonadal dysgenesis [10–12]. Caution must be exercised in the evaluation of OCT3/4 expression in biopsies performed in the first year of life because of the presence of residual OCT3/4-positive germ cells unrelated to malignant transformation [12, 13]. *TSPY* is a multicopy gene expressed in spermatogonia, CIS, and gonadoblastoma [14, 15]. It regulates cell progression by interacting with cyclin B1. Loss of *TSPY* can be observed in CIS cells adjacent to an invasive component [16], but actual proof that *TSPY* is related to the pathogenesis of GCC is still lacking [9, 16].

Genes that are upregulated in CIS compared with normal testis are markers of primordial germ cell/gonocyte and/or stem cell phenotypes and include *OCT3/4*, *NANOG*, *XBP1*, *XIST*, *LIN28*, *SOX17*, and *KIT*, among others [17, 18].

C-kit (CD117), a tyrosine kinase receptor, is downregulated during normal germ cell development and overexpressed in a large percentage of CIS and seminomas, but not in other GCTs. Despite the overexpression of this antigen, care must be taken when interpreting c-kit in CIS, since it is known that low-intensity c-kit expression is present in spermatogonia and normal human germ cells [19]. Analysis of c-kit expression in seminoma and CIS revealed significantly downregulated expression in seminomas with respect to CIS, suggesting a role in the initiation of oncogenesis of GCTs, but not in the progression from precursor lesion to seminoma [20]. Different conclusions were drawn by McIntyre et al. [21], who claimed that *KIT* amplification and overexpression were associated with progression in seminoma. There is more consensus about frequent *c-KIT* mutations that seem predictive of bilateral seminomas [20, 22]. It appears that in invasive tumors, genes associated with "stemness" are expressed by both seminoma and EC and include *OCT3/4*, *NANOG*, and *GDF3* [23]. For other genes such as *SOX2*, *TDGF1*, and *FGF4*, expression is limited to EC [18, 24]. SOX17 is found to be present instead of SOX2 in early germ cells and their malignant counterparts, CIS and seminoma [24]. The differential expression of SOX17 and SOX2 could be useful in routine diagnostics, but the lack of standardization of laboratory protocols is a hindrance to their use in everyday practice [25].

Progression from Precursor Lesion to Invasiveness: Role of Chromosome 12

No consistent gain of chromosome 12 has been detected in CIS, while the consistent gain of 12p was first described in GCT by Atkin and Baker [26]. More than 80 % of testicular GCTs have one or more copies of isochromosome 12p (i[12p]), and less than 20 % without i(12p) show a high level of amplification. The abnormal chromosome comprises 2 fused short arms of chromosome 12 and occurs irrespective of the histologic subtype of GCT [27].

The remaining i(12p)-negative GCTs have also been shown to contain gain of chromosome 12p sequences as tandem duplications located in situ or transposed elsewhere in the genome [26]. In a small proportion of GCTs, amplification of subregions of chromosome 12p (12p11.2-p12.1 and 12p12~13) has been identified [28]. The amplification was initially observed in metastatic seminoma and is frequently found in i(12p)-negative GCTs [5]. Mostert et al. [29] observed the shortest region of overlap of amplification, where some genes including *KRAS2*, *JAW1*, and *SOX5* are located. The consistent gain of chromosome 12p sequences in all testicular GCTs suggests that gain of one or more genes on 12p is important in the development of GCTs. The genes associated with gain of chromosome 12p sequences are *CCND2*, *KRAS*, *DAD-R*, *β-CAT*, *E-KIT*, *NANOG*, *STELLA*, and *GDF3*, but the exact nature of the development of invasiveness is still unclear [30–34].

All the results suggest a role of the gain of 12p sequences in the progression to invasiveness of GCTs. Many studies have investigated the potential role of i(12p) in the diagnosis of testicular CGTs by establishing its presence using interphase fluorescent in situ hybridization (FISH) on paraffin-embedded tissues [35]. Generally a library probe covering 12p is used in combination with a chromosome 12 centromeric probe in a 2-color probe [35, 36]; this is an important tool to demonstrate the germ cell nature of somatic malignancies arising in metastatic teratomas as well [37, 38].

The Pathogenesis of Spermatocytic Tumor

In the 2016 WHO classification, the previously used term *spermatocytic seminoma* changes to *spermatocytic tumor* (ST), to underline that this tumor is not a variant of seminoma and has a good prognosis (see Chap. 6). It has been widely agreed that ST differs from other types of GCTs; however, the identity of the progenitor cells remains controversial. Looijenga et al. have suggested that ST derives from an adult germ cell lineage that lacks any residual embryonic traits, postulating primary spermatocytes as tumorigenic precursors [39]. The pathogenesis is unclear, and it was suggested that amplification of the DMRT1 locus on chromosome 9 could be involved [39], and gain of chromosome 9 has been reported as the only consistent chromosomal anomaly [39, 40]. The origin from a distinctive subpopulation of spermatogonia was described by Lim et al. [41], who analyzed the expression pattern of the spermatogonial markers OCT2, SSX, and SAGE1 in subpopulations of spermatogonia including dark spermatogonia, considered to be the reserve stem cell populations; pale spermatogonia; and mature B spermatogonia, which give rise to primary spermatocytes that enter meiosis and lead to the formation of spermatids. According to the authors, the different expression in 36 tested STs supports the origin from spermatogonia and provides evidence for the heterogeneity of this tumor [41]. All studies have confirmed by genomic profiling, cytogenetics, and immunohistochemistry [42] that ST is distinct from classical seminoma and from the other nonseminomatous GCTs and is the only postpubertal neoplasm of the testis lacking i(12p) overexpression [43].

Other Genetic Alterations

CIS, seminoma, and all variants of nonseminomatous GCT show marked aneuploidy [44] as well as specific chromosome gains and losses. High-level amplification of 12p has been observed in particular in seminomas and in other GCTs as well, but with lower expression levels, while gain of proximal 17q and loss of 10q have been detected in nonseminomas [45].

Compared with chromosomal abnormalities, specific gene mutations are more difficult to assess because studies of clinical and molecular genetic features of GCT histology are often limited by the fact that 60 % of GCTs are mixed tumors with 2 or more histologic components. In a gene expression profiling study of 84 nonseminomatous GCTs, Korkola et al. [46] investigated transcripts predictive of EC histology that included stem-cell-specific genes such as *OCT3/4*, *DPPA4*, and *NANOG*, while downregulation of these genes was associated with differentiation into different lineages belonging to YST, choriocarcinoma, and teratoma subtypes. Another cluster of genes (*CENPA*, *CDCA1*, *CCNB1*, *CDC20*, and *MCM5*) was found to be downregulated in teratomas, while *hCG*, *CGA*, *CGB*, and *PLAC6*, genes that are associated with placenta and trophoblasts, were restricted to choriocarcinoma. A number of genes implicated

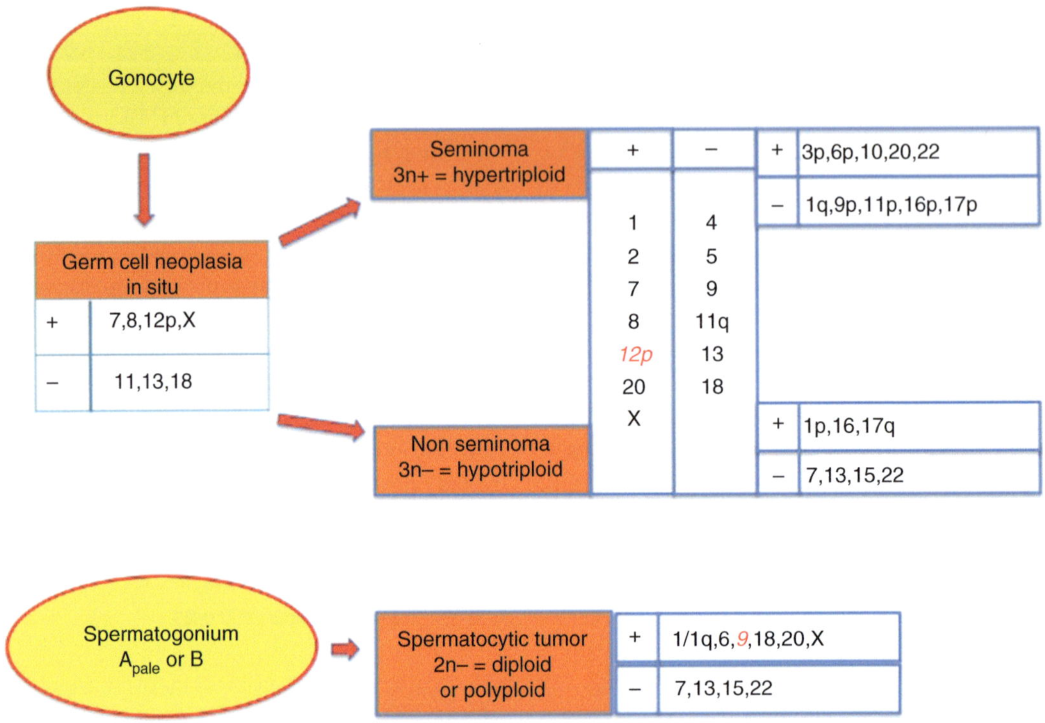

Fig. 5.1 Synopsis of chromosomal changes in the germ cell tumors of the testis (+ gain, – loss). In the vertical columns gains and losses common both to seminoma and nonseminoma, in the horizontal one specific aberrations for the respective tumor. The gain of 12p (*red*) is observed in seminoma and nonseminoma, but not in spermatocytic tumor. The gain of chromosome 9 (*red*) is specific for spermatocytic tumor

in differentiation into endodermal (*AFP*, *VTN*, *OTX1*, *OTX2*, *BMP2*, *FOX A2*, *PAX6*) or mesodermal (*EOMES*) lineages are most predictive of YST histology. The most frequent single genes involved in GCTs but with low mutation percentages (ranging from 1 to 8 %) are *KIT*, *KRAS*, *NRAS*, and *BRAF* [47].

Using targeted next-generation sequencing in 32 testicular GCTs, approximately 60 different gene mutations were recently detected in both pure and mixed GCTs, the majority of which were associated with signal transduction genes. Besides the gene mutations already described (*KIT*, *KRAS*, etc.), mutations were frequently seen in oncogenes, transcription factors, and genes associated with tyrosine kinase receptors, such as *CREBBP*, *FGFR*, *FLT1/3*, *JAK3*, *NFKB*, and *PDGFR* [48]. A synopsis of chromosomal changes in the germ cell tumors of the testis is reported in Fig. 5.1 [49, 50].

References

1. Ulbright TM, Young RH. Tumours of the testis and adjacent structures. Fourth Series fascicle 18. Silver Spring: American Registry of Pathology; 2013.
2. Pierce GB, Abell MR. Embryonal carcinoma of the testis. Pathol Annu. 1970;5:27–60.
3. Sonne SB, Almstrup K, Dalgaard M, Juncker AS, Edsgard D, Ruban L, Harrison NJ, Schwage C, Abdollahi A, Huber PE, Brunak S, Gjerdrum LM, Moore HD, Andrews PW, Skakkebaek NE, Rajpert-De Meyts E, Leffers H. Analysis of gene expression profiles of microdissected cell populations indicates that testicular carcinoma in situ is an arrested gonocyte. Cancer Res. 2009;69:5241–50.
4. Oosterhuis JW, Looijenga LH. Testicular germ-cell tumours in a broader perspective. Nat Rev Cancer. 2005;5:210–22.
5. Looijenga LH, Zafarana G, Grygalewicz B, Summersgill B, Debiec-Rychter M, Veltman J, Schoenmakers EF, Rodriguez S, Jafer O, Clark J, van Kessel AG, Shipley J, van Gurp RJ, Gillis AJ, Oosterhuis JW. Role of gain of 12p in germ cell tumour development. APMIS. 2003;111:161–73.

6. Friedman NB, Moore RA. Tumors of the testis; a report on 922 cases. Mil Surg. 1946;99:573–93.
7. Bredael JJ, Vugrin D, Whitmore Jr WF. Autopsy findings in 154 patients with germ cell tumors of the testis. Cancer. 1982;50:548–51.
8. Looijenga LH, Stoop H, de Leeuw HP, de Gouveia Brazao CA, Gillis AJ, van Roozendaal KE, van Zoelen EJ, Weber RF, Wolffenbuttel KP, van Dekken H, Honecker F, Bokemeyer C, Perlman EJ, Schneider DT, Kononen J, Sauter G, Oosterhuis JW. POU5F1 (OCT3/4) identifies cells with pluripotent potential in human germ cell tumors. Cancer Res. 2003;63:2244–50.
9. Li Y, Tabatabai ZL, Lee TL, Hatakeyama S, Ohyama C, Chan WY, Looijenga LH, Lau YF. The Y-encoded TSPY protein: a significant marker potentially plays a role in the pathogenesis of testicular germ cell tumors. Hum Pathol. 2007;38:1470–81.
10. Cheng L, Sung MT, Cossu-Rocca P, Jones TD, MacLennan GT, De Jong J, Lopez-Beltran A, Montironi R, Looijenga LH. OCT4: biological functions and clinical applications as a marker of germ cell neoplasia. J Pathol. 2007;211:1–9.
11. Jones TD, Ulbright TM, Eble JN, Cheng L. OCT4: a sensitive and specific biomarker for intratubular germ cell neoplasia of the testis. Clin Cancer Res. 2004;10:8544–7.
12. Jones TD, MacLennan GT, Bonnin JM, Varsegi MF, Blair JE, Cheng L. Screening for intratubular germ cell neoplasia of the testis using OCT4 immunohistochemistry. Am J Surg Pathol. 2006;30:1427–31.
13. de Jong J, Stoop H, Dohle GR, Bangma CH, Kliffen M, van Esser JW, van den Bent M, Kros JM, Oosterhuis JW, Looijenga LH. Diagnostic value of OCT3/4 for pre-invasive and invasive testicular germ cell tumours. J Pathol. 2005;206:242–9.
14. Hildenbrand R, Schröder W, Brude E, Schepler A, König R, Stutte HJ, Arnemann J. Detection of TSPY protein in a unilateral microscopic gonadoblastoma of a Turner mosaic patient with a Y-derived marker chromosome. J Pathol. 1999;189:623–6.
15. Kersemaekers AM, Honecker F, Stoop H, Cools M, Molier M, Wolffenbuttel K, Bokemeyer C, Li Y, Lau YF, Oosterhuis JW, Looijenga LH. Identification of germ cells at risk for neoplastic transformation in gonadoblastoma: an immunohistochemical study for OCT3/4 and TSPY. Hum Pathol. 2005;36:512–21.
16. Looijenga LH, Stoop H, Biermann K. Testicular cancer: biology and biomarkers. Virchows Arch. 2014;464:301–13.
17. Almstrup K, Hoei-Hansen CE, Wirkner U, Blake J, Schwager C, Ansorge W, Nielsen JE, Skakkebaek NE, Rajpert-De Meyts E, Leffers H. Embryonic stem cell-like features of testicular carcinoma in situ revealed by genome-wide gene expression profiling. Cancer Res. 2004;64:4736–43.
18. Houldsworth J, Korkola JE, Bosl GJ, Chaganti RS. Biology and genetics of adult male germ cell tumors. J Clin Oncol. 2006;24:5512–8.
19. Biermann K, Stoop H, Looijenga L. c-KIT protein expression does not discriminate neoplastic from non-neoplastic intratubular germ cells. Histopathology. 2012;60:1017–9.
20. Biermann K, Göke F, Nettersheim D, Eckert D, Zhou H, Kahl P, Gashaw I, Schorle H, Büttner R. c-KIT is frequently mutated in bilateral germ cell tumours and down-regulated during progression from intratubular germ cell neoplasia to seminoma. J Pathol. 2007;213:311–8.
21. McIntyre A, Summersgill B, Grygalewicz B, Gillis AJ, Stoop J, van Gurp RJ, Dennis N, Fisher C, Huddart R, Cooper C, Clark J, Oosterhuis JW, Looijenga LH, Shipley J. Amplification and overexpression of the KIT gene is associated with progression in the seminoma subtype of testicular germ cell tumors of adolescents and adults. Cancer Res. 2005;65:8085–9.
22. Looijenga LH, de Leeuw H, van Oorschot M, van Gurp RJ, Stoop H, Gillis AJ, de Gouveia Brazao CA, Weber RF, Kirkels WJ, van Dijk T, von Lindern M, Valk P, Lajos G, Olah E, Nesland JM, Fosså SD, Oosterhuis JW. Stem cell factor receptor (c-KIT) codon 816 mutations predict development of bilateral testicular germ-cell tumors. Cancer Res. 2003;63:7674–8.
23. Port M, Schmelz HU, Stockinger M, Sparwasser C, Albers P, Pottek T, Abend M. Gene expression profiling in seminoma and nonseminoma. J Clin Oncol. 2005;23:58–69.
24. de Jong J, Stoop H, Gillis AJ, van Gurp RJ, van de Geijn GJ, Boer M, Hersmus R, Saunders PT, Anderson RA, Oosterhuis JW, Looijenga LH. Differential expression of SOX17 and SOX2 in germ cells and stem cells has biological and clinical implications. J Pathol. 2008;215:21–30.
25. Ulbright TM, Tickoo SK, Berney DM, Members of the ISUP Immunohistochemistry in Diagnostic Urologic Pathology Group, Srigley JR. Best practices recommendations in the application of immunohistochemistry in testicular tumors: report from the International Society of Urological Pathology consensus conference. Am J Surg Pathol. 2014;38:e50–9.
26. Atkin NB, Baker MC. Specific chromosome change, i(12p), in testicular tumours? Lancet. 1982;2:1349.
27. Rodriguez E, Houldsworth J, Reuter VE, Meltzer P, Zhang J, Trent JM, Bosl GJ, Chaganti RS. Molecular cytogenetic analysis of i(12p)-negative human male germ cell tumors. Genes Chromosomes Cancer. 1993;8:230–6.
28. Roelofs H, Mostert MC, Pompe K, Zafarana G, van Oorschot M, van Gurp RJ, Gillis AJ, Stoop H, Beverloo B, Oosterhuis JW, Bokemeyer C, Looijenga LH. Restricted 12p amplification and RAS mutation in human germ cell tumors of the adult testis. Am J Pathol. 2000;157:1155–66.
29. Mostert MC, Verkerk AJ, van de Pol M, Heighway J, Marynen P, Rosenberg C, van Kessel AG, van Echten J, de Jong B, Oosterhuis JW, Looijenga LH. Identification of the critical region of 12p over-representation in testicular germ cell tumors of adolescents and adults. Oncogene. 1998;16:2617–27.
30. Rodriguez S, Jafer O, Goker H, Summersgill BM, Zafarana G, Gillis AJ, van Gurp RJ, Oosterhuis JW,

Lu YJ, Huddart R, Cooper CS, Clark J, Looijenga LH, Shipley JM. Expression profile of genes from 12p in testicular germ cell tumors of adolescents and adults associated with i(12p) and amplification at 12p11. 2-p12.1. Oncogene. 2003;22:1880–91.

31. Bourdon V, Naef F, Rao PH, Reuter V, Mok SC, Bosl GJ, Koul S, Murty VV, Kucherlapati RS, Chaganti RS. Genomic and expression analysis of the 12p11-p12 amplicon using EST arrays identifies two novel amplified and overexpressed genes. Cancer Res. 2002;62:6218–23.
32. Korkola JE, Houldsworth J, Chadalavada RS, Olshen AB, Dobrzynski D, Reuter VE, Bosl GJ, Chaganti RS. Down-regulation of stem cell genes, including those in a 200-kb gene cluster at 12p13.31, is associated with in vivo differentiation of human male germ cell tumors. Cancer Res. 2006;66:820–7.
33. Vos A, Oosterhuis JW, de Jong B, Buist J, Schraffordt Koops H. Cytogenetics of carcinoma in situ of the testis. Cancer Genet Cytogenet. 1990;46:75–81.
34. Hussain SA, Ma YT, Palmer DH, Hutton P, Cullen MH. Biology of testicular germ cell tumors. Expert Rev Anticancer Ther. 2008;8:1659–73.
35. Kernek KM, Brunelli M, Ulbright TM, Eble JN, Martignoni G, Zhang S, Michael H, Cummings OW, Cheng L. Fluorescence in situ hybridization analysis of chromosome 12p in paraffin-embedded tissue is useful for establishing germ cell origin of metastatic tumors. Mod Pathol. 2004;17:1309–13.
36. Kum JB, Ulbright TM, Williamson SR, Wang M, Zhang S, Foster RS, Grignon DJ, Eble JN, Beck SD, Cheng L. Molecular genetic evidence supporting the origin of somatic-type malignancy and teratoma from the same progenitor cell. Am J Pathol. 2012;36:1849–56.
37. Mikuz G, Colecchia M. Teratoma with somatic-type malignant components of the testis. A review and an update. Virchows Arch. 2012;461:27–32.
38. Motzer RJ, Amsterdam A, Prieto V, Sheinfeld J, Murty VV, Mazumdar M, Bosl GJ, Chaganti RS, Reuter VE. Teratoma with malignant transformation: diverse malignant histologies arising in men with germ cell tumors. J Urol. 1998;159:133–8.
39. Looijenga LH, Hersmus R, Gillis AJ, Pfundt R, Stoop HJ, van Gurp RJ, Veltman J, Beverloo HB, van Drunen E, van Kessel AG, Pera RR, Schneider DT, Summersgill B, Shipley J, McIntyre A, van der Spek P, Schoenmakers E, Oosterhuis JW. Genomic and expression profiling of human spermatocytic seminomas: primary spermatocyte as tumorigenic precursor and DMRT1 as candidate chromosome 9 gene. Cancer Res. 2006;66:290–302.
40. Verdorfer I, Rogatsch H, Tzankov A, Steiner H, Mikuz G. Molecular cytogenetic analysis of human spermatocytic seminomas. J Pathol. 2004;204:277–81.
41. Lim J, Goriely A, Turner GD, Ewen KA, Jacobsen GK, Graem N, Wilkie AO, Rajpert-De Meyts E. OCT2, SSX and SAGE1 reveal the phenotypic heterogeneity of spermatocytic seminoma reflecting distinct subpopulations of spermatogonia. J Pathol. 2011;224:473–83.
42. Kao CS, Badve SS, Ulbright TM. The utility of immunostaining for NUT, GAGE7 and NY-ESO-1 in the diagnosis of spermatocytic seminoma. Histopathology. 2014;65:35–44.
43. Looijenga LH, Stoop H, Hersmus R, Gillis AJ, Wolter Oosterhuis J. Genomic and expression profiling of human spermatocytic seminomas: pathogenetic implications. Int J Androl. 2007;30:328–36.
44. Mayer F, Stoop H, Sen S, Bokemeyer C, Oosterhuis JW, Looijenga LH. Aneuploidy of human testicular germ cell tumors is associated with amplification of centrosomes. Oncogene. 2003;22:3859–66.
45. Mohamed GH, Gelfond JA, Nicolas MM, Brand TC, Sarvis JA, Leach RJ, Johnson-Pais TL. Genomic characterization of testis cancer: association of alterations with outcome of clinical stage 1 mixed germ cell nonseminomatous germ cell tumor of the testis. Urology. 2012;80:485.e1–5.
46. Korkola JE, Houldsworth J, Dobrzynski D, Olshen AB, Reuter VE, Bosl GJ, Chaganti RS. Gene expression-based classification of nonseminomatous male germ cell tumors. Oncogene. 2005;24:5101–7.
47. Sheikine Y, Genega E, Melamed J, Lee P, Reuter VE, Ye H. Molecular genetics of testicular germ cell tumors. Am J Cancer Res. 2012;2:153–67.
48. Coulson H, Loda M, O'Donnell E, Sweeney C, Hirsch M. Targeted next generation sequencing of testicular germ cell tumors. Mod Pathol. 2015;28 Suppl 2:213A.
49. Verdorfer I. Genetic of testicular germ cell tumors. Pathologe. 2014;35:218–23.
50. Mikuz G. Update on the pathology of testicular tumors. Anal Quant Cytopathol Histopathol. 2015;37:75–85.

6 Tumors of the Testis

Gregor Mikuz and Maurizio Colecchia

Introduction

The clinical term "testicular tumor" is an umbrella term for all intrascrotal masses regardless of their actual anatomic location. In fact, some 90 % of tumors in the scrotum arise in the testis [1], and at least 90 % of them belong to the group of germ cell tumors (GCTs), the incidence of which is continuously increasing in western industrialized countries, especially in central and northern Europe. Although rare, GCTs have been of great interest to the pathologist because of their peculiar biology and morphology and also to the clinician, as they used to be deadly tumors, but nowadays can be cured in more than 90 % of cases. It took a long time before a comprehensive, histogenetically based classification was available, the classification proposed by Mostofi and Sobin in 1977 [2]. The discovery of a precursor lesion [3], originally called "carcinoma in situ of the testis", supported the theoretical background of this classification.

G. Mikuz
Institute of Pathology, Medical University of Innsbruck, Innsbruck, Austria
e-mail: Gregor.Mikuz@i-med.ac.at

M. Colecchia (✉)
Uropathology Unit, Department of Pathology, Fondazione IRCCS Istituto Nazionale dei Tumori di Milano, Milan, Italy
e-mail: maurizio.colecchia@istitutotumori.mi.it

Classification

According to the WHO classification of 2004 [4], testicular tumors are grouped into tumors of germ cell origin and those arising from specialized testicular stroma (sex cord/stromal tumors) and tumors containing both germ cell and sex cord/gonadal stromal elements. Furthermore, the classification includes tumors of the collecting ducts, paratesticular tumors (epididymis and tunics), miscellaneous neoplasms mostly of unclear origin, tumors of nonspecialized stroma (soft tissue tumors), metastases, and hematopoietic tumors, which are rather frequent in older men. In the revised WHO classification of 2016 [5], the names of the precursor lesion and of spermatocytic seminoma were changed, while yolk sac tumor (YST) and teratoma were divided into a prepubertal and postpubertal type because of the different histogenesis and prognosis of these tumors in childhood.

Germ Cell Tumors

As already mentioned, GCTs account for 90 % of all intratesticular tumors. The 2004 WHO classification [4] (modified in Table 6.1) distinguish between GCTs of one histologic type (pure forms) and those with a mixture of two or more different histologic patterns (mixed forms) (Table 6.1). Almost half (40–50 %) of all GCTs

M. Colecchia (ed.), *Pathology of Testicular and Penile Neoplasms*,
DOI 10.1007/978-3-319-27617-5_6

Table 6.1 Classification of testicular tumors (only tumors arising in the testis are listed) (modified from [4])

Germ cell tumors
Germ cell neoplasia in situ
Tumors of one histologic type (pure forms)
Seminoma
Seminoma with syncytiotrophoblastic cells
Spermatocytic tumor
Spermatocytic tumor with sarcoma*
Embryonal carcinoma
Yolk sac tumor
Prepubertal
Postpubertal
Trophoblastic tumors
Choriocarcinoma
Non-choriocarcinomatous trophoblastic tumors
Epithelioid trophoblastic tumor
Placental site trophoblastic tumor
Cystic trophoblastic tumor
Teratoma
Prepubertal
Postpubertal
Dermoid cyst
Well-differentiated neuroendocrine tumour (monodermal teratoma)
Teratoma with somatic-type malignancies
Germ cell tumors of unknown type
Regressed germ cell tumors
Tumors of more than one histologic type (mixed forms)
Mixed embryonal carcinoma and teratoma*
Mixed teratoma and seminoma*
Choriocarcinoma and teratoma/embryonal carcinoma*
Mixed teratoma and yolk-sac tumor, pre-pubertal-type
Sex cord/gonadal stromal tumors
Pure forms
Leydig cell tumor
Malignant Leydig cell tumor
Sertoli cell tumor
Intratubular large cell hyalizing Sertoli cell neoplasia
Large-cell calcifying Sertoli cell tumor
Malignant Sertoli cell tumor
Granulosa cell tumor
Adult-type granulosa cell tumor
Juvenile-type granulosa cell tumor
Tumors of the thecoma/fibroma group
Unclassified sex cord-stromal tumor
Sex cord/gonadal stromal tumor, mixed forms
Malignant sex cord/gonadal stromal tumor
Myoid gonadal stromal tumor*
Tumors containing both germ cell and sex cord/ gonadal stromal element
Gonadoblastoma
Germ cell-sex cord/gonadal stromal tumor, unclassified
Miscellaneous
Wilms' tumor
Hematopoietic tumors
Metastases

*Not included in the WHO 2016 classification as a distinct tumor

are pure seminomas; a third are mixed forms of nonseminomatous germ cell tumors (NSGCTs) including combinations with seminomas; and only 14–16 % are pure NSGCTs [6–9].

Germ Cell Neoplasia in Situ

In 1972 Skakkebaek [3] described the forerunner of all GCTs in biopsies of infertile men and called it "carcinoma in situ." The name was subsequently changed to "intratubular germ cell neoplasia, unclassified" (IGCNU) [4]. The adjective *unclassified* was used to emphasize that the morphology of the tumor cells does not permit the assignment to a definite type of GCT. In analogy to other intraepithelial neoplasia types, in German-speaking countries, the term "testicular intratubular neoplasia" (TIN) is still the most used. The new WHO classification of 2016 returns more or less to Skakkebaek's original phrasing and names the lesion "germ cell neoplasia in situ" (GCNIS). In this chapter, we adopt the term CIS to remember the first proposed terminology [3].

Epidemiology

The prevalence of these lesions can be roughly estimated to account for 0.4–0.8 % of healthy men and approximately 1 % of the infertile male population [10]. The frequency in cryptorchid testes of adults is 2–4 %, while in those of children, it is significantly lower (0.5 %). However, the identification of atypical germ cells in prepubertal testis is rather difficult because these cells are morphologically and immunophenotypically very similar to prepubertal gonocytes [11]. Maturation delay of germ cells and their progression to CIS frequently occurs in intersex patients (about 10 %). A developmentally delayed germ cell resembles a CIS cell and displays prolonged expression of immunohistochemical markers used for the diagnosis of CIS [11].

In patients with unilateral GCTs in situ, neoplasia is encountered in 4–6 % of contralateral testes [12], while in tissue surrounding GCT, it appears in more than 90 % of cases [13]. In retroperitoneal "extragonadal" GCTs, atypical germ cells can be found in the testes of about half of all cases, whereas in mediastinal GCTs, the testes only rarely show such cells [14] (Table 6.2).

Table 6.2 Prevalence of germ cell neoplasia in situ

Prevalence of germ cell neoplasia in situ	
Healthy men	0.4–0.8 %
Infertile men	1.0 %
Cryptorchid testis of adults	2–4 %
Intersex	20 %
Contralateral testis of patients with GCT	4–6 %
Retroperitoneal "extragonadal" GCT	50 %

Morphology

Macroscopically, the affected testes can be normal or atrophic. They have a firm consistency as a result of atrophy and fibrosis. Microscopically, the atypical germ cells are not uniformly distributed in the parenchyma but show focal or segmental accumulation. The seminiferous tubules containing these cells are narrowed and have a thickened, hyalinized wall. The atypical germ cells are attached to the usually thickened basement membrane and push the Sertoli cells toward the lumen of the seminiferous tubules (Fig. 6.1). The cytoplasm is clear because of the large amount of glycogen, which stains purple with PAS. The nuclei are larger ($\varnothing \approx 9.7$ μm) than those of spermatogonia ($\varnothing \approx 6.5$ μm) and contain 1 or more nucleoli. Mitoses (including abnormal ones) are abundant. The interstitium surrounding the affected tubules is frequently infiltrated by lymphocytes, and microcalcifications are frequent (40 %). These cells can spread with a "pagetoid" pattern to the epithelia of the rete testis or infiltrate the interstitium already in the

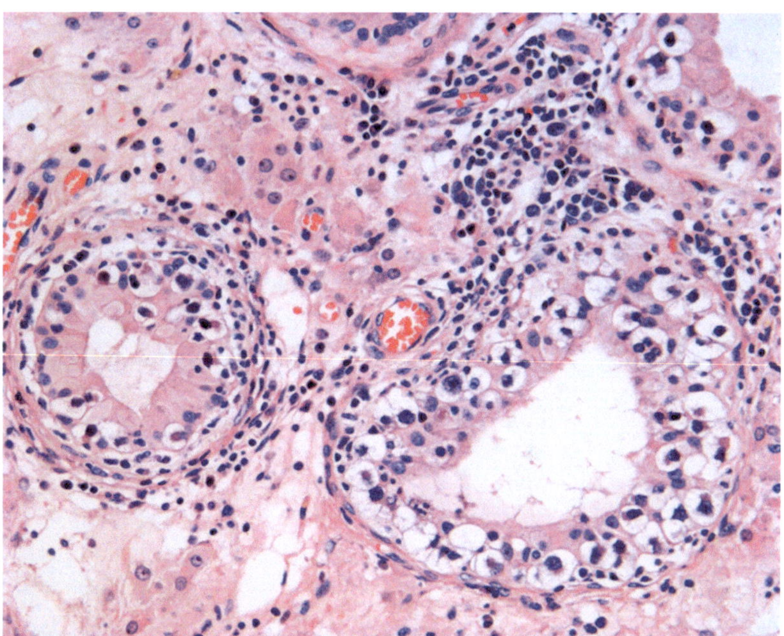

Fig. 6.1 Germ cell neoplasia. Narrowed seminiferous tubules lined with atypical germ cells with clear cytoplasm. The atypical cells push the Sertoli cells toward the lumen. Lymphocytic infiltrates are common in the interstitium

undifferentiated stage. Intratubularly growing GCTs (mostly seminomas or embryonal carcinomas [ECs]) should not be mistaken for CIS.

Immunohistochemistry

Atypical germ cells commonly react with PLAP (Fig. 6.2), CD117 (c-kit), OCT3/4, NANOG, AP-2γ, SALL4, and SOX17, but not with SOX2 [15, 16]. OCT3/4, NANOG, and AP-2γ are the most sensitive markers and are detected also in cases in which PLAP and other markers are absent [17]. Some of these markers, especially CD117, are expressed also in normal spermatogenesis or in cases of delayed maturation.

DNA Ploidy and Cytogenetic Analysis

Atypical germ cells are aneuploid [18] and the chromosomal aberrations correspond to those of invasive GCTs, with the typical differences between seminoma and NSGCTs [19]. The isochromosome i(12p) appears only shortly before CIS turns invasive [20].

Differential Diagnosis

Intratubular seminoma, EC and especially spermatocytic tumors, which always show areas of intratubular growth, can be mistaken for CIS. By extensive sampling, invasive growth areas can be found almost in every such tumor, and in ambiguous cases, the use of immunohistochemical algorithms leads to the correct diagnosis.

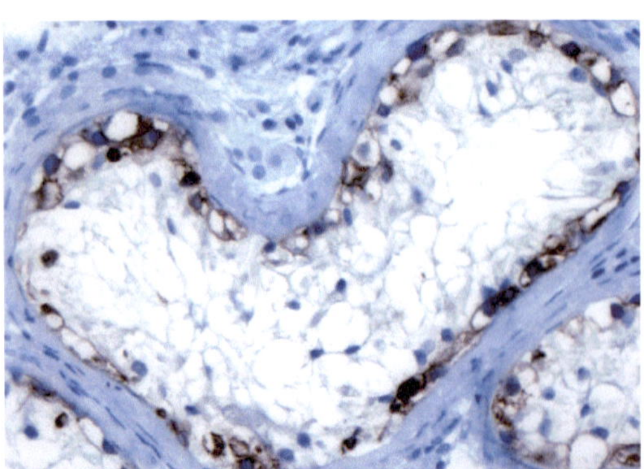

Fig. 6.2 Intratubular germ cell neoplasia. Immunohistochemistry with antibody to PLAP shows strong reactivity of the neoplastic cells

In biopsies of infertile men, it was found that early maturation arrest of spermatogenesis can mimic CIS. The spermatogonia on the basement membrane are isolated from the other cells, and their nuclei have an atypical, worrisome appearance. Moreover, the basement membrane may be thickened and the cells are CD117 positive.

Clinical Features

There is no doubt that with an interval of 5–7 years, 90 % of CIS will evolve into overt invasive GCT. For this reason, European urologists and oncologists advocate biopsy of the healthy contralateral testis in patients with GCTs [21–23]. In case such a biopsy is positive for CIS, the gonad will be treated with radiotherapy at a dose of 18–20 Gy (because with lower doses the lesion persists). Chemotherapy is completely useless to treat CIS [24]. Urologists in the USA are more skeptical about or even contrary to biopsy of the contralateral testis. They argue that a biopsy is positive in only about 5.5 % of cases, and bilateral GCTs are even rarer (3 %) and can be easily cured when they do occur [25].

Seminoma

Epidemiology

Seminoma comprises 40–50 % of all GCTs. In white American men, its incidence has increased over the last 20 years by more than 60 %, whereas the incidence of NSGCTs has risen only by 24 % [26]. It occurs commonly between the ages of 25–50, with a peak incidence at about 34 years [26] (Table 6.3). Seminoma is virtually nonexistent before puberty and it is rare in adolescence (1 %) [1, 27]. About 10 % of seminoma patients have a history of cryptorchidism [1].

Morphology

Macroscopically, small seminomas are homogeneous, well-circumscribed tumors, whereas large seminomas cause marked testicular enlargement; the tunica albuginea is, however, mostly intact and the epididymis uninvolved. On section the tumor bulges above the testicular parenchyma and is lobulated and well circumscribed but without a

Table 6.3 Typical ages of patients with various GCT

Typical ages of patients with various GCT	
Seminoma	Average age 30–40 Extremely rare before puberty and after 70
Spermatocytic tumor	>40
Embryonal carcinoma	Average age 30 Rare before puberty and after 50
Yolk sac tumor	
Prepubertal	3–39 months
Postpubertal	25–30 years
Choriocarcinoma	20–30 years
Teratoma	
Prepubertal	20 months
Postpubertal	20–30 years
Mixed GCT	28 years if NSGCT component prevails 33 years if SE prevails

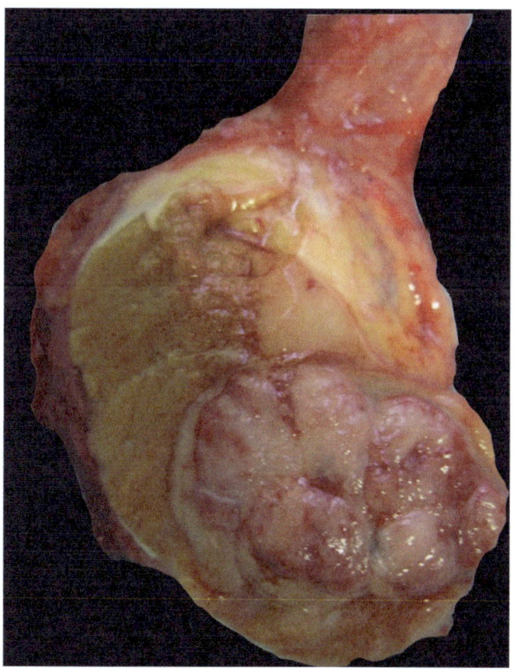

Fig. 6.3 Seminoma. Macroscopic features with typical lobulated pinkish-white cut surface with punctate foci of hemorrhage

capsule (Fig. 6.3). The color is white to pinkish white or tan in cases with heavy lymphocytic infiltration. In large tumors, small necrotic areas and small dot-like hemorrhages are present, but large hemorrhagic, firm, or cystic areas are strongly suggestive of an NSGCT component. If the tumor shows these features or has a diameter >4 cm, extensive sampling is required.

The typical microscopic pattern of seminoma shows lobules composed of a few dozen to roughly 100 cells, which are separated by thin fibrous septa. The cells resemble immature spermatogonia and are rather monomorphous. The cytoplasm is rich in glycogen and fat and therefore appears water-clear in formalin-fixed material (Fig. 6.4). In well-fixed specimens, mitoses are abundant.

More than 80 % of seminomas show lymphocytic infiltration (CD8+ and CD4+ T lymphocytes and some NK cells) [1, 28] ranging in appearance from uniform peppering or clumps scattered in stroma to formation of lymphoid follicles in about 18 % of cases [1] (Fig. 6.5). Macrophages and (in lesser amount) B lymphocytes are also present. Some 10 % of seminomas develop a marked noncaseating granulomatous reaction with epithelioid cells and a few Langhans-type giant cells (granulomatous seminoma) [1] (Fig. 6.6). The reaction is usually patchy but may involve the entire tumor.

Beside this "classical" morphology, there are some variants (Table 6.4). Because they do not have any prognostic or therapeutic importance, these variants have not been listed in the WHO classification [4]. In pseudoglandular and tubular seminoma, tumor cells form small gland-like clefts (Fig. 6.7). Accumulation of edematous fluid in interstitial tissue gives the tumor a microcystic or cribriform appearance (Fig. 6.8). The name *intratubular* or *interstitial seminoma* derives from the predominant way the tumor cells spread (Figs. 6.9 and 6.10). Also seminomas with a high mitotic rate (formerly anaplastic or atypical seminomas) are not considered as an entity in their own right because the high mitotic count does not negatively influence the course of the disease.

Seminoma with syncytiotrophoblastic cells is a separate entity in the WHO classification [4]. On H&E-stained slides, multinucleated giant cells are detected in about 7 % of seminomas, mostly close to vessels (Fig. 6.11). With the use of antibodies against human chorionic gonadotropin (hCG), however, positive cells

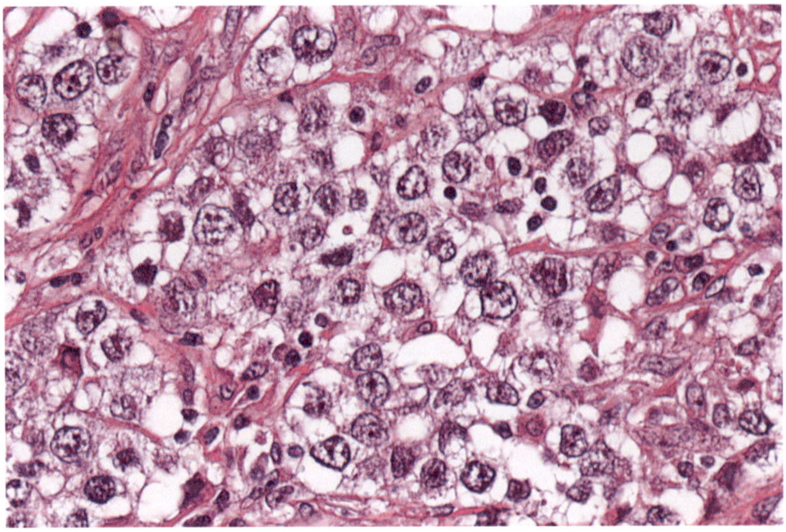

Fig. 6.4 Seminoma. The tumor is composed of cells that have abundant clear cytoplasm and round nuclei with prominent central nucleoli

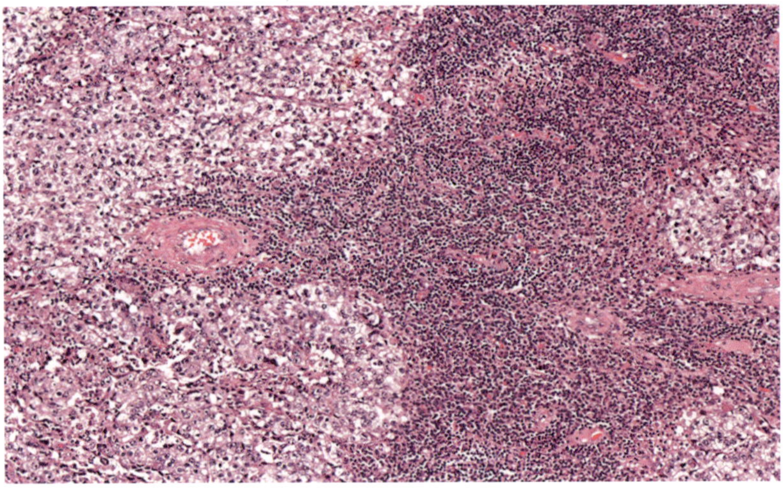

Fig. 6.5 Seminoma. A dense lymphocytic infiltrate (right) is seen at low magnification

are detectable in about one-quarter of all cases [29]. In some cases also mononucleated cells are hCG positive. Syncytiotrophoblastic giant cells also appear in other NSGCTs, and such tumors must not be confused with true choriocarcinomas.

Immunohistochemistry

Seminoma is positive for all markers of embryonic stem cells: PLAP, OCT3/4, NANOG, CD117 (c-kit), and AP-2γ as well as the transcription factor SALL4, which stains all GCTs

Table 6.4 Morphological variants of seminoma non-listed in the WHO classification

Morphological variants of seminoma non-listed in the WHO classification
Intratubular seminoma
Interstitial seminoma
Tubular seminoma
Pseudoglandular seminoma
Microcystic/cribriform seminoma
Granulomatous seminoma
Seminoma with high mitotic rate ("anaplastic seminoma")

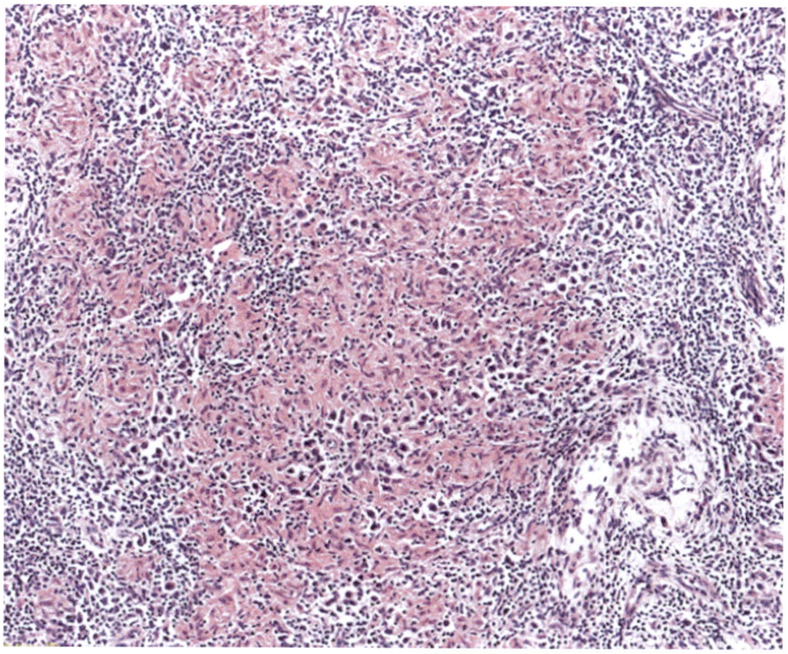

Fig. 6.6 Seminoma. Epitheloid-cell reaction in a so-called granulomatous seminoma

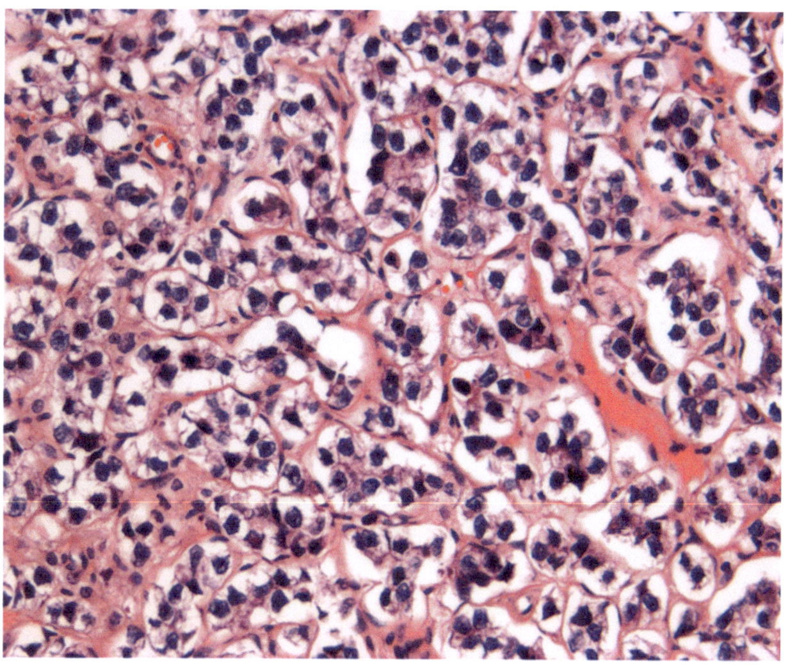

Fig. 6.7 Seminoma. This "tubular" seminoma is composed of tumor cells forming tubular or gland-like structures (With permission of the editor from Gregor Mikuz, Peter Mazal "Hoden und Infertilität beim Mann" Springer-Verlag Berlin Heidelberg, 2016)

[30]. Novel markers are the membrane glycoprotein of podocytes podoplanin (D2-40) and SOX17, an essential factor for inducing the primordial germ cell lineage in humans [30, 31] (Table 6.5). In some seminomas, single tumor cells are positive for cytokeratin and CD30, perhaps as a sign of beginning transition from seminoma to EC [32].

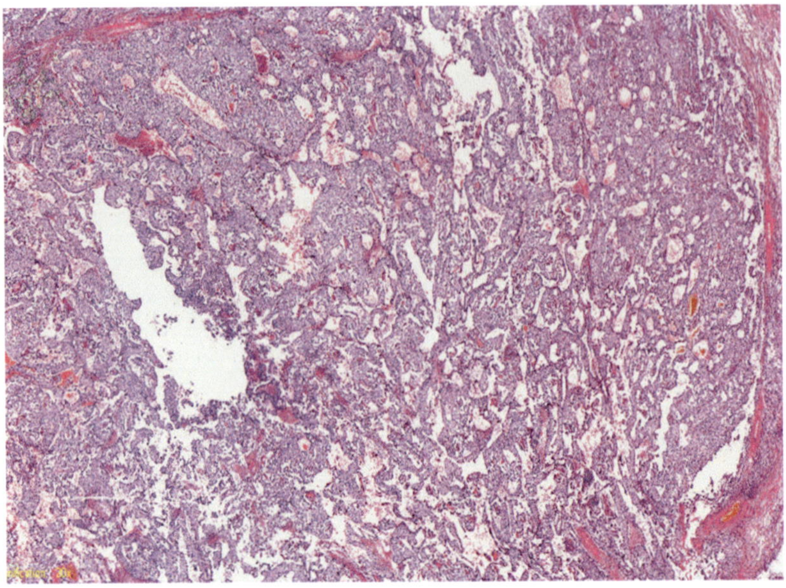

Fig. 6.8 Interstitial edema gives a cribriform, microcystic appearance to seminoma

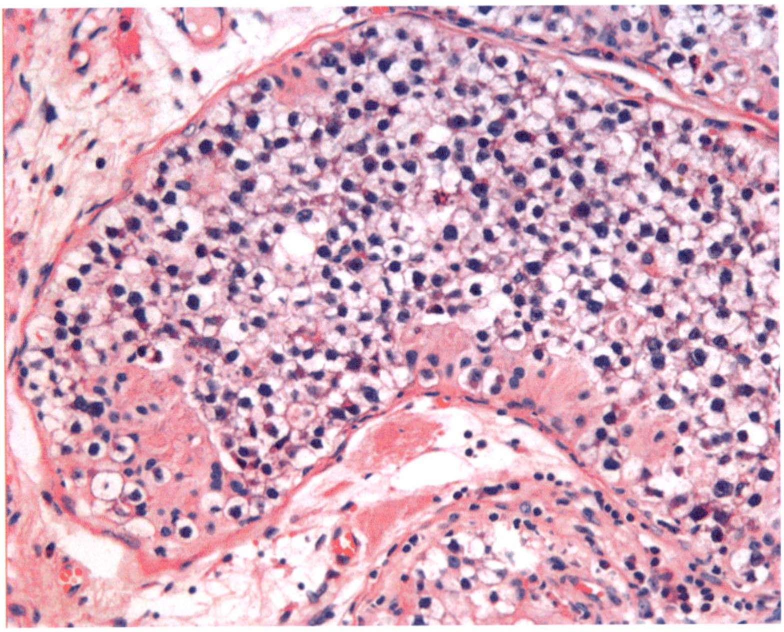

Fig. 6.9 Intratubular seminoma. Tumoral cells fill the seminiferous tubules

DNA Ploidy and Cytogenetic Analysis

All seminomas are aneuploid, mostly with a hypertetraploid stem line [33, 34]. Sporadic reports on diploid seminomas are the result of measurement errors. In flow cytometric measurements, the diploid stem line is not derived from the tumor cells but from the many lymphocytes present in the tumor [33].

Like all GCTs, also seminomas show gain of isochromosome i(12p); the number of copies is, however, lower than in NSGCTs [35]. Gain of chromosomes 1, 2, 7, 8, 20, and X and loss of chromosomes 4, 5, 9, 11q, 13, and 18 are typical of seminoma and NSGCT. Additionally, seminomas can show gain of chromosomes 3p, 6p, 10, and 22 and loss of 1q, 9p, 11p, 16p, and 17p [34].

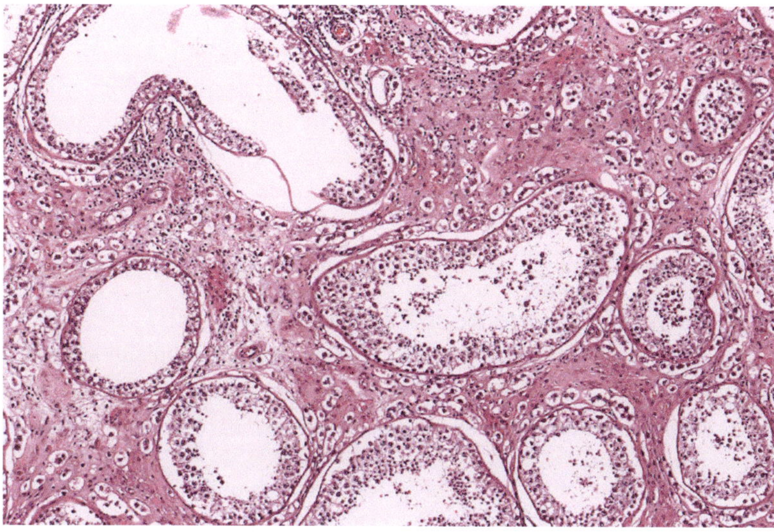

Fig. 6.10 Intertubular seminoma. Tumors with exclusively intertubular growth are susceptible to being overlooked. Sometimes it is a component of a typical seminoma

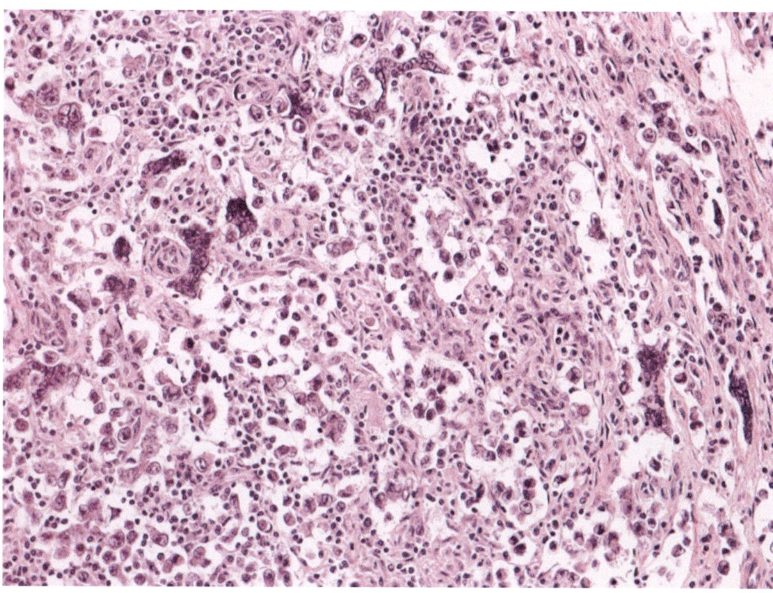

Fig. 6.11 Seminoma with syncytiophoblastic giant cells. This tumor shows edema separating the tumor cells and multinucleated cells

Differential Diagnosis

The cytomorphology of seminoma cells strongly depends on the proper fixation of the surgical specimen. In insufficiently fixed autolytic tissue, the cytoplasm of the tumor cells turns dark and eosinophilic, and the nuclei may swell or shrink. This leads to diagnostic difficulties; in the worst case, the tumor is mistaken for an EC, and as a consequence, the patient will receive totally different and inadequate therapy. If marked lymphocytic infiltration or a granulomatous reaction is present, the tumor is probably a seminoma. By contrast, glandular and papillary structures are highly suggestive of an EC. PLAP stains seminoma cells delicately and perimembranously, while it stains EC cells diffusely and very strongly. To avoid errors, the use of immunohistochemistry is mandatory: seminomas are CD117 and SOX17 positive and AE1/AE2, CD30, and SOX2 negative, whereas ECs are CD117 and

SOX17 negative and AE1/AE2, CD30, and SOX2 positive (Table 6.5) [30].

YSTs with a solid growth pattern can be mistaken for seminoma too (Fig. 6.12). YSTs are strongly pancytokeratin positive and OCT3/4 negative, but the most specific marker is glypican-3, which stains only YST cells [30]. Since alpha fetoprotein (AFP) expression in YST cells is not evenly distributed, absolutely negative areas can occur; therefore, the use of glypican-3 should be preferred. Seminoma cells do not produce AFP, so a high AFP level in serum means that the sampling was insufficient and NSGCT areas were missed; it can also result from an error in laboratory measurements.

Table 6.5 Immunohistochemical reactions useful for the differential diagnosis of seminoma, embryonal carcinoma and spermatocytic tumor

Antibody	Seminoma	Embryonal carcinoma	Spermatocytic tumor
PLAP	++	+	–
CD30	–	++	–
AE1/AE3	±	++	*Dot-like*
CD117	+	±	±
OCT3/4	+	+	–
SALL4	+	+	+
SOX2	–-	+	–
SOX17	+	–	–

Other possible pitfalls are caused by Sertoli cell tumors and malignant lymphomas, which are, however, tumors of aged men. With the use of SALL4 antibodies, which stain exclusively GCTs, such mistakes can be easily avoided [36].

Clinical Features

The presenting complaint associated with seminoma is mostly testicular swelling, while about 10 % of patients experience local discomfort and pain. Symptoms due to metastases include supraclavicular lymph node swelling and abdominal pain due to enlarged retroperitoneal lymph nodes, which can also obstruct the ureters and cause hydronephrosis. Gynecomastia can be a symptom in patients affected by seminoma with syncytiotrophoblastic giant cells.

The main unfavorable morphologic prognostic factors are a tumor diameter >4 cm and tumor pagetoid infiltration of the epithelium of the rete testis (Fig. 6.13) or the rete testis stromal infiltration, whereas vascular invasion is prognostically not as important as in NSGCTs [37]. In a recent publication, it was reported that the risk of tumor relapse was directly proportional to the tumor

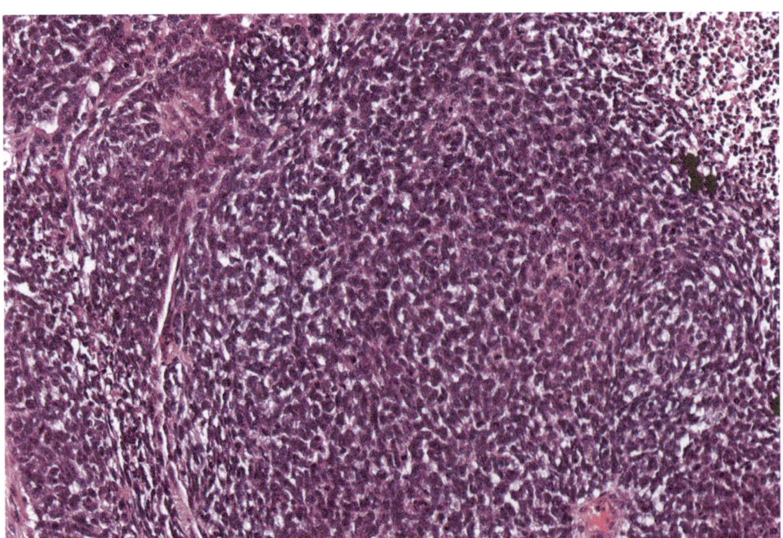

Fig. 6.12 Solid yolk sac tumor resembling seminomatous proliferation

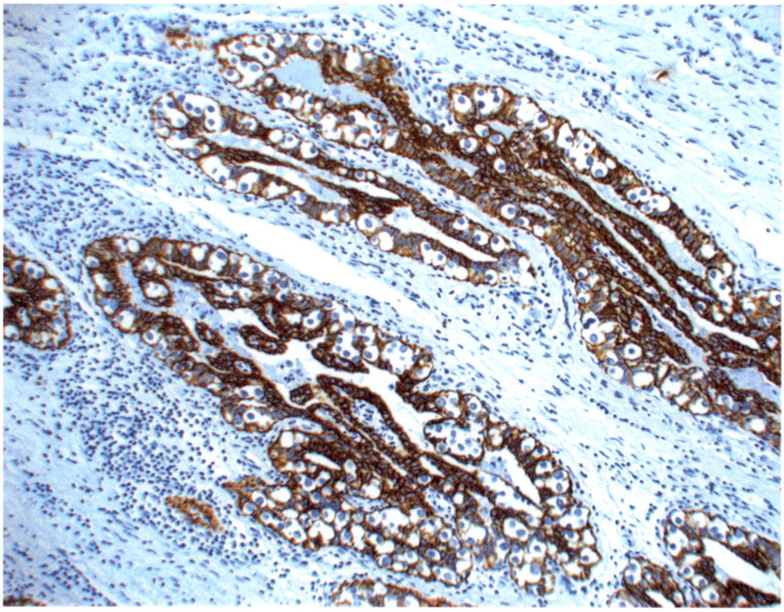

Fig. 6.13 Pagetoid invasion of unstained seminoma cells in the epithelium of the rete testis immunohistochemically positive for cytokeratin antibodies

diameter; this can be used in therapeutic decision-making, i.e., in the choice between surveillance and adjuvant radio- or chemotherapy [38]. Following inguinal orchiectomy, the management options for patients with stage I seminoma are initial surveillance or adjuvant treatment. The recommendation for patients with two risk factors (tumor size and rete testis invasion) is treatment with carboplatin, while for patients with 0–1 risk factor, surveillance is recommended [39]. It should be mentioned that patients treated with chemotherapy often experience late complications such as metabolic syndrome, myocardial infarction, and secondary neoplasms [37].

Spermatocytic Tumor

In 1946 the renowned French-Canadian pathologist Pierre Masson described a novel GCT composed of tumor cells with filamentous nuclear chromatin resembling spermatocytes and therefore named it "spermatocytic seminoma" [40]. In the 2016 WHO classification, the name has been changed to "spermatocytic tumor" (ST) to stress the fact that this tumor is not a variant of seminoma [5]. However, it does not originate from spermatocytes but from spermatogonia [41]. The pathogenesis seems to be quite different from that of the other GCTs because ST does not develop from the CIS precursor and the common chromosomal aberration i(12p) is missing. Moreover, it is the only GCT that does not occur in the ovary [42] (Table 6.6).

ST is an extremely rare tumor and accounts for only 0.61 % of all GCTs. The incidence is 0.3/1 million in men younger than 55 years of age and 0.8/1 million in older men [43]. With an average age of 55 years, patients are older than those with seminoma; nevertheless, in one-quarter of reported cases, patients were younger than 40 years. Young age, even under 30 years, is therefore not an exclusion criterion for this diagnosis.

There are no known risk factors for ST, not even cryptorchidism. There are also no differences in incidence between races.

Morphology

Because of the gelatinous and mucinous cut surface and/or the presence of small mucoid

Table 6.6 The main differences between seminoma and spermatocytic tumor

Characteristics	Spermatocytic tumor	Seminoma
Site of primary	Only testis	Testis, ovary, mediastinum, retroperitoneum, CNS
Cryptorchidism	No	10 %
Mean age	53 (19–92)[a]	36 (8–82)
Genetic predisposition	Unknown	Unknown
Incidence	0.4/1 million	2–5/100,000
Metastases	Extremely rare	Frequent
Combined with other GCT	Never	≈15 %
Combined with GCNIS	Never	>90 %
Combined with sarcoma	Occasionally	Never
Cytoplasmic glycogen	Missed	Abundant
Chromosome	+9	i(p12)

[a]Caveat, young age does not exclude the diagnosis of spermatocytic tumor

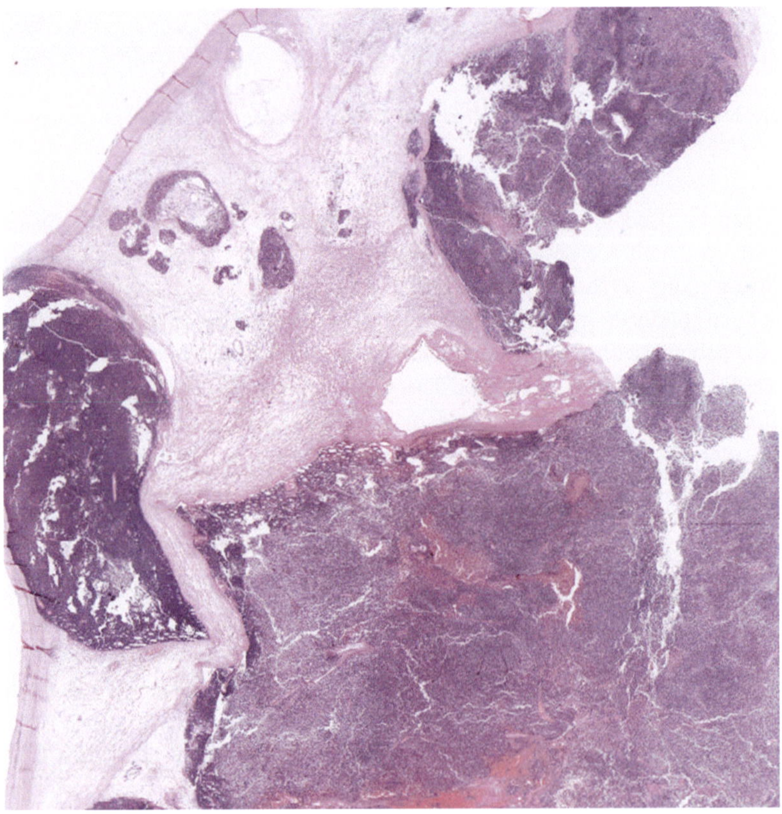

Fig. 6.14 Spermatocytic tumor. A multinodular pattern is apparent on scanning magnification

cysts, the macroscopic appearance of ST is unique and would permit a diagnosis "at first glance." The tumors are usually rather large with a mean diameter of 4–5 cm, but sizes up to 15 cm have been reported. The outline of the tumor is well delineated, the color grayish white, and the consistency soft with typical multinodular pattern of growth (Fig. 6.14).

ST is microscopically composed of three distinct cell types: medium-sized cells (diameter,

15–20 μm) with a rather regular, round nucleus; small cells (diameter, 6–8 μm) resembling lymphocytes; and scattered single mono- or multinucleated giant cells (diameter, 50–150 μm) whose nuclei have coarse chromatin similar to the spireme of spermatocytes in meiotic division (Fig. 6.15) [44]. The main part of the tumor shows an expansive growth pattern, and the surrounding tubules are greatly extended and filled with neoplastic cells (Fig. 6.16). Tubular rupture in more than one area explains the occurrence of multiple distinct tumor nodules in one testis. In contrast to other GCTs, no CIS can be detected in the adjacent tubules; they may show completely normal spermatogenesis with mature spermatozoa. The stroma is inconspicuous and there are no lymphocytic infiltrates. Large edematous areas similar to those of microcystic seminomas are also often observed.

So far 18 cases of ST combined with sarcoma have been described [42, 45]. Eight of these sarcomas were rhabdomyosarcomas, and the others

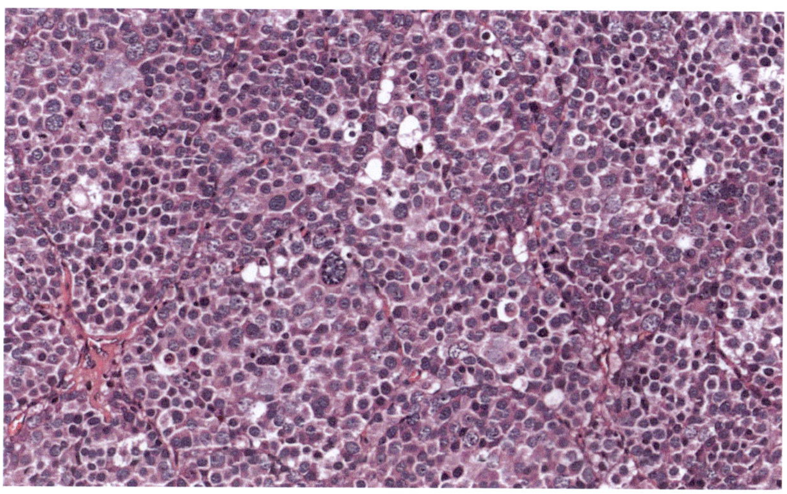

Fig. 6.15 Spermatocytic tumor composed of three distinct cell types: predominant large cells, scattered small, lymphocyte-like cells, and a single giant cell

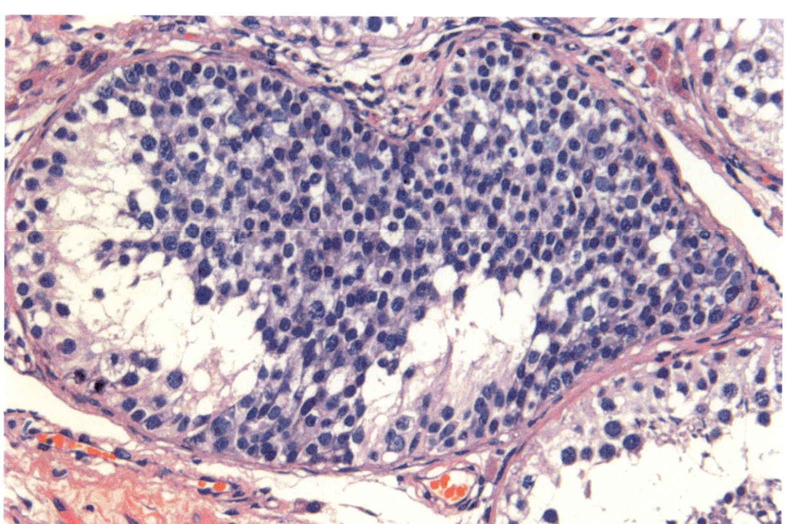

Fig. 6.16 Intratubular growth of spermatocytic tumor. The adjacent tubules shows almost normal spermatogenesis

were defined as undifferentiated spindled or epithelioid.

In 1996 Albores Saavedra et al. [46] described four cases of a variant of ST named "anaplastic spermatocytic seminoma" (ASS). More recently, four additional cases were described [47]. In contrast to ST, ASS contains only the medium-sized cell type characterized by large nucleoli, causing the cells to resemble those of an EC. Moreover, mitotic activity is brisk and areas of necrosis are frequently observed, and there are usually many apoptotic tumor cells (Figs. 6.17 and 6.18).

Immunohistochemistry

STs are negative for the classical markers of GCT: PLAP and OCT3/4. They stain positively for SALL4 and CD117, but not in all cases [47], and the cytoplasm of single cells shows a dot-like reaction for pancytokeratin (AE1/AE3; CAM5.2) (Fig. 6.19). The novel markers NUT, GAGE7, and NY-ESO-1 are variably sensitive to ST, and

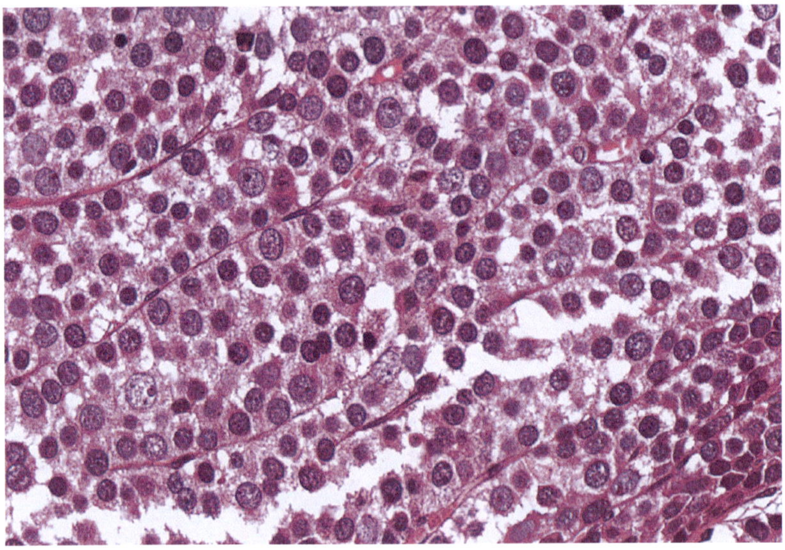

Fig. 6.17 Spermatocytic tumor with many apoptotic tumor cells

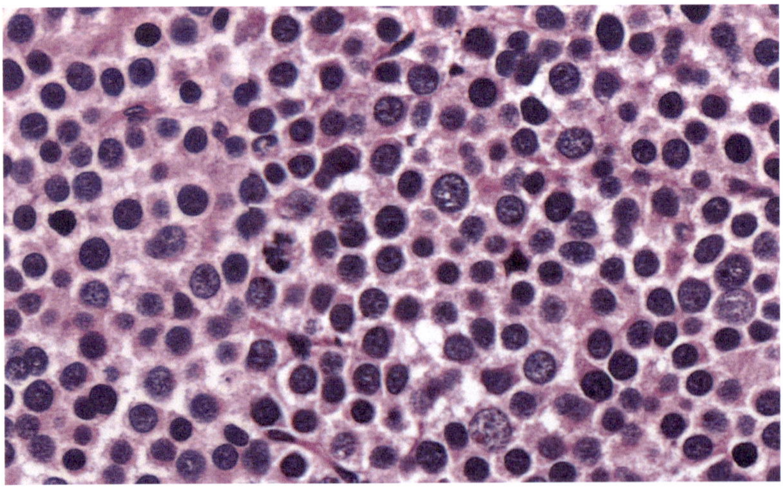

Fig. 6.18 Anaplastic spermatocytic tumor composed only of large cells undergoing mitosis and apoptosis

high specificity is attained when there is multifocal and strong nuclear staining [48].

DNA Ploidy and Cytogenetic Analysis

The ploidy of ST depends on the cell type: the small lymphocyte-like tumor cells are diploid, while the other types are hyperploid with single values up to 42c [49–51].

Gain of chromosome 9 and the absence of the i(12q) isochromosome are almost specific for ST. However, in one "hybrid" case, the isochromosome and gain of chromosome 7, which are characteristic of the other GCTs, were observed [47].

Differential Diagnosis

In our experience, ST is one of the most frequently misdiagnosed tumors due to its rarity. The polymorphous and harmful-looking tumor cells and the lack of stroma make the tumor similar to malignant lymphomas. "Anaplastic seminoma" and even YST are other "popular" misdiagnoses. Immunohistochemistry is not very helpful unless a lymphoma should be confirmed or excluded. The macroscopic features of the tumor and recognition of the three cell types as well as the spireme-like structure of the nuclear chromatin will guide the pathologist to the correct diagnosis.

Clinical Features

Like in other GCTs, the main symptom is painless swelling of the testicle. Serum markers are negative. Pure STs do not need any therapy after orchiectomy. Most cases of metastasizing ST diagnosed in the pre-immunohistochemistry era turned out to be malignant lymphomas [45]. After critical reevaluation, only six cases could be confirmed as metastasizing ST; five of these patients died and one is alive without disease after chemotherapy [42]. The patient with the hybrid tumor died of widespread organ metastases [47]. Metastasizing STs are therefore chemotherapy resistant. All patients with ST combined with sarcoma died of sarcoma metastases.

Embryonal Carcinoma

EC is a highly malignant tumor composed of primitive cells that retain the ability to differentiate toward somatic or extraembryonic structures.

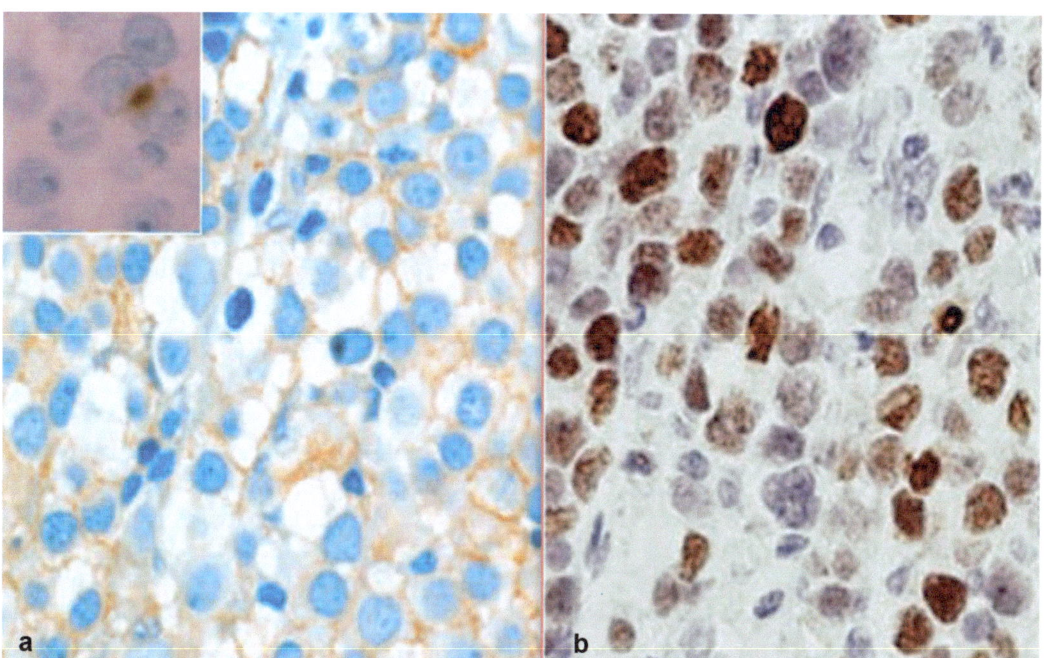

Fig. 6.19 Spermatocytic tumor immunohistochemistry: (**a**) CD117 (c-kit). (**b**) SALL4. Insert: dot-like positivity for CAM5.2

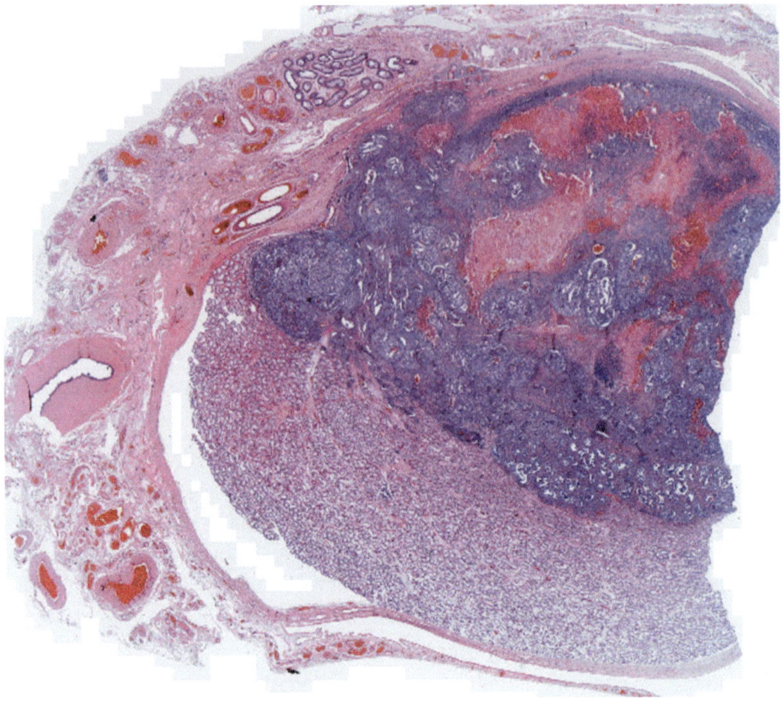

Fig. 6.20 Overview of embryonal carcinoma with a large area of hemorrhage and necrosis

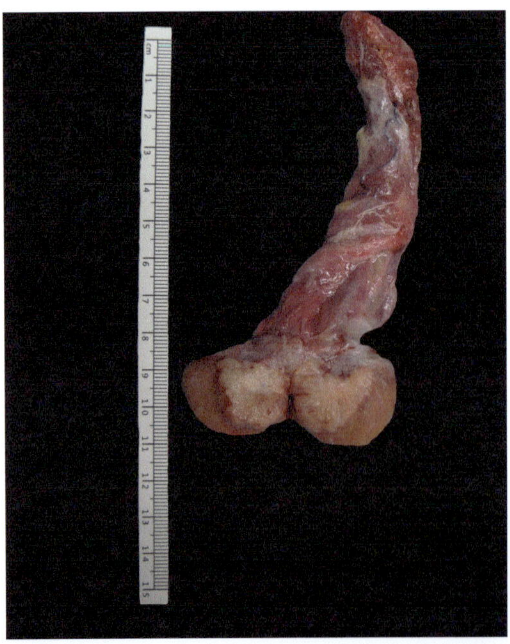

Fig. 6.21 Embryonal carcinoma. A solid yellow-tan tumor occurring in an atrophic adult testis

Epidemiology

The pure form of EC accounts for only 2–10 % of all testicular GCTs, but is very frequent (80 %) in mixed neoplasms with more than one germ cell component. Patients are on average 30 years of age, which is nearly as old as those with seminoma; around 5 % have a history of cryptorchidism [1]. EC in childhood and after age 50 is rare.

Morphology

Macroscopically, ECs are mostly smaller and not as well circumscribed as seminomas. The cut surface is soft, grayish, and focally hemorrhagic or necrotic (Figs. 6.20 and 6.21). Microscopically, EC grows as a true epithelial neoplasm in solid sheets with or without clefting (Fig. 6.22) or in a papillary (Fig. 6.23) or adenomatous formation resembling an adenocarcinoma. It is frequent in the solid sheets to find darkly staining, degenerate-appearing cells that show the tendency to "apply" themselves to adjacent cells ("appliqué pattern of

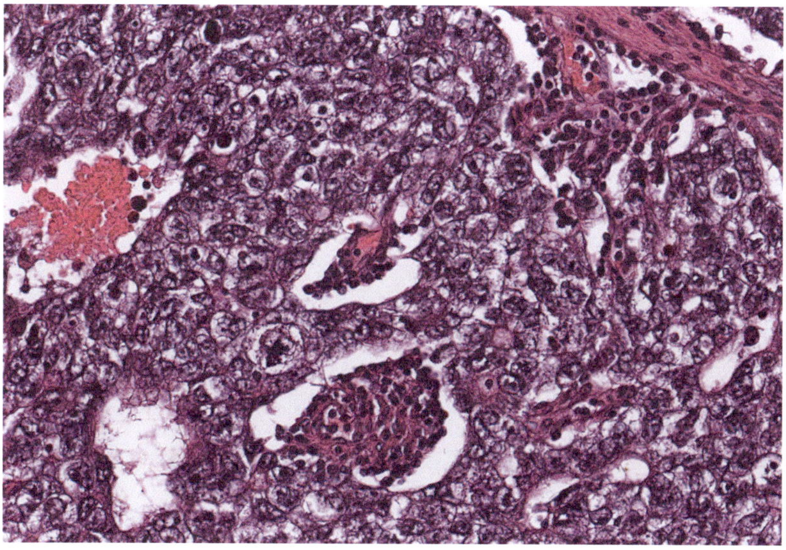

Fig. 6.22 Embryonal carcinoma. The tumor is composed of undifferentiated cells that have overlapping nuclei and scant cytoplasm. Tumor cells form solid nests with some slit spaces

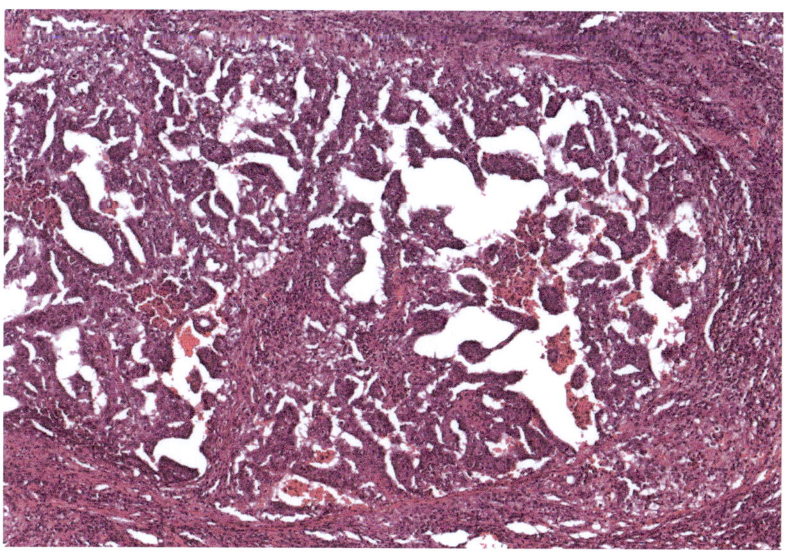

Fig. 6.23 Embryonal carcinoma. This tumor has a papillary pattern lacking fibrovascular cores

embryonal carcinoma") (Fig. 6.24). Intratubular ECs form comedo structures with central necrosis as in breast cancer (Fig. 6.25). Lymphocytes are mostly absent. The tumor cells are very polymorphous and can have a polygonal, cuboid, or columnar shape. The color of the cytoplasm changes from clear to eosinophilic, amphiphilic, or basophilic. The nuclei have coarse chromatin and large single or multiple nucleoli. The mitotic activity is brisk, and vascular invasion is easily detected (Fig. 6.26). As in seminoma also in EC syncytiotrophoblastic giant cells can be scattered all over the tumor (Fig. 6.27). Rete testis involvement is of unclear prognostic significance (Fig. 6.28).

Immunohistochemistry

In contrast to seminoma cells, the cells of EC show a strongly positive reaction to various

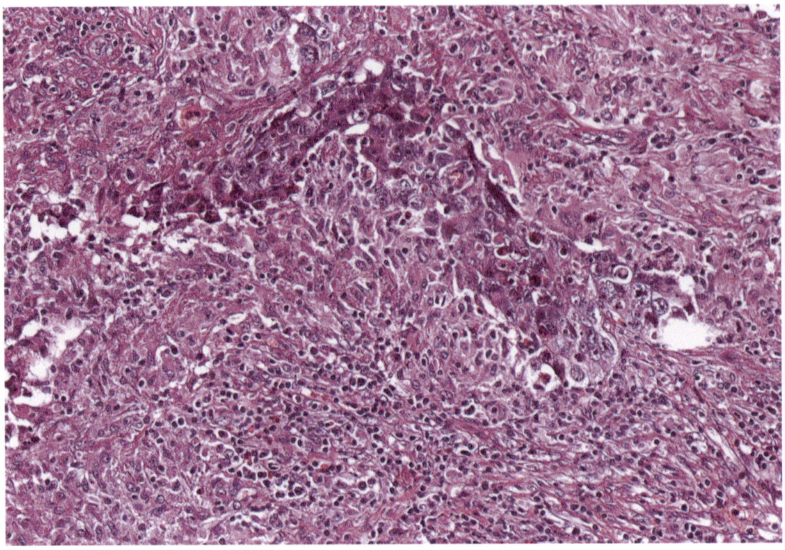

Fig. 6.24 Embryonal carcinoma. Smudged cells "apply" themselves to adjacent cells in this so-called appliqué pattern (Published with kind permission of ©Maurizio Colecchia 2015. All Rights Reserved)

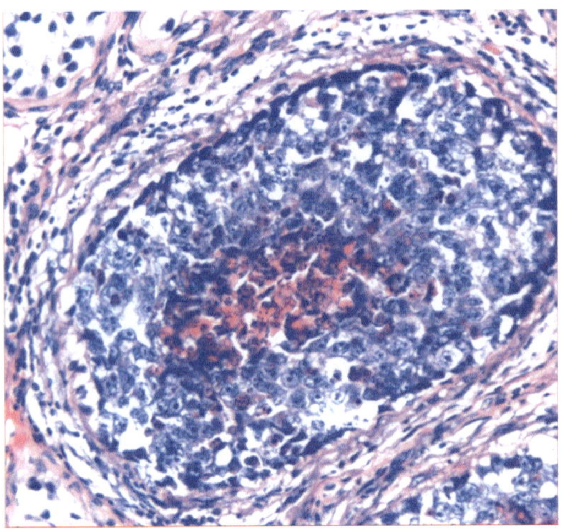

Fig. 6.25 Intratubular embryonal carcinoma. The tubules are expanded by viable tumor cells with central comedo necrosis

cytokeratins (AE1/AE3, CAM5.2, CK7), CD30, SOX2, and OCT3/4, and are negative for CD117, SOX17, and D2-40. PLAP occurs only focally not only as a membranous but also cytoplasmic stain. AFP may be present in scattered cells, and hCG obviously stains the syncytiotrophoblastic giant cells [4, 15, 16, 30, 52].

Caveat: In multiple-relapse/chemoresistant cases, the persistence of CD30 expression is associated with a significantly poorer prognosis and is an independent prognostic factor for survival [53] (Fig. 6.29).

DNA Ploidy and Cytogenetic Analysis

ECs are triploid or hypotriploid tumors [34]. Cytogenetic analysis shows unspecific anomalies, and only i(12p) is present in most cases. There is a correlation between the aggressiveness of the tumor and the number of isochromosome copies [54].

Differential Diagnosis

EC should be differentiated from seminoma (see section on seminoma) because of the therapeutic consequences; any confusion with YST is, however, absolutely unimportant. The diagnosis of YST is based on its peculiar morphology and not on AFP positivity. EC may be confounded with large-cell B-cell lymphoma, especially if it is CD30 positive. In such cases, the use of PLAP and/or cytokeratin antibodies is recommended.

Clinical Features

The main symptom is a testicular mass that causes pain and discomfort. Ten percent of patients suffer from systemic symptoms such as weight loss, fever, night sweats, and headaches

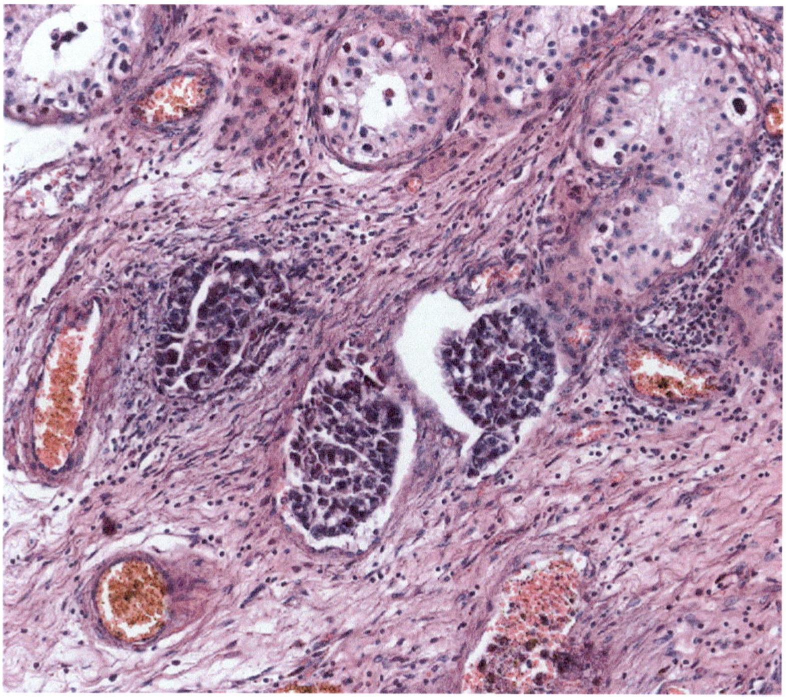

Fig. 6.26 Vascular invasion is a frequent event in embryonal carcinoma with tumor cells conformed to the shape of the vessels

or have brain or lung metastases. AFP in serum may be elevated even in histologically pure EC, and hCG is detectable in cases with syncytiotrophoblastic giant cells. Less than half of the patients have localized disease at presentation, 40 % have retroperitoneal lymph node involvement, and 20 % have supradiaphragmatic lymph node and/or visceral metastases [55]. Even though pure EC is an extremely aggressive tumor, it can be cured with modern chemotherapy.

Yolk Sac Tumor

YST is a tumor composed of structures resembling the embryonal yolk sac, allantois, and embryonal mesenchyme. Teilum first described this entity in 1959 and named it "endodermal sinus tumor" [56], while in the so-called British classification, the name was "orchioblastoma" [1].

Since with few exceptions the pure form occurs only in children and the oncogenesis in childhood and adults seems to be quite different, in the new WHO classification, a prepubertal and a postpubertal type are distinguished [5].

Epidemiolology

According to the Prepubertal Testis Tumor Registry of the Urologic Section of the American Academy of Pediatrics, YST accounts for 62 % of all testicular GCTs and 70 % of all GCTs [57]. The median age of affected children is about 19 months (range, 3–39) [58]. The incidence is the same in Afro-American and Caucasian children [59]. In almost 40 % of adult cases, YST is a component of a mixed GCT [4].

Morphology

YST's gross and microscopic appearance is identical in children and adults. Macroscopically, the tumor is grayish white and soft, with a mucoid surface and hemorrhagic and necrotic areas. The microscopic impression is that of a confusing variety of cells and patterns, but in sporadic cases, the tumor is composed of a single cell type or only one histologic pattern. The microcystic (reticular) and solid patterns are the

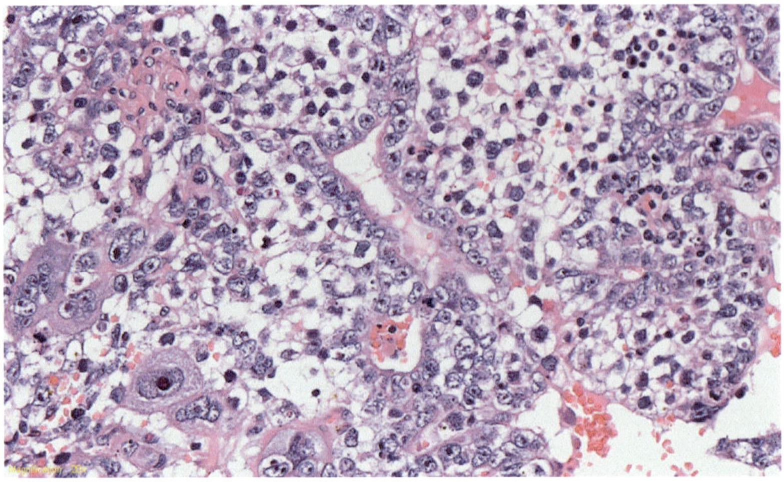

Fig. 6.27 Mixed germ cells tumor. Seminoma with a rim of cuboidal embryonal carcinoma cells and scattered syncytiotrophoblastic giant cells

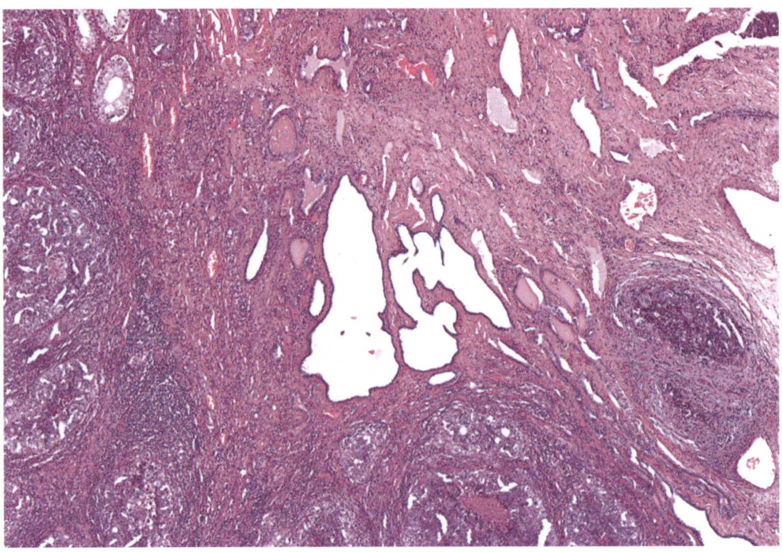

Fig. 6.28 Embryonal carcinoma. The tumor infiltrates the rete testis

most common and are present in more than 80 % of cases (Fig. 6.30) [4]. The solid pattern has intercellular basement membrane deposits. The papillary and even the eponymous polyvesicular vitelline pattern as well as many others are not so frequently encountered (Table 6.7). Such patterns can blend into enteric-type glands, which focally show hepatic-like differentiation or the unusual endometrioid pattern (Fig. 6.31). Also the diagnostic Schiller-Duval bodies (Fig. 6.32), perivascular structures resembling the endodermal sinus of rat placenta, are scarce in most cases. Tumor cells can contain hyaline globules ($\varnothing \leq 1$ μm) staining positively with diastase-resistant PAS, which are absent in other GCTs (Fig. 6.33). Longitudinally and transversely sectioned endodermal sinus-like structures could be difficult to recognize to correctly identify yolk sac tumor subtype (Fig. 6.34). Rare cases occur with solid pattern yolk sac tumor with a blastema-like appearance (Fig. 6.35).

Immunohistochemistry

The most reliable markers of YST are AE1/AE3 cytokeratin and glypican-3 (Fig. 6.36), whereas AFP is negative in about one-third of cases [60]. PLAP and OCT3/4 are always negative, but CD117 is positive in almost half of cases and therefore cannot be used as a discriminator between seminoma and YST (Table 6.8).

DNA Ploidy and Cytogenetic Analysis

The DNA stem line of YST is peritetraploid and occasionally even diploid [18, 61]. Anomalies of chromosomes 1p, 6q, and 13q are common in pediatric tumors, whereas i(12p) is missing [62].

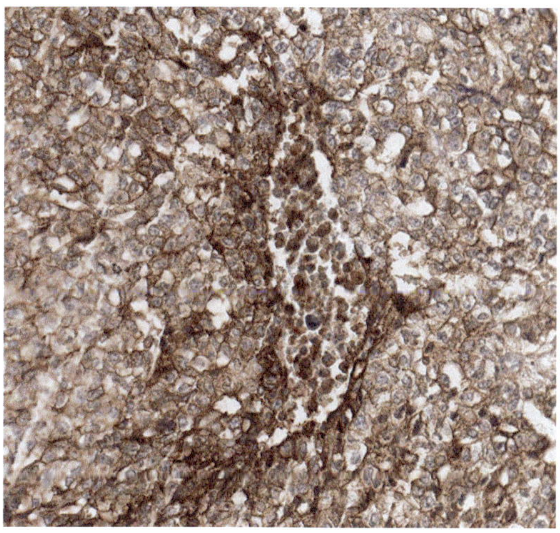

Fig. 6.29 CD 30 immunoreactivity observed in this chemoresistant embryonal carcinoma

Differential Diagnosis

As already mentioned, YST with a solid pattern can be mistaken for seminoma, but thorough analysis of the slides will reveal papillary or microcystic structures or hyaline globules in many cases, which will lead to the correct diagnosis [60]. The diagnosis of YST should be based on morphology and not on AFP positivity. In adults confusion with other NSGCTs is unimportant because the therapy is the same.

Clinical Features

A painless testicular tumor and high AFP in serum are the main features of YST in childhood. Eighty percent of prepubertal patients present with stage I disease. Following surgical resection, they can be safely monitored, and chemotherapy is necessary only when the tumor recurs [57]. Retroperitoneal lymph node dissection (RPLND) is no longer performed in children [57].

Polyembryoma

This tumor never occurs in a pure form and is only microscopically detectable in NSGCTs, mostly YSTs and teratomas. The characteristic embryoid

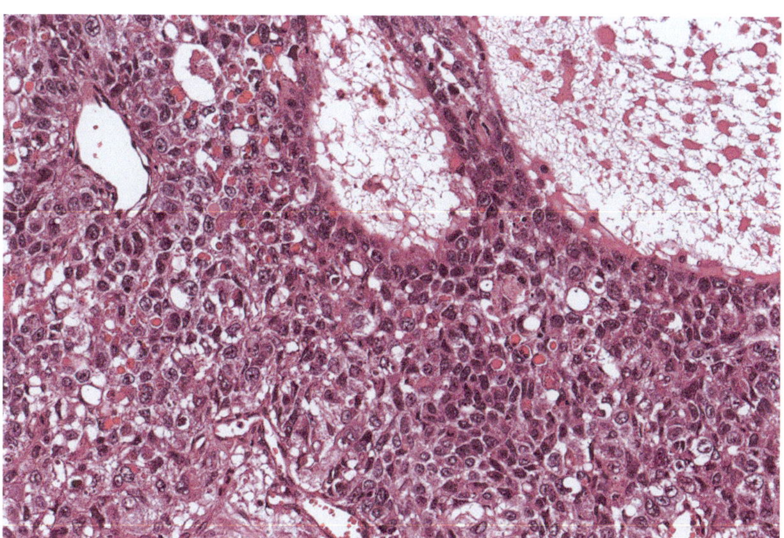

Fig. 6.30 Yolk sac tumor. Microcystic and solid patterns are admixed in this area

bodies are composed of two or three layers of primitive embryonal cells with an amnion-like cyst on the convex side and a yolk saclike vesicle on the concave side (Fig. 6.37). These structures surrounded by a myxomatous stroma do not have any prognostic or therapeutic importance.

Choriocarcinoma

Choriocarcinoma is composed of syncytiotrophoblasts, cytotrophoblasts, and intermediate trophoblasts.

Epidemiology

Pure choriocarcinoma is an extremely rare tumor with an incidence of 0.8/100,000 in countries with a high incidence of GCTs. Even in mixed GCTs, choriocarcinoma elements can be found only in 8 % of cases [4].

Table 6.7 Histologic pattern of yolk sac tumors

Endodermal sinus
Endometrioid
Glandular-alveolar
Hepatoid
Macrocystic
Microcystic-reticular
Myxomatous
Papillary
Parietal
Sarcomatoid-spindle cell
Solid pattern
Vitelline

Morphology

Macroscopically, these mostly small-sized tumors present as a hemorrhagic nodule surrounded by a whitish rim. Also in mixed GCTs, hemorrhagic nodules are highly suspicious for choriocarcinoma. Microscopically, syncytiotrophoblast and cytotrophoblast cells grow in solid sheets and are intermixed in a random fashion (Fig. 6.38). Occasionally syncytiotrophoblastic giant cells cover the proliferated cytotrophoblast like a cap, giving the impression of a placenta villus (Fig. 6.39). The cytotrophoblast cells have a distinct cell membrane, clear cytoplasm, and a vesicular nucleus. Similar cells with eosinophilic cytoplasm represent the intermediate trophoblast. Since the tumor does not have its own stroma, the syncytiotrophoblastic giant cells directly invade the local vessels.

Other Trophoblastic Tumors

Tumors exclusively composed of cytotrophoblast are called "epithelioid choriocarcinoma" (formerly monophasic choriocarcinoma). The pure proliferation of intermediate trophoblast cells is called "placental site trophoblastic tumor",

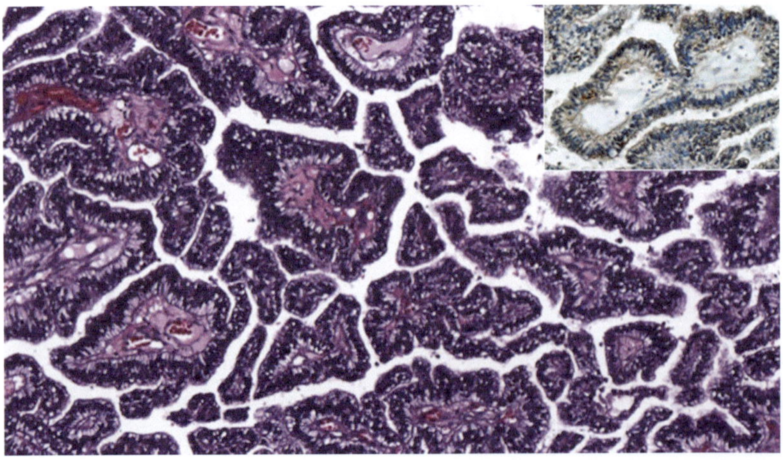

Fig. 6.31 Yolk sac tumor with endometrioid pattern. This pattern is extremely rare in the testis. Insert: AFP positive tumor cells (Courtesy of Prof. Wittekind, Leipzig)

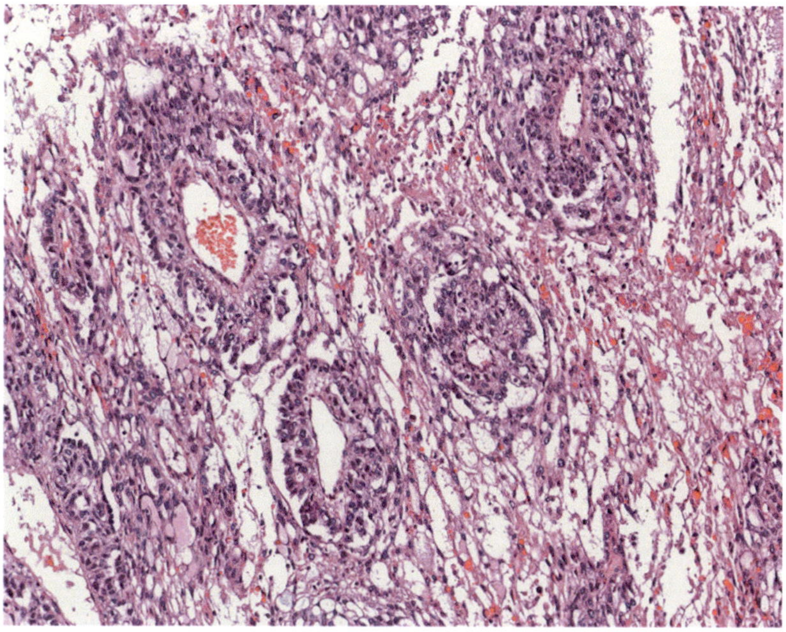

Fig. 6.32 Yolk sac tumor. Typical Schiller-Duval bodies

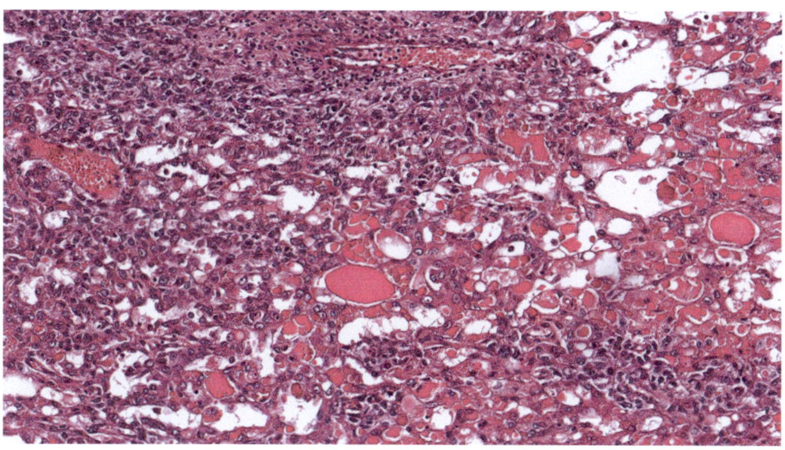

Fig. 6.33 Yolk sac tumor. Mostly macrocystic pattern with intracytoplasmic hyaline globules

because it is morphologically identical to its counterpart in the uterus (Fig. 6.40) [63].

Immunohistochemistry

All three cell types are strongly reactive for cytokeratin antibodies (CK7, 8, 18, 19, CAM5.2, AE1/AE3) and α-inhibin. hCG and EMA stain the syncytiotrophoblastic giant cells [4, 64–66]. Human placental lactogen and pregnancy-specific β1-glycoprotein are reactive to syncytiotrophoblastic giant cells and intermediate trophoblast but not cytotrophoblast. SALL4 reacts only with mononuclear tumor cells [36]. Cytotrophoblast cells proliferate, whereas syncytiotrophoblast giant cells do not [67]. Proliferation markers (MIB-1) can therefore be used to distinguish the two cell types.

DNA Ploidy and Cytogenetic Analysis

Due to the rarity of these tumors, ploidy studies and cytogenetic analysis have rarely been carried out, but i(12p) has been detected also in choriocarcinoma [68].

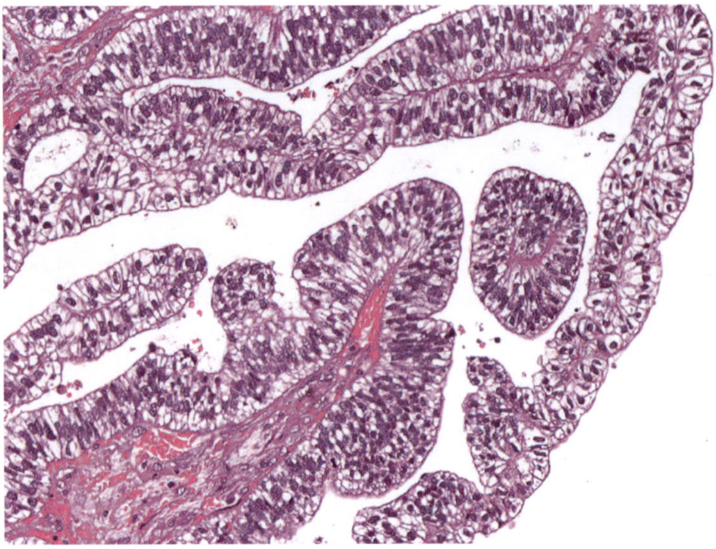

Fig. 6.34 Yolk sac tumor. Endodermal sinus-like structures longitudinally and transversely sectioned

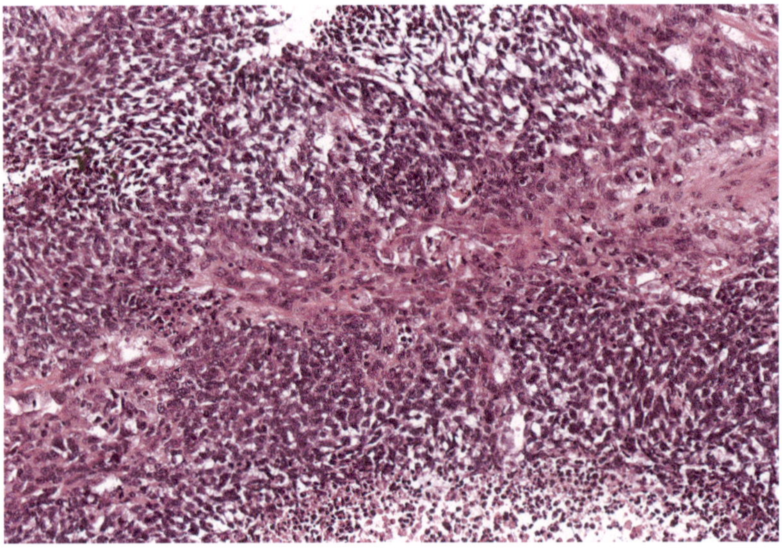

Fig. 6.35 Yolk sac tumor. Solid pattern of blastema-like cells with oval to fusiform nuclei and scant cytoplasm (Published with kind permission of ©Maurizio Colecchia 2015. All Rights Reserved)

Differential Diagnosis

Choriocarcinoma should not be confused with hemorrhagic necrosis of another origin (torsion, trauma, coagulopathy). In such conditions, testicular swelling is sudden and painful.

The main source of misdiagnosis is EC with syncytiotrophoblastic giant cells. For a correct choriocarcinoma diagnosis, cytotrophoblast cells have to be detected, which can, however, be similar to EC cells. The hemorrhagic background and lack of stroma are features not seen in EC. The diagnosis can be difficult in intratubular EC with comedo necrosis, where the necrotic cells squeezed against the tubule wall can mimic syncytiotrophoblastic giant cells. In doubtful cases, the use of hCG immunohistochemistry is mandatory.

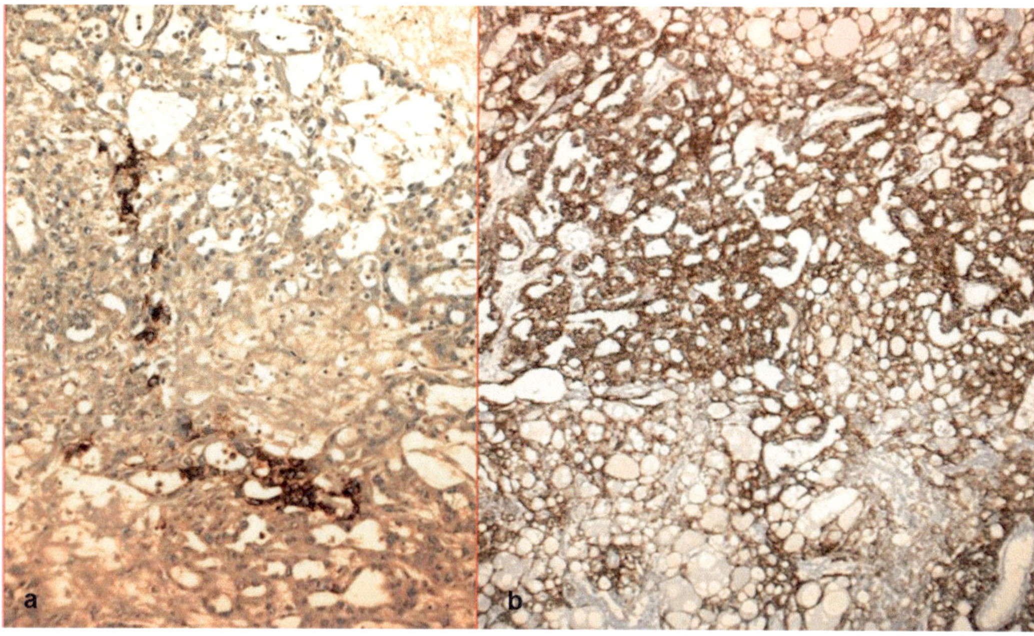

Fig. 6.36 Yolk sac tumor immunohistochemistry. (**a**) Patchy positivity for AFP. (**b**) Marked reactivity with pancytokeratin

Clinical Features

The first symptoms of the disease are mainly caused by organ metastases. Due to the hematogenous spread, the retroperitoneal lymph nodes are not involved. Metastases arise in the lung (100 %), liver (86 %), brain (56 %), and gastrointestinal tract (70 %) [69]. The high serum hCG levels (often >100,000 IU/L) cause gynecomastia.

Choriocarcinoma is a very aggressive tumor: up to the late 1970s, 90 % of patients died within a year. Nowadays it can be cured with energetic chemotherapy, but compared with the other GCTs, the mortality is still high [69]. Profuse intestinal and intracranial bleeding is referred to as "choriocarcinoma syndrome."

Table 6.8 Immunohistochemical reactions useful for the differential diagnosis seminoma vs. yolk sac tumor

Antibody	Seminoma	Yolk sac tumor
AFP	–	+
AE1/AE3	±	+
OCT3/4	+	–
SALL4	+	+
Glypican 3	–	+

Teratoma

Teratoma is composed of tissue components deriving from all three germinal layers: endoderm, ectoderm, and mesoderm. The name, given by Virchow [70], derives from *teras* (τεραα), which in ancient Greek means marvel or monster. Because of the different histogenesis and prognosis, the new WHO classification distinguishes a pre- and a postpubertal form [5]. The use of the old denomination "mature" and "immature" teratoma should be avoided because clinicians understand these adjectives as synonyms for "benign" and "malignant."

Epidemiology

After YSTs, teratomas are the second most frequent testicular tumors (14–20 %) in childhood [27]; about two-thirds of teratomas occur before the age of 2 years (mean age at onset, 20 months). In adults pure teratomas account for only 3–7 % of GCTs. Teratoma is, however, present as a tumor component in nearly half of all mixed GCTs [4, 34] (Figs. 6.41 and 6.42).

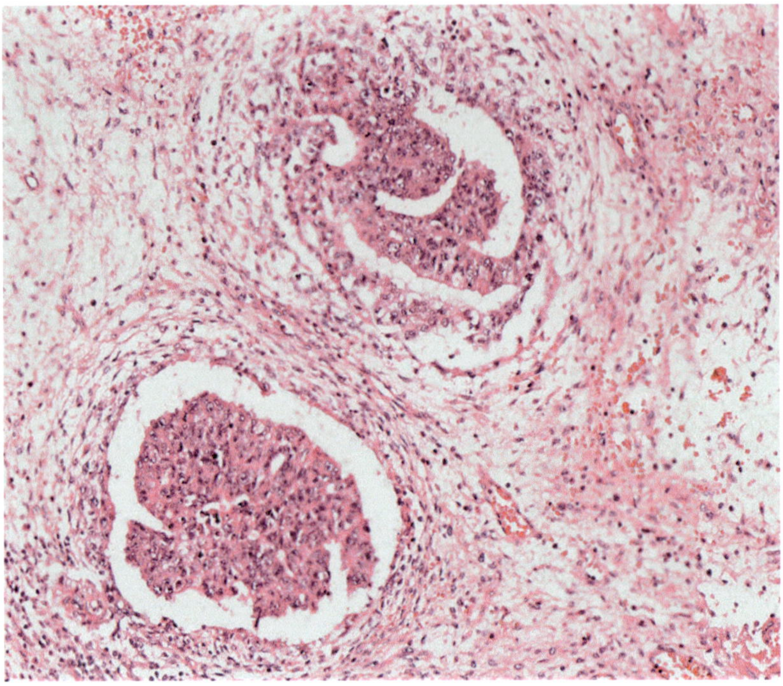

Fig. 6.37 Polyembryoma with "embryoid bodies" resembling a 14-day-old presomite embryo

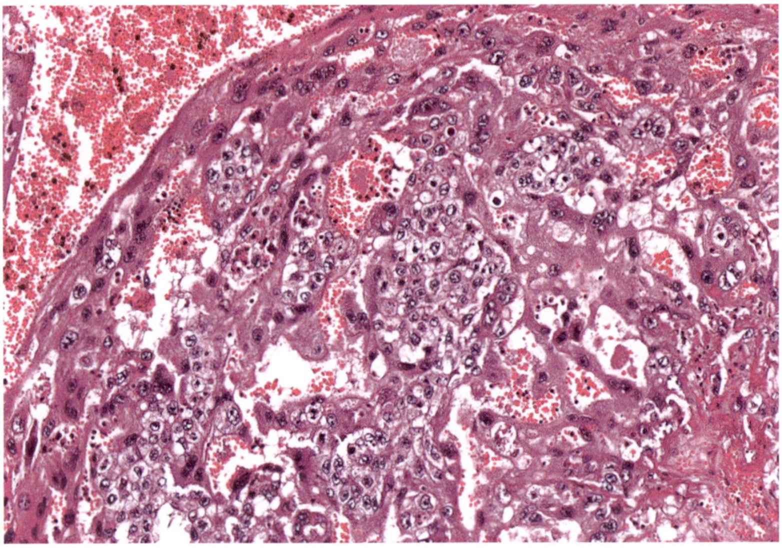

Fig. 6.38 Choriocarcinoma. Pale mononucleated trophoblast cells are surrounded by multinucleated syncytiotrophoblasts with eosinophilic cytoplasm

Morphology

The macroscopic and microscopic appearance depend on the amounts of different tissues present in the tumor. The cut surface has a variegated appearance with cysts filled with hair, mucus, or sebaceous material. Cartilage takes the shape of a glassy nodule. Pigmented areas derive from tissue simulating the retina.

Microscopically, the well-differentiated "mature" areas contain cysts lined with squamous

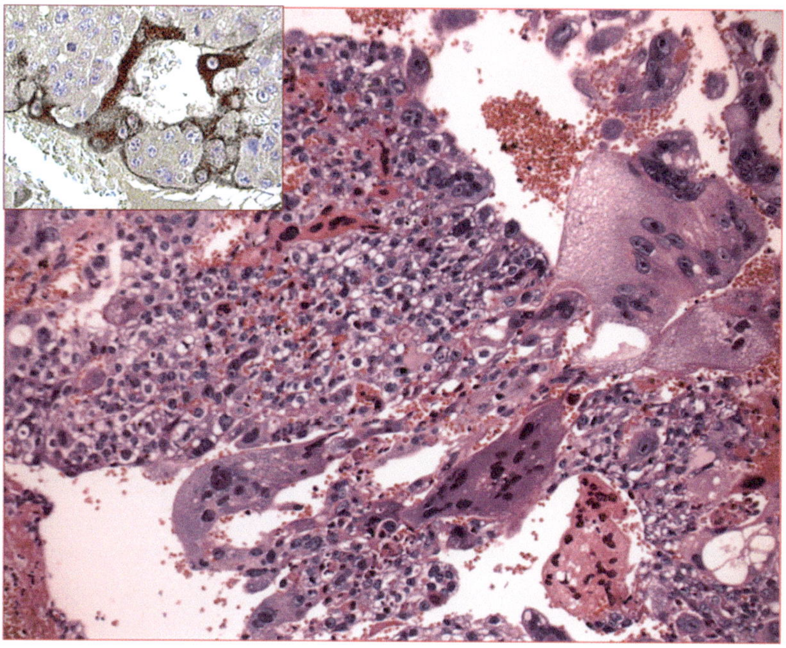

Fig. 6.39 Choriocarcinoma. This tumor is composed of cytotrophoblastic clear cells covered with syncytiotrophoblastic giant cells. Insert: hCG positive giant cells

or glandular epithelium of the enteric-type or ciliated respiratory-type epithelium (Fig. 6.43). The cysts can be filled with mucus or keratin. Organoid structures mimicking gut or bronchus are composed of the corresponding epithelium encircled by smooth muscle. In these organoid structures, neuroendocrine cells producing all kinds of hormones (gastrin, bombesin, somatostatin, etc.) are scattered among the columnar epithelia [71]. Mesodermal tissue is always represented by smooth muscle and sometimes by cartilage; bone with or without hematopoietic marrow is less common. Neuroglia with ependymal differentiation is also a rather common component. Pigmented retinal epithelium can occasionally be present. Differentiated liver, prostate, pancreas, and thyroid are rare (Fig. 6.44).

Less differentiated "immature" tissues are represented by a mesenchymal stroma composed of undifferentiated spindle cells and small immature glands. Also the squamous epithelium is arranged in solid nests without keratinization. Other components are primitive neuroepithelium, renal blastema, rhabdomyoblasts, and fetal adipose tissue with lipoblasts (Fig. 6.45). Interestingly, "immature" tissue is more often encountered in adult patients than in children.

In the 2004 WHO classification, the rare "dermoid cyst" of the testis was listed as a separate category, because this tumor never metastasizes [4]. As in the ovary, the cyst is lined with epidermis, skin, hair follicles, and sebaceous glands.

In monodermal teratomas, a tissue component deriving from one germinal layer overgrows the other components present in the teratoma. The most frequent type is primitive neuroectodermal tumor (PNET), but also chondroma, nephroblastoma, and carcinoid have been described.

The epidermoid cyst, which accounts for 1 % of all intrascrotal tumors and can arise at any age, is the most common monodermal differentiated teratoma [72]. These tumors are easily recognizable with ultrasound and by the naked eye because they have a thin whitish wall and are filled with horny material arranged in a laminated layer similar to onion skin. An epidermis-like layer of squamous epithelium without skin

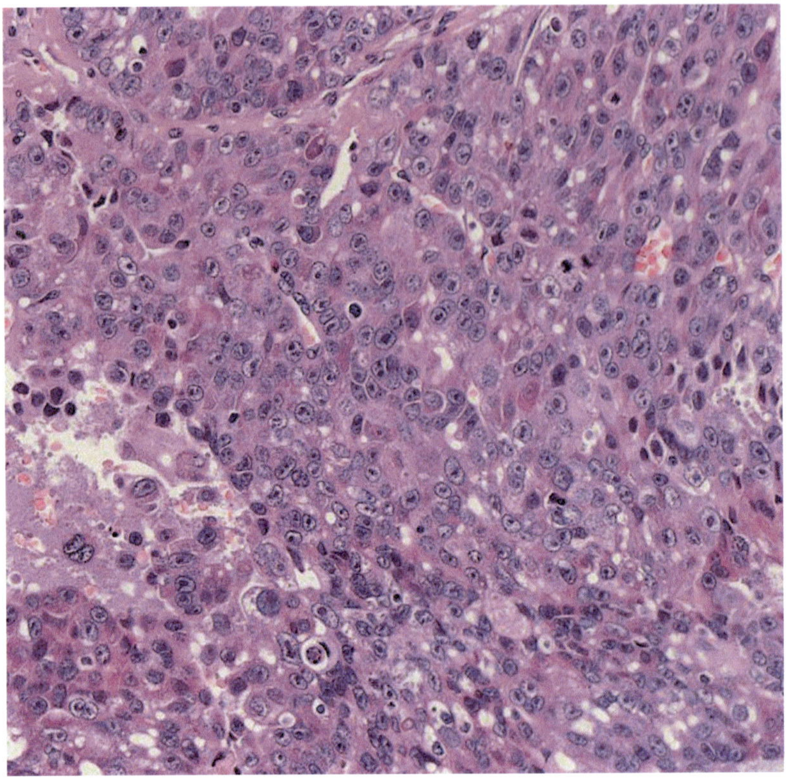

Fig. 6.40 Epitheloid trophoblast in a choriocarcinoma metastasis (Published with kind permission of ©Maurizio Colecchia 2015. All Rights Reserved)

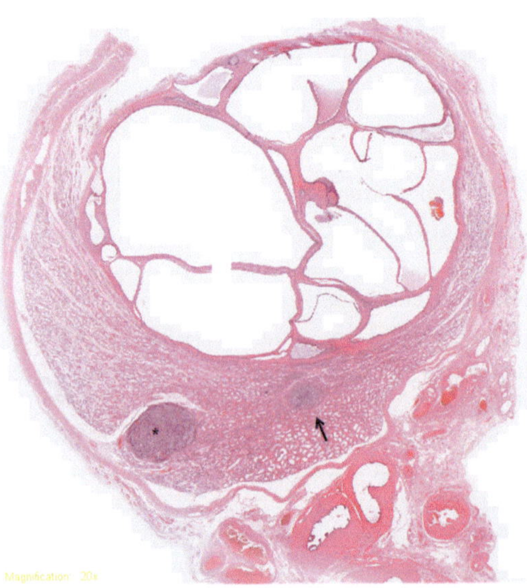

Fig. 6.41 Cystic teratoma with a small embryonal carcinoma (*) and seminoma component (*arrow*)

appendages lines the cyst (Fig. 6.46). It has been discussed for many years whether this tumor is really a teratoma or only an inclusion cyst. Since this tumor is perfectly benign, in the new WHO classification, it will be classified as prepubertal teratoma, even when it arises in adults.

Teratoma with Somatic-Type Malignancy

Transformation of a GCT into a somatic malignancy is uncommon. Its presentation differs from series to series, with almost half of adult cases identified within the primary tumor and the remainder in recurrences or metastases [73]. The most frequent somatic malignancies are sarcomas, especially rhabdomyosarcomas (Figs. 6.47 and 6.48). Among the epithelial

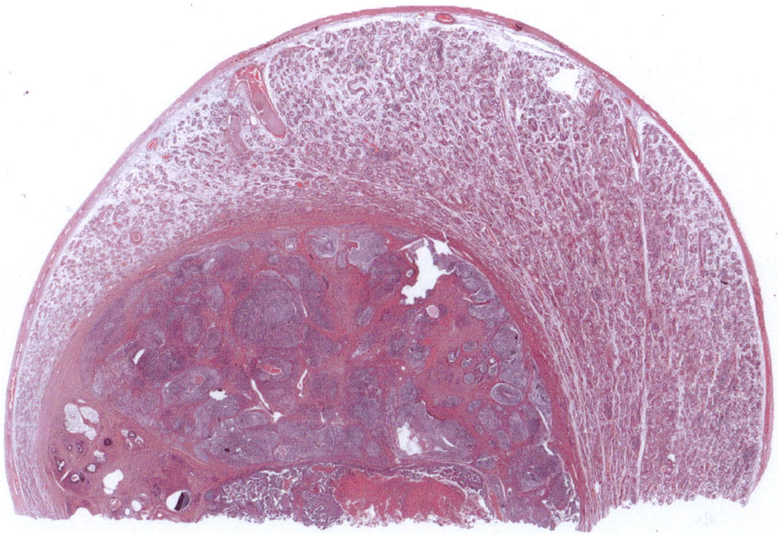

Fig. 6.42 Mixed germ cell tumor. Small mature teratoma and a prevalent component of embryonal carcinoma

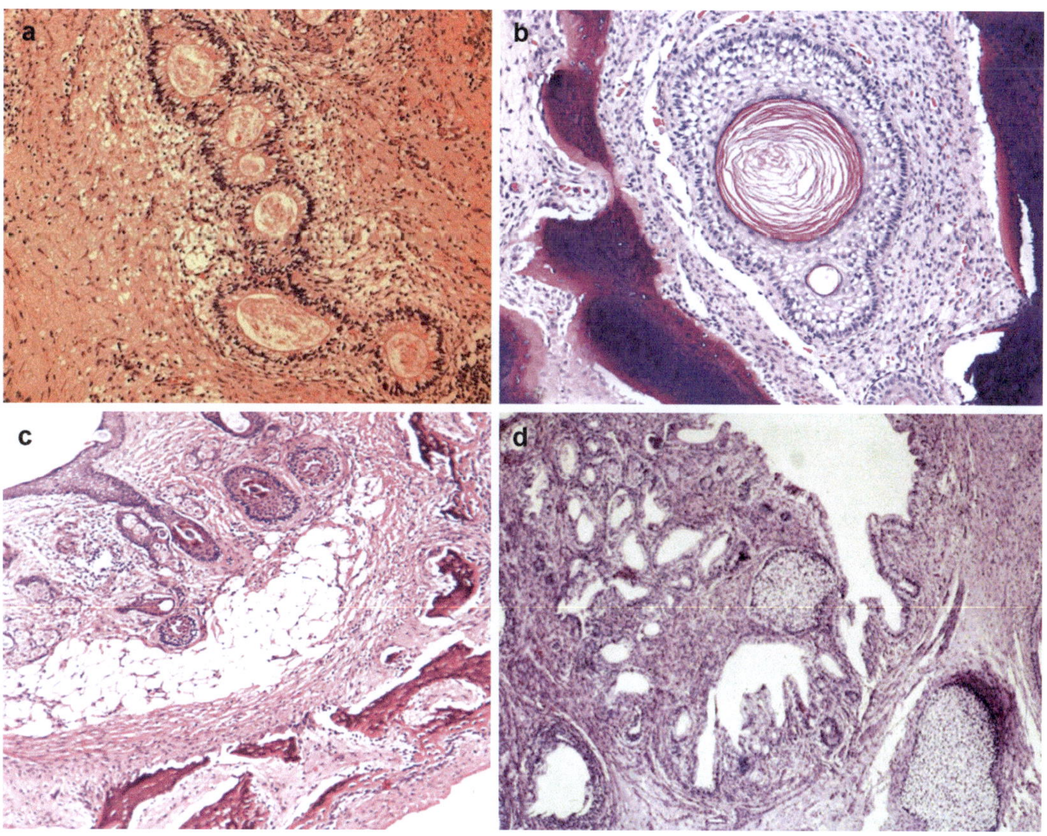

Fig. 6.43 Teratoma. (**a**) Small glands lined with cylindrical intestinal epithelium. (**b**) Squamous epithelium and mature bone. (**c**) Cyst lined with dermis with hair follicle and sebaceous glands. (**d**) Cysts lined with respiratory epithelium and immature cartilage

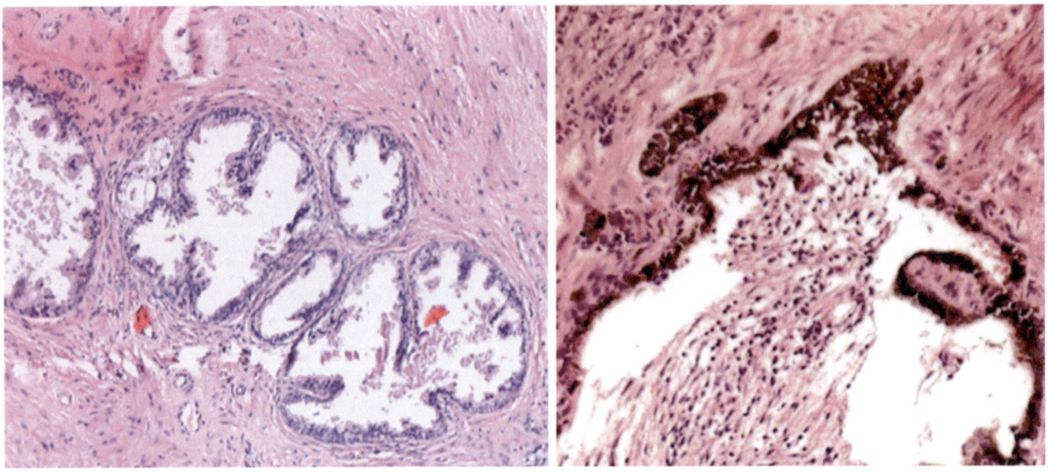

Fig. 6.44 Teratoma containing prostate gland tissue (*left*) and retinal pigment epithelium (*right*)

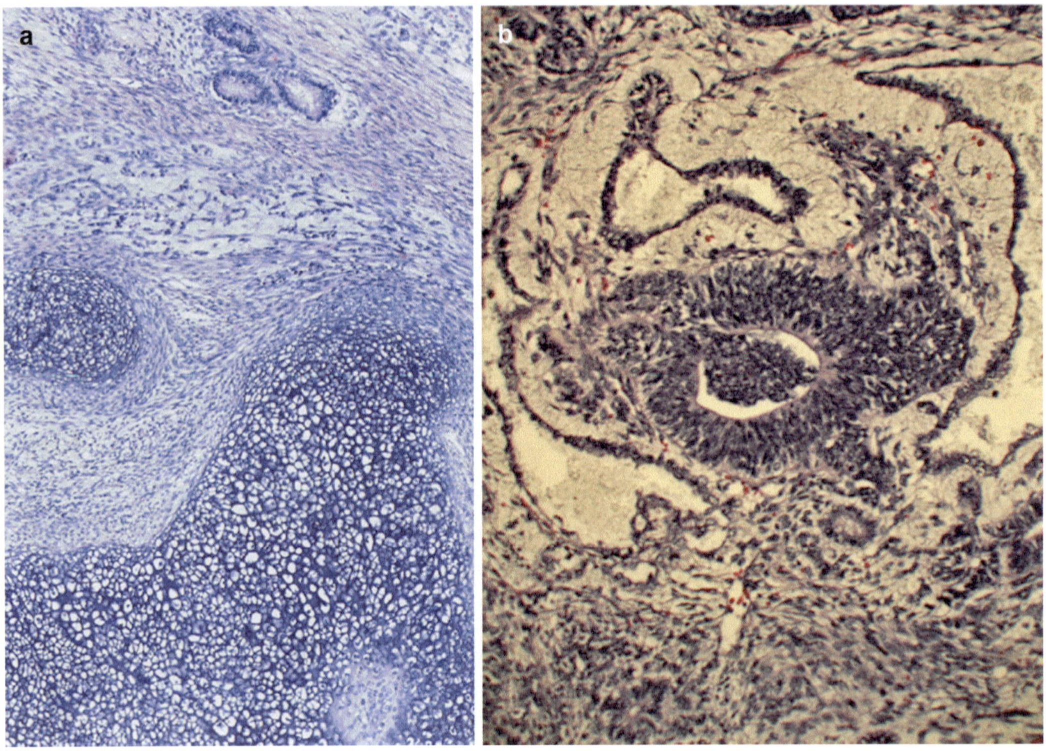

Fig. 6.45 Teratoma with immature tissue. (**a**) Immature cartilage and some immature cysts. (**b**) Neural tubelike structure

neoplasms, adenocarcinomas and squamous cell carcinomas predominate. Such malignancies are clinically important only if the somatic malignancy fills a field of view at low magnification (×4) (Fig. 6.49) [74], although this criterion is still under debate.

Immunohistochemistry

The different tissues in the tumor react with the same antibodies as their normal counterparts. SALL4 is positive in the epithelia of enteric-type glands [36] and is sometimes observed in a few tumor cells in PNET.

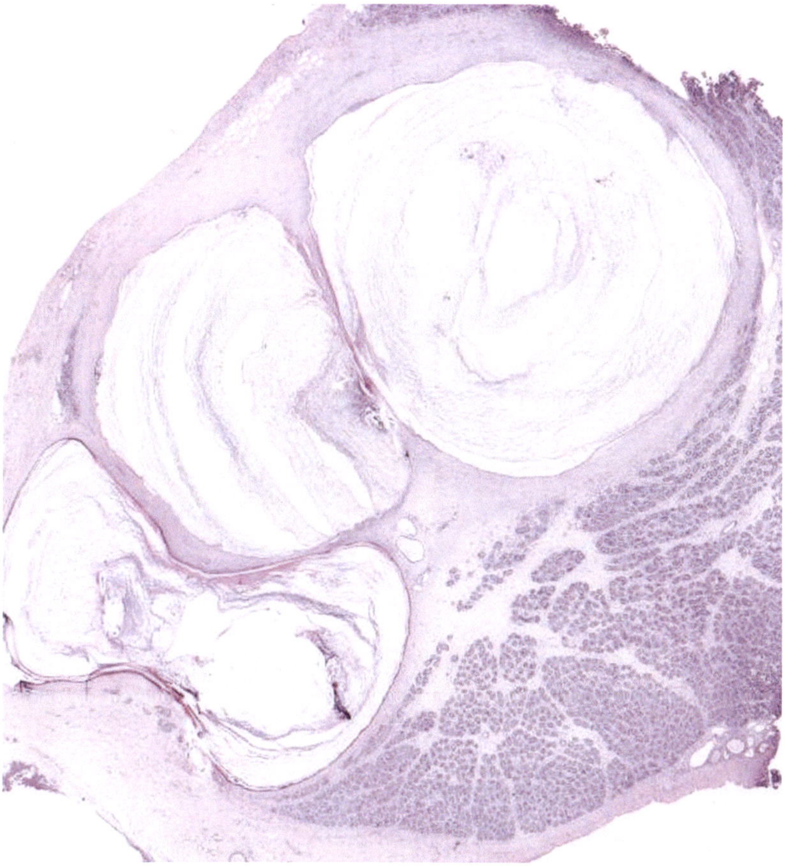

Fig. 6.46 Epidermoid cyst lined with squamous epithelium and filled with abundant amounts of keratin. No teratomatous or adnexal structures are present

DNA Ploidy and Cytogenetic Analysis

Teratomas are diploid in prepubertal and hypotriploid in postpubertal patients [75]. The i(12p) isochromosome is present in adults. Somatic-type malignancies can show aberrations typical of the respective somatic tumor (mostly translocations) as well as the i(12p) isochromosome that is specific for GCTs [76].

Differential Diagnosis

The histology of teratoma is characteristic insofar as the tumor cannot be mistaken for any other GCT. It is important, however, that in epidermoid and dermoid cysts with accurate sampling, other tissue components can be excluded. Moreover, there are several other, also benign cystic testicular lesions in childhood, which should be ruled out (Table 6.9).

Clinical Features

Painless testicular swelling is the main symptom. Since prepubertal teratoma does not metastasize, surgery, and for small tumors even parenchyma-sparing surgery, is the only necessary treatment [77]. Postpubertal teratomas metastasize first to the retroperitoneal lymph nodes and are resistant to chemotherapy and radiotherapy. Surgical removal of the lymph node and organ metastases is the only therapeutic option.

If in a somatic-type malignancy arising within a teratoma the tumor is limited to the testis, the prognosis is not negatively affected. In metastatic sites, somatic-type malignancies have a dismal prognosis. Colecchia et al. [78] reported a stage-specific survival of 100 % for patients with stage I tumors, 87.5 % for stage II, and 53 % for stage III.

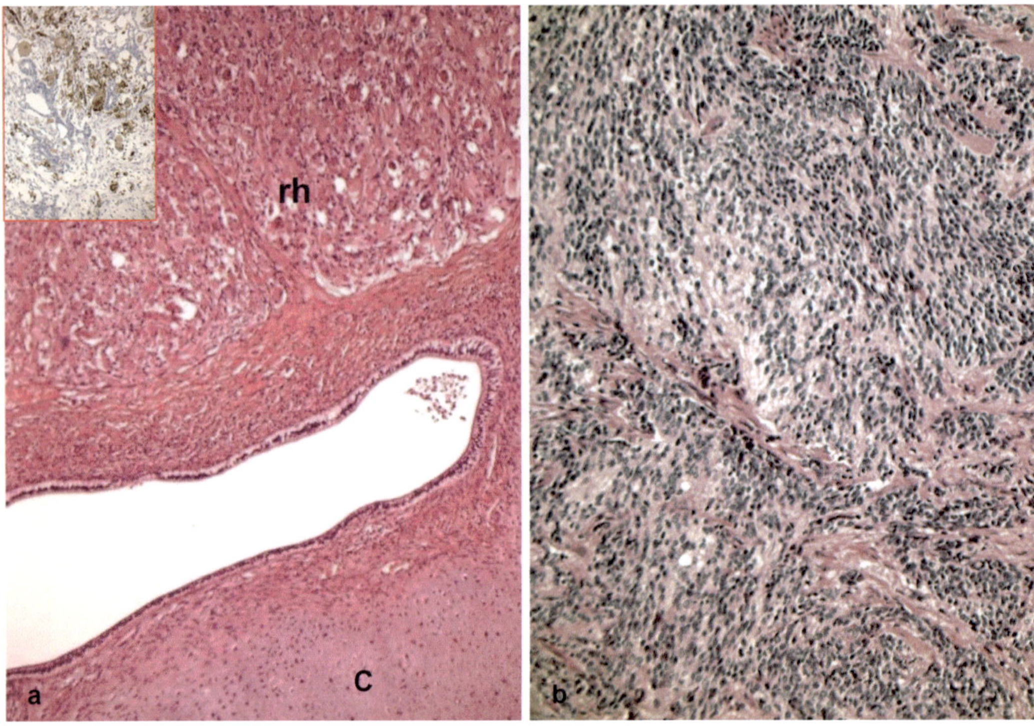

Fig. 6.47 Teratoma with somatic-type malignancy. (**a**) Differentiated cyst with rhabdomyosarcoma and a small cartilage component (*c*). Insert: Desmin-stained rhabdomyoblasts. (**b**) Primitive neuroectodermal tumor

Tumors of More Than One Histologic Type: Mixed Forms

Mixed forms account for 30–54 % of all GCTs and are about as frequent as seminomas. The macro- and micromorphology are dependent on the amount of the different components. Although the various types are randomly mixed, certain combinations are more frequent than others (Table 6.10) [79]. EC is with 80 % the most frequent component, and seminoma is present in about 15 % of mixed GCTs.

For the choice of treatment, it is important that seminomas are extensively sampled to rule out a nonseminomatous component (Fig. 6.50). High AFP in seminoma means that a nonseminomatous component has been overlooked. Unfortunately, serum AFP is meaningless for the pathologist because 15 % of NSGCTs are AFP negative.

The invasion of lymph or blood vessels is the most powerful predictor of relapse or metastases. A large EC component also negatively influences prognosis, whereas the presence of teratoma is a marker of favorable prognosis [80, 81]. The combination of percentage EC and vascular invasion allows correct prediction of the final pathologic stage in 88 % of patients [80].

Burned-Out Germ Cell Tumors (pT0)

Many old reports suggested that GCTs could regress spontaneously. Conclusive evidence for spontaneous GCT regression was established by Azzopardi et al. who examined autopsy material from patients who died of metastatic GCT but lacked testicular masses [82]. Retroperitoneal so-called extragonadal GCTs are almost always associated with a burned-out tumor in the testis, whereas GCT located in the mediastinum only rarely shows such an association. Intracranial GCTs growing in the pineal region do not have any relationship with testicular tumors. Our experience but also other studies [83] show that regression of testicular GCT is mostly associated with seminoma.

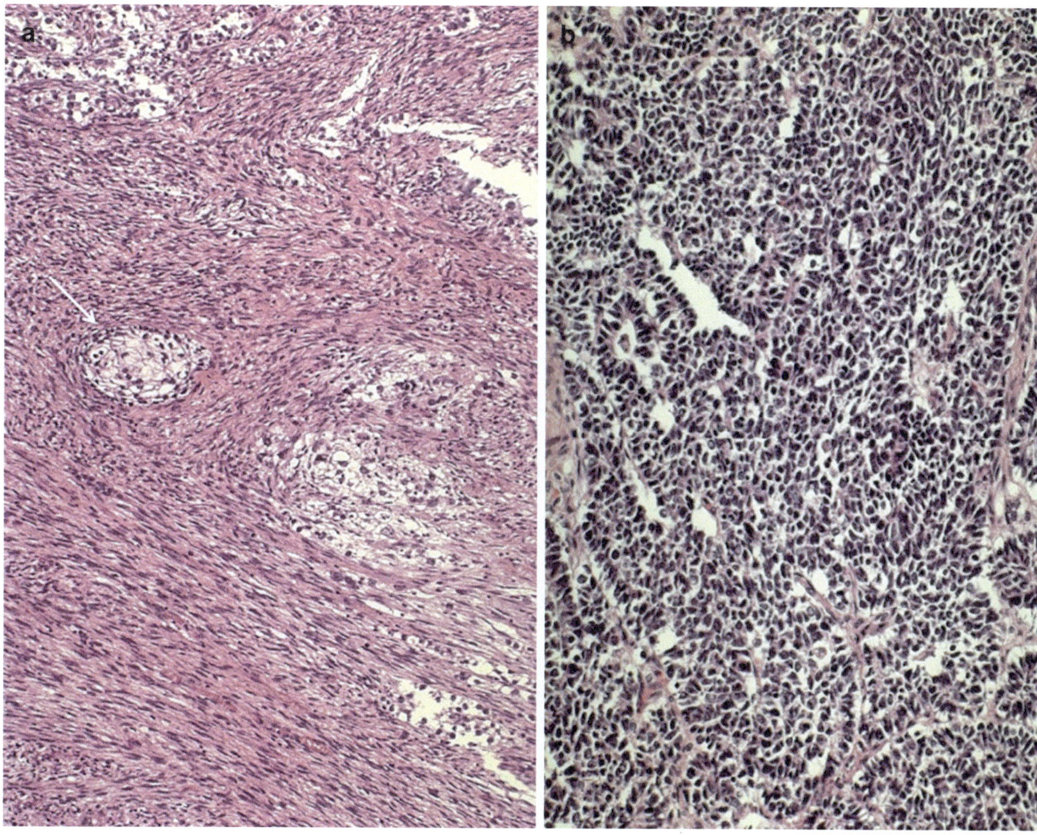

Fig. 6.48 Teratoma with somatic-type malignancy. (**a**) Leiomyosarcoma with entrapped immature squamous epithelium and scattered seminoma cells. (**b**) Nephroblastoma (Wilms' tumor) with immature blastematous cells and tubule formations

Morphology

Macroscopically, burned-out tumors consist of single or multiple scars (Fig. 6.51), and sometimes of cysts or cartilaginous areas. A well-demarcated, nodular scar with aggregates of proliferated Leydig cells in the surrounding atrophic testis is the main microscopic feature. The scar can show coarse calcification and scattered siderophages or foamy cells. The tubules of the surrounding parenchyma are atrophic with hyalinized or completely collapsed walls or may contain microliths (Fig. 6.52). In many cases, CIS can be detected [84].

Differential Diagnosis

One should keep in mind that also trauma or vascular disease may cause a testicular scar. Scars in a testicular biopsy without a retroperitoneal tumor are not a priori burned-out tumors, unless the scar is associated with CIS in the surrounding tubules.

Clinical Features

The prognosis and treatment of regressed GCT depend on the morphology of the primary tumor. Retroperitoneal metastases in young men are always suspicious for a primary tumor in the testis. A biopsy or surgical exploration with intraoperative frozen section is helpful for reaching a correct diagnosis. The detection of the tumor in the testis can be difficult even with ultrasound.

The pseudotubular pattern observed in Leydig tumor could represent in the intraoperative examination a pitfall about the stromal origin of the tumor (Fig. 6.53)

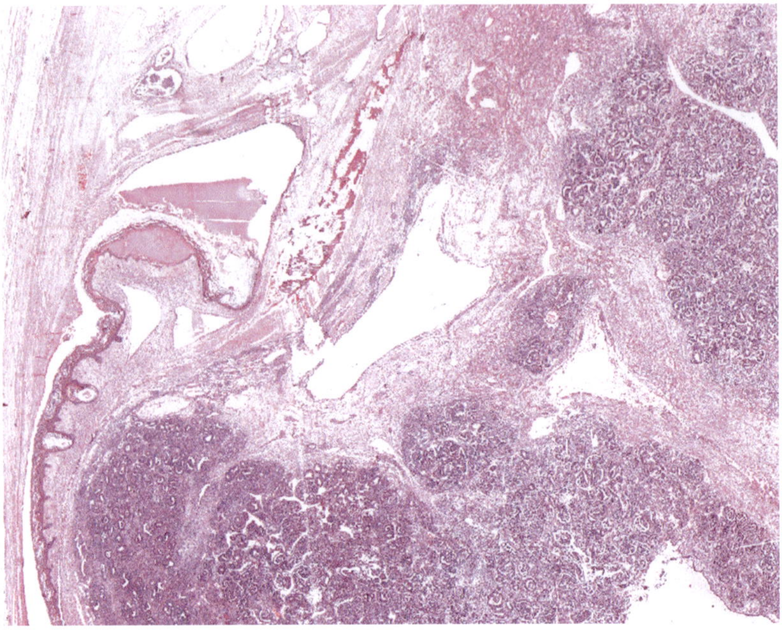

Fig. 6.49 The low-power field (x4) is entirely occupied by Wilms' tumor in an otherwise mature teratoma (Published with kind permission of ©Maurizio Colecchia 2015. All Rights Reserved)

Table 6.9 Cystic lesions occurring in the testis in childhood

Teratoma
Epidermoid cyst
Dermoid cyst
Yolk sac tumor
Cystadenoma of ovarian type
Granulosa cell tumor-juvenile type
Cystic lymphangioma
Cystic dysplasia of rete testis
Simple cyst

Table 6.10 Mixed germ cell tumors: some preferred combinations

Combination		OR	P value
Teratoma	Embryonal Ca	0.48	0.001
Teratoma	Chorioca	1.47	0.002
Teratoma	Yolk sac tumor	2.58	0.001
Teratoma	Seminoma	0.71	0.001
Embryonal Ca	Chorioca	1.23	0.149
Embryonal Ca	Yolk sac tumor	1.42	0.001
Embryonal Ca	Seminoma	0.55	0.001
Chorioca	Yolk sac tumor	1.38	0.007
Chorioca	Seminoma	0.65	0.002
Yolk sac tumor	Seminoma	0.95	0.552

Modified after Mosharafa et al. [79]

Retroperitoneal Lymph Node Dissection

RPLND is a standard procedure in the treatment of GCT. Because of the prognostic and therapeutic importance of retroperitoneal metastases, clinicians prefer to use staging systems (Table 6.11) and not the TNM algorithm (Table 6.12).

For adequate management of the disease, thorough sampling and histologic workup of the dissected lymph nodes is mandatory. Overlooked residual tumor can severely reduce the survival chances of the patient. Markers of unfavorable prognosis after chemotherapy include viable residual tumor, teratoma remnants, and the development of a somatic-type neoplasm.

Sex Cord/Gonadal Stromal Tumors

The name was chosen in analogy to the name given by Teilum [85] to the same type of tumors of the ovaries. These tumors arise in the gonads of both genders and only differ in the frequency of the individual subtypes. In the testis, Leydig and Sertoli cell tumors predominate, whereas in

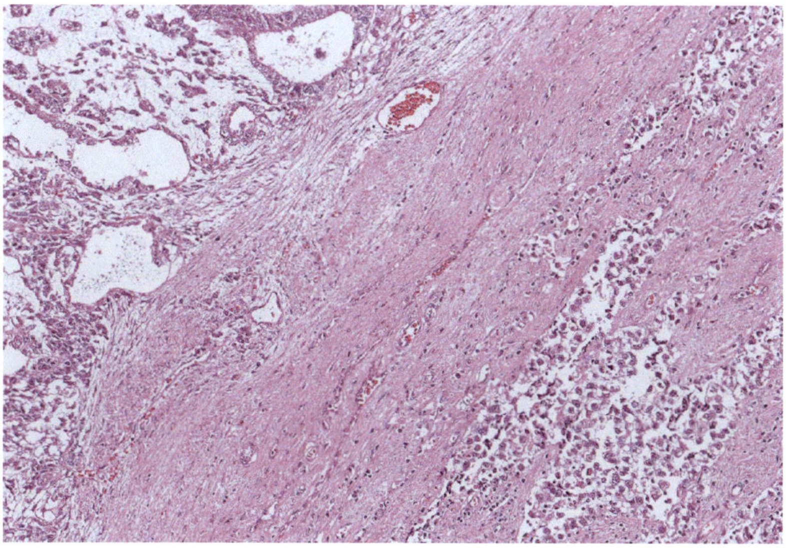

Fig. 6.50 Mixed germ cell tumor. Seminoma (*lower right*) and yolk sac tumor (*left*)

the ovary, granulosa cell and theca-fibroma-type tumors are the most frequent. In addition to differentiated, "pure-form" tumors, also mixed types and poorly differentiated or completely undifferentiated tumors exist.

In large series, these tumors account for only 3–6 % of adult testicular tumors but over 30 % of infant and childhood tumors. About 10 % of sex cord tumors metastasize and do so predominantly in adults. Nothing is known about the causes and pathohistogenesis of these tumors [4].

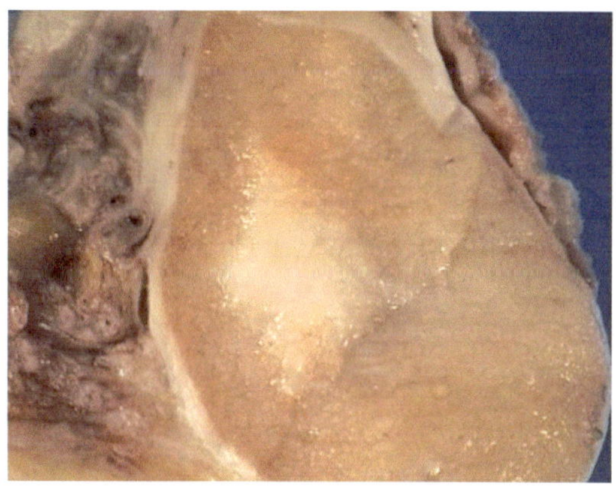

Fig. 6.51 Burned-out germ cell tumor. A whitish scar with the irregular contour in the testicular parenchyma

Leydig Cell Tumor

Leydig cell tumors (LCTs) are composed of more or less well-differentiated Leydig cells.

Epidemiology

LCT is the most frequent sex cord tumor, accounting for up to 3 % of testicular tumors. The average age at diagnosis is between 30 and 50 years; in 20 % of cases, patients are younger than 10 years of age, and in 25 %, they are older than 50 (range, 2–90 years) [4]. Three percent of LCTs are bilateral, and 5–10 % of patients have a history of cryptorchidism [86]. In a few cases, LCT was found to be associated with Klinefelter syndrome [87].

Morphology

On gross examination, LCTs are on average 2–3 cm in diameter (range, 0.5–10 cm). They have a thin fibrous capsule and a brown color of different shades (yellowish, reddish, and dark brown) as observed in metastatic localization too (Fig. 6.54). Tumors with a diameter ≥5 cm are almost without exception malignant.

Microscopically, the tumor is composed of nests or sheets of polyhedral cells with eosinophilic cytoplasm and big round to oval nuclei with prominent nucleoli (Fig. 6.55). Multinucleated nuclei may occur. Reinke

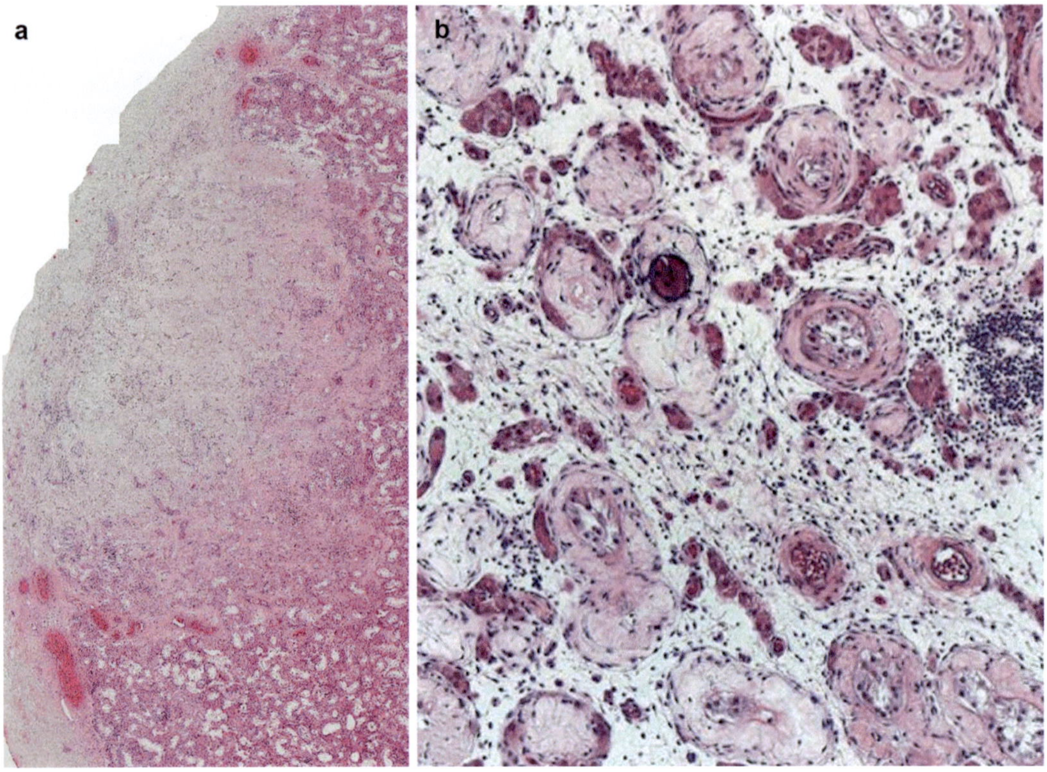

Fig. 6.52 Burned-out germ cell tumor. (**a**) Large scar surrounded by atrophic testicular parenchyma. (**b**) Atrophic tissue surrounding the scar with hyalinized tubules, lymphocytic infiltration, and intratubular calcification (microlithiasis)

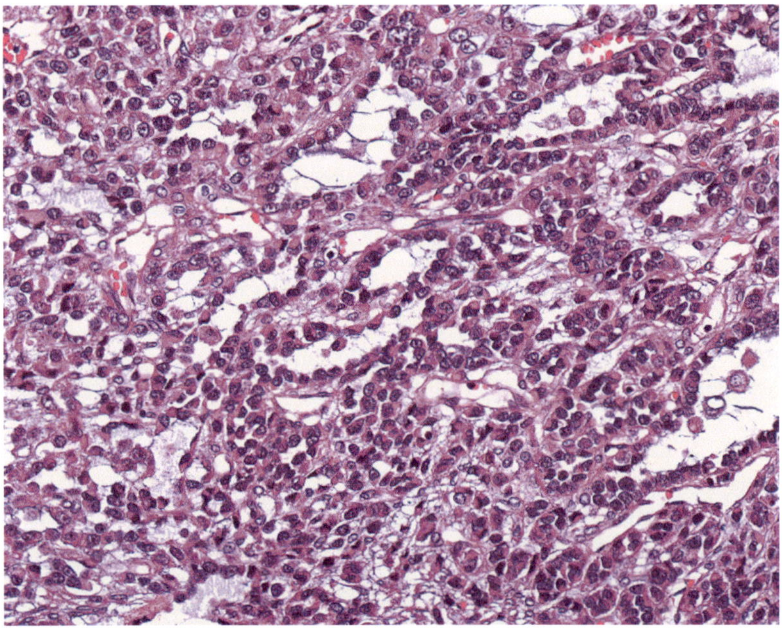

Fig. 6.53 Leydig cell tumor showing pseudotubular structures (Published with kind permission of ©Maurizio Colecchia 2015. All Rights Reserved)

Table 6.11 Prognostic factors of seminoma and nonseminomatous germ cell tumors

Features	Seminoma	Nonseminomatous GCT
Size	>4 cm *unfavorable*	Insignificant
Rete testis invasion	*Unfavorable*	Insignificant
Vascular invasion	Insignificant	*Unfavorable*
High amount (%) of EC		*Unfavorable*
In absence of EC S-phase fraction >29 %	Insignificant	*Unfavorable*
Presence of teratoma		Favorable

Table 6.12 Clinical tumor stages and corresponding TNM stages

Clinical staging AJCC	TNM
Stage 0 Tis	N0, M0, S0
Stage IA	T1, N0, M0, S0
Stage IB	T2–T4, N0, M0, S0
Stage IC	Any T, N0, M0, S1–S3
Stage IIA	Any T, N1, M0, S0–S1
Stage IIB	Any T, N2, M0, S0 S1
Stage IIC	Any T, N2, M0, S0–S1
Stage IIIA	Any T, any N, M1a, S0–S1
Stage IIIB	Any T, any N, M0–M1a, S2
Stage IIIC	Any T, any N, M0–M1a, S3 or any T, any N,M1b, any S

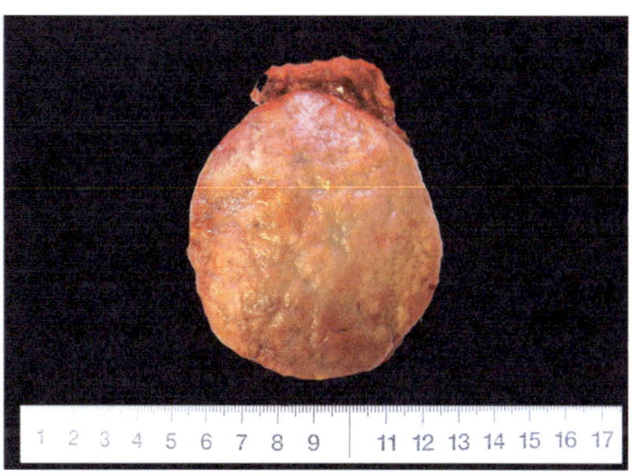

Fig. 6.54 Metastatic Leydig cell tumor. A para-aortic nodule with brownish color and small necrotic areas (Published with kind permission of ©Maurizio Colecchia 2015. All Rights Reserved)

crystalloids are visible in about one-third and lipofuscin in 15 % of cases. The stroma is scanty with a network of capillaries typical of endocrine tumors. Some tumors are composed of spindle cells (sarcoma-like) or cells with a large quantity of intracytoplasmic lipids (Fig. 6.56). Even psammoma bodies and calcifications have been described [88].

The most important feature of malignant LCT is its size, which on average is about 7 cm versus <3 cm in benign LCT. Mitoses are obviously also more frequent in malignant than benign tumors 13.9/HPF vs. 1.9/HPF. Further microscopic indi cators of malignancy are a spindled cell shape, nuclear atypia and polymorphism (Fig. 6.57), necrosis (Fig. 6.58), vascular invasion, and invasion of surrounding tissue [86, 89]. The number of proliferating cells (Ki67/MIB-1) is also greater in malignant LCT [89]. However, to predict a malignant course, at least two of these features should be present. In fact, only metastases provide the conclusive evidence of malignancy; one should therefore be somewhat restrictive in the histopathologic diagnosis of malignancy (Table 6.13).

Immunohistochemistry

There are a number of antibodies that react more or less with all sex cord tumors (see Table 6.14); however, only rarely are 100 % of the cells of a given tumor type positive, and a negative result therefore does not exclude such a tumor [90].

Over 90 % of LCTs are positive for calretinin, α-inhibin, melan-A, and steroidogenic factor 1 (SF1). But they also stain with β-catenin, CD99, FOXL2, and synaptophysin and in 20 % of cases with CK and S100. In some cases, the use of androgen receptor antibodies can be helpful. The only antibody that does not react with this tumor is WT1 [90].

DNA Ploidy and Cytogenetic Analysis

As is well known, also benign endocrine tumors can have an aneuploid stem line [91]. It is therefore not surprising that all metastasizing LCTs but also 30 % of benign LCTs are aneuploid. For this reason, ploidy cannot be used as an absolute marker of malignancy.

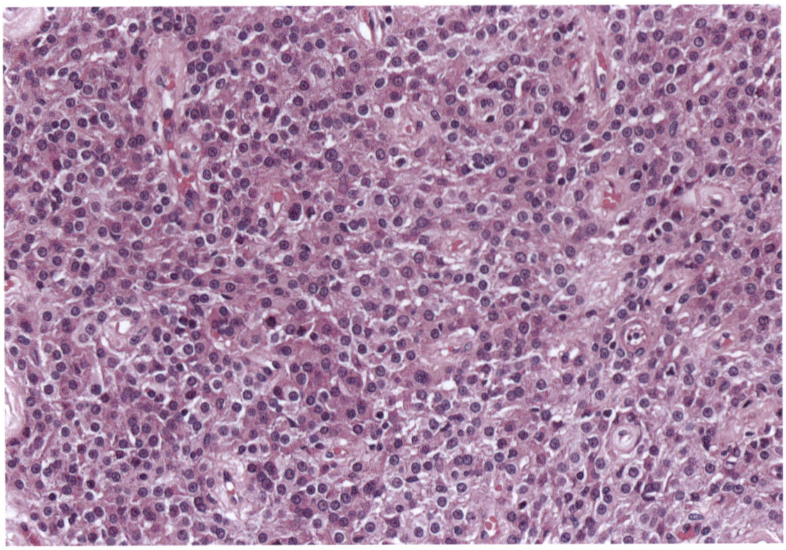

Fig. 6.55 Leydig cell tumor. The tumor cells have abundant eosinophilic cytoplasm and regular round nuclei with inconspicuous nucleoli

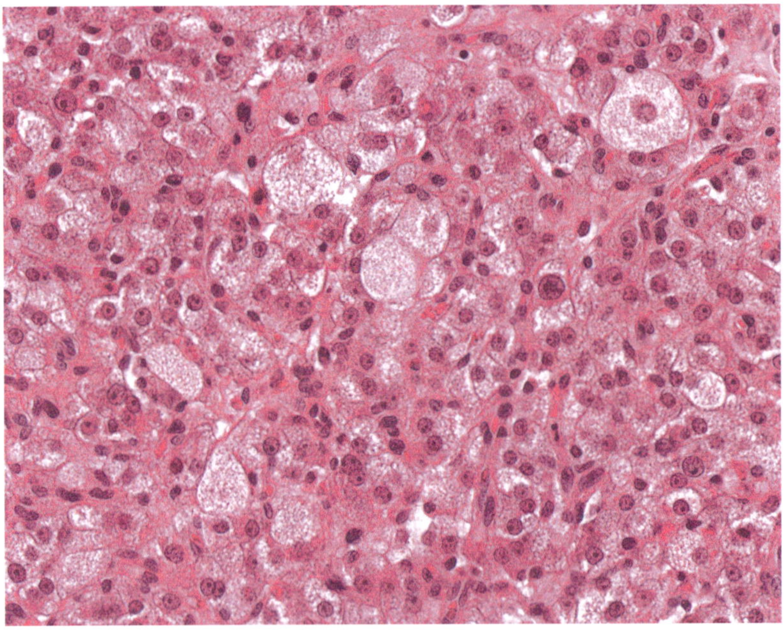

Fig. 6.56 Leydig cell tumor. The cytoplasm is extensively vacuolated or spongy due to abundant lipid

The genetic features of the uncommon sex cord tumors are largely unknown. FISH analysis showed in 21/25 (84 %) of LCTs gain of chromosome X (Fig. 6.59), 19 or 19p, and loss of chromosomes 8 and 16 [92]. In two boys with LCT, LH-receptor gene mutations were detected [93].

Differential Diagnosis

Three benign diseases can be mistaken for LCT. The most common is Leydig cell hyperplasia, which is commonly detected in cryptorchid testes and in Klinefelter syndrome. Unlike LCT, the hyperplasia is nodular and multifocal. Among

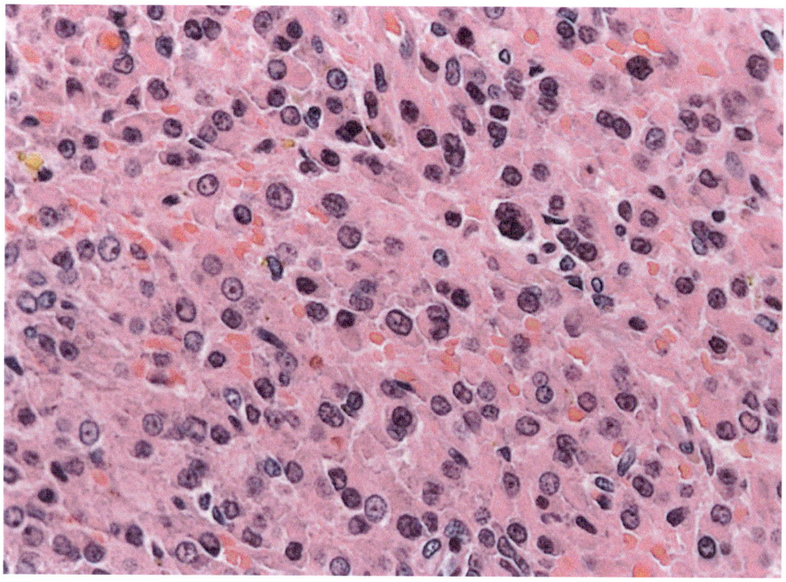

Fig. 6.57 Malignant Leydig cell tumor. Slight cellular and nuclear polymorphism

the hyperplastic nodules, well-preserved or atrophic tubules can be observed, a feature which excludes a tumor diagnosis.

On the inner surface of the nuclear membrane, one Barr body (sex chromatin) is visible at higher magnification in Klinefelter syndrome. In humans with more than one X chromosome, the number of visible Barr bodies is always one less than the total number of X chromosomes.

In rare malacoplakia of the testis, large macrophages with eosinophilic granular cytoplasm show some similarity to Leydig cells. These inflammatory cells contain basophilic inclusions called Michaelis-Gutmann bodies and are strongly reactive for the macrophage marker CD68 and negative for α-inhibin.

Testicular tumor of adrenogenital syndrome (TTAGS) is a rare, mostly bilateral neoplasm, the cells of which resemble Leydig cells. Misdiagnosis of this tumor may have as its consequence an absolutely unnecessary bilateral orchiectomy. TTAGS regresses "spontaneously" under steroid therapy. Like in hyperplasia, tubules are entrapped among the proliferated tumor cells. The tumor cells are larger than those of LCT and are filled with dark-brown lipochrome pigment. Immunohistochemically, TTAGS shows diffuse and strong positivity for CD56 (NCAM) and negative reactivity for androgen receptor. In contrast, LCT displays focal weak to moderate (or negative) reactivity for CD56 and positive reactivity for androgen receptor [94].

Even melanoma metastases can mimic an LCT and, like LCT, they are melan-A positive [95].

Clinical Features

In about half of the patients, unilateral testicular swelling is the presenting symptom; another frequent symptom is gynecomastia, which may also precede the swelling. Twenty-five percent of adults suffer from loss of libido and impotence because the tumor produces estrogen [86]. Prepubertal LCT produces testosterone and can cause pubertas praecox, in which case penile growth and pubic hair growth are the most common symptoms, followed by facial acne and a deep voice. Precocious closure of the growth plates arrests the longitudinal growth of the bones. Boys affected by LCT are aggressive and withdrawn. Twenty percent of malignant LCTs have already metastasized at the time of diagnosis. The average age at diagnosis is 67 years, which is significantly older than in benign tumors [41]. Prepubertal malignancy is rare.

Metastases first appear in the retroperitoneal lymph nodes (72 %); the tumor then spreads by

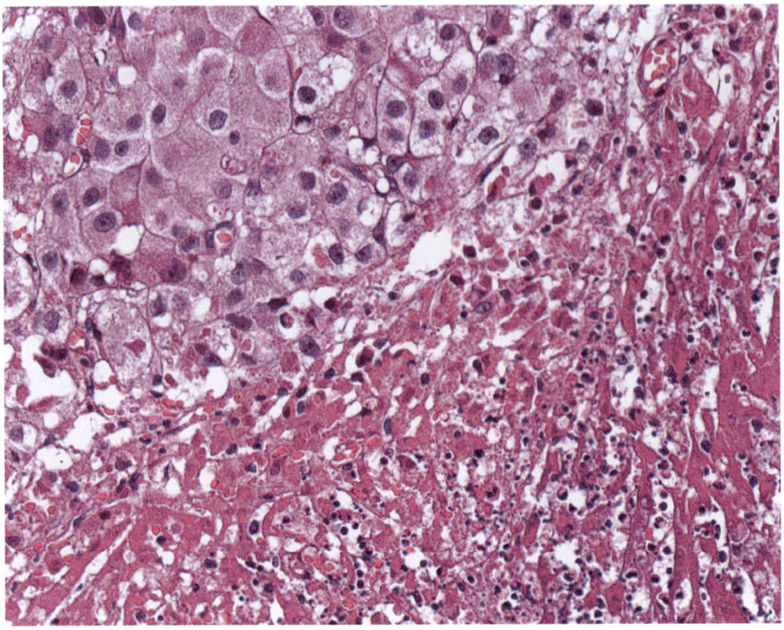

Fig. 6.58 Malignant Leydig cell tumor. Microscopic findings in a necrotic area of the metastatic tumor reported in Fig. 6.53 (Published with kind permission of ©Maurizio Colecchia 2015. All Rights Reserved)

Table 6.13 Malignancy criteria of Leydig- and Sertoli-cell tumors

Leydig cell tumor		Sertoli cell tumor
Only adults; never in infants		At any age; >30 % gynecomastia
	Diameter >5 cm	
	High mitotic count (normal average 1.9/HPF)	
	Spindled cell shape	
	Nuclear atypia and polymorphism	
	Necrosis	
	Vascular invasion	
	Invasion of surrounding tissue	

Only the diameter is a very reliable single prognostic factor. The other listed features are as a single criterion unreliable. For the prediction of malignancy, more of them must be present

the hematogenous route to the lungs (43 %), liver (38 %), and bones (28 %) [96]. Since LCTs are resistant to chemotherapy, orchiectomy with RPLND and radiotherapy is the only therapeutic option. The prognosis is dismal, and on average, patients do not survive more than 5 years.

Sertoli Cell Tumor

Sertoli cell tumor (SCT) is a tumor of the gonadal stroma; it is composed of cells resembling embryonal, prepubertal, and adult Sertoli cells.

Epidemiology

SCTs are rare and account for only 1 % of testicular tumors. The average age at diagnosis is 45 years. Before the age of 20, SCT is even rarer, unless it is associated with Peutz-Jeghers syndrome or Carney's complex. The occurrence of bilateral tumors is also extremely rare.

Morphology

The tumor is encapsulated and rather small (average, 3.5 cm). The color of the cut surface may contain various shades of yellowish (yellowish white, gray, or tan). The tumor cells form well or poorly shaped tubular structures

Table 6.14 Immunohistochemistry useful for the diagnostic of sex cord/gonadal stroma tumors [90]

Antibody	LCT	SCT	USCST	GCT	LCCST	TTAG
SF-1	92	75	57	50	50	100
FOXL2	21	83	67	100	–	–
B-catenin	50	83	60	100	50	100
Inhibin	97	67	38	67	75	100
Melan-A	94	67	75	50	50	100
Calretinin	97	56	75	44	75	100
WT1	0	82	57	50	75	50
CD99	74	56	25	86	0	0
Synaptophysin	65	24	29	0	0	50
CK	22	78	17	43	67	–
S100	28	28	43	38	75	0

LCT Leydig CT, *SCT* Sertoli CT, *USCST* unclassified CST, *GCT* granulosa CT, *LCCST* large-cell calcifying SCT, *TTAG* testicular tumor of adrenogenital syndrome

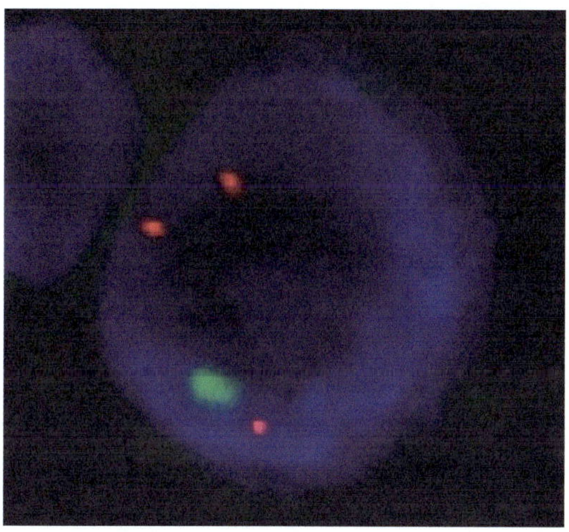

Fig. 6.59 Interphase FISH of Leydig cell tumor: three signals (*red*) for chromosome X

(Fig. 6.60). The cytoplasm is usually eosinophilic but sometimes contains a large amount of lipids (the lipid-rich variant listed in the WHO classification of 2004 [4], though not as an entity of its own). The tubules can be highly differentiated with a clearly visible basement membrane lined with rather well-differentiated Sertoli cells having oval vesicular nuclei and prominent reddish nucleoli. Less differentiated tumors are composed of spindle-shaped cells growing in solid sheets, which are barely recognizable as Sertoli cells. Between the well- and less differentiated tumors, all possible transitional forms are possible. Heterologous carcinosarcomatous components were observed in one case [97].

Among the tumor cell formations, bands of fibrous tissue can be present in various amounts. The exuberant sclerotic stroma is the hallmark of sclerosing SCT [98] (Fig. 6.61).

Like other malignant sex cord tumors, malignant SCTs are quite large (7–15 cm) and show nuclear pleomorphism and occasionally invasion of the lymph vessels.

Immunohistochemistry

The best markers are β-catenin, FOXL2, and WT1, although they stain no more than 80 % of SCTs. The reactivity of all other markers ranges between 28 and 75 % [90]. In many cases, immunohistochemistry is not very helpful for reaching a correct diagnosis.

DNA Ploidy and Cytogenetic Analysis

The genetic features of these uncommon tumors are largely unknown. In a small series, five of 11 patients showed gain of chromosome X, and two patients showed complete loss of chromosome 2 [99]. The importance of these findings for tumor pathohistogenesis is unclear. Mutations of the *CTNNB1* (cadherin-associated protein β1) gene were reported in a recent study, and the authors argued that this mutation was likely to be involved in the pathogenesis of SCT, causing nuclear accumulation of β-catenin and affecting the expression of cyclin D1 (Fig. 6.62) [100].

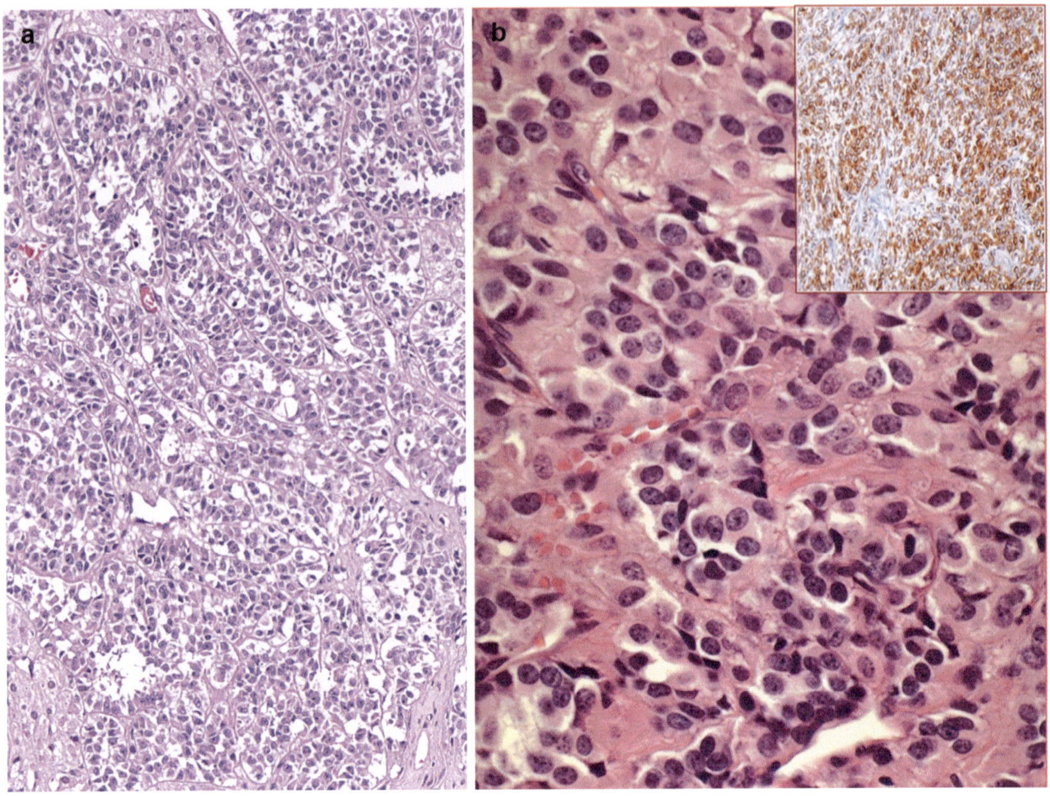

Fig. 6.60 Sertoli cell tumor. (**a**) Sertoli cell tumor with tubular structures lined with well-differentiated Sertoli cells; (**b**) Solid-growing less differentiated Sertoli cell tumor. Insert: α-inhibin positive tumor cells

Differential Diagnosis

Hypoplastic zones (Sertoli cell nodules), a very common feature of cryptorchid testes, should not be mistaken for SCT. Such nodules are well circumscribed and are composed of prepubertal seminiferous tubules with a prominent basement membrane and lined with immature Sertoli cells. In testicular feminization, Sertoli "microadenomas" are a characteristic feature; it is, however, not clear whether these are true neoplasms or reactive hyperplastic nodules.

The tubular variant of seminoma can easily be mistaken for SCT, but in the surrounding tubules, CIS is present. If necessary, PLAP immunohistochemistry will bring clarity.

Adenomatoid tumors (which are positive for calretinin, CK, and vimentin and negative for α-inhibin) are rarely located in the testis. Intracytoplasmic vacuoles and the spindle shape of the tumor cells distinguish adenomatoid tumor from SCT.

Clinical Features

The main symptom is testicular swelling. If the tumor produces estrogen, gynecomastia, loss of libido, and impotence are likely to occur. Gynecomastia seems to be more frequent in malignant cases.

About 12 % of SCTs are malignant; malignant cases have also been reported in children [101, 102]. The distribution of organ metastases is very similar to that of LCT. Orchiectomy is the only therapeutic option, because radiotherapy and chemotherapy have been unsuccessful to date.

Large-Cell Calcifying Sertoli Cell Tumor (LCCSCT)

LCCSCT is a morphologic but also nosologic variant of SCT, morphologically characterized by coarse calcifications and clinically by its possible

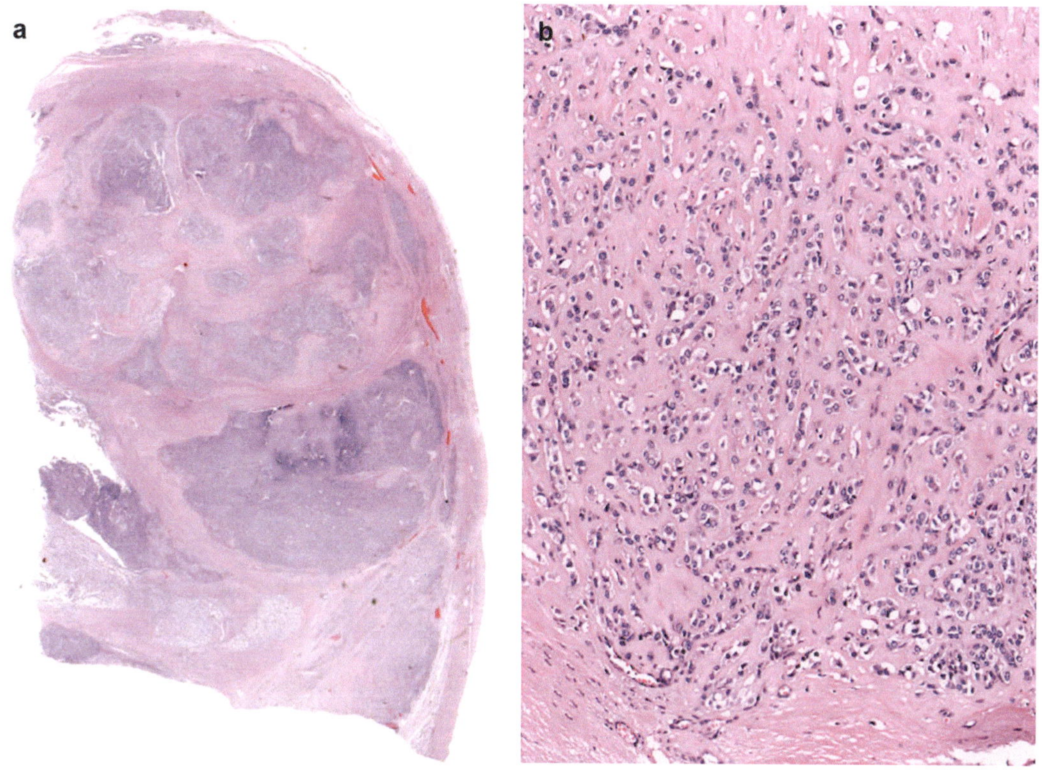

Fig. 6.61 Sclerosing Sertoli cell tumor. (**a**) Overview shows broad hyaline bands dissecting the tumor. (**b**) Tumor cells entrapped in an abundant hyaline stroma

association with Peutz-Jeghers syndrome and Carney's complex (syndromic LCCSCT).

Epidemiology

LCCSCT was first described in adolescents and later also in adult and aged men. In young men (mean age, 17 years; range, 2–38 years), the tumor is mostly benign, bilateral, and multifocal. Thirty-six of benign tumors in adolescents are associated with other endocrine disorders (mostly Carney's complex) [103]. Malignant LCCSCT occurs in adults (mean age, 39 years; range, 28–73 years), is unilateral and solitary, and is usually not associated with endocrine syndromes, although an exception has been described in the literature [104, 105] (Table 6.15).

Morphology

LCCSCT is typically yellow or tan white on section (Fig. 6.63). Due to calcifications, the surface is gritty. Benign tumors are confined to the testis, while malignant tumors can extend to the neighboring organs. Benign LCCSCTs are smaller (range, 0.8–2.3 cm) than malignant ones (range, 2–15 cm), which can replace the entire testicular parenchyma. Foci of necrosis and hemorrhage are typical for malignant LCCSCTs [104, 105].

Large, irregular, and confluent calcifications are the microscopic hallmark and the namegiver of these tumors, regardless of the tumor's biologic behavior. The tumor cells are large with eosinophilic, finely granular cytoplasm and oval nuclei with one or two small to occasionally prominent nucleoli (Fig. 6.64). The tumor cells resemble Leydig cells more than Sertoli cells; in fact, their true origin was revealed by electron microscopy [106]. They are growing in tubules, cords, or trabeculae embedded in a myxoid (Fig. 6.65) or fibrous stroma with lymphocytic infiltrates. Intratubular growth is not rare.

Except for the cellular polymorphism, the cytomorphology of malignant LCCSCT is not

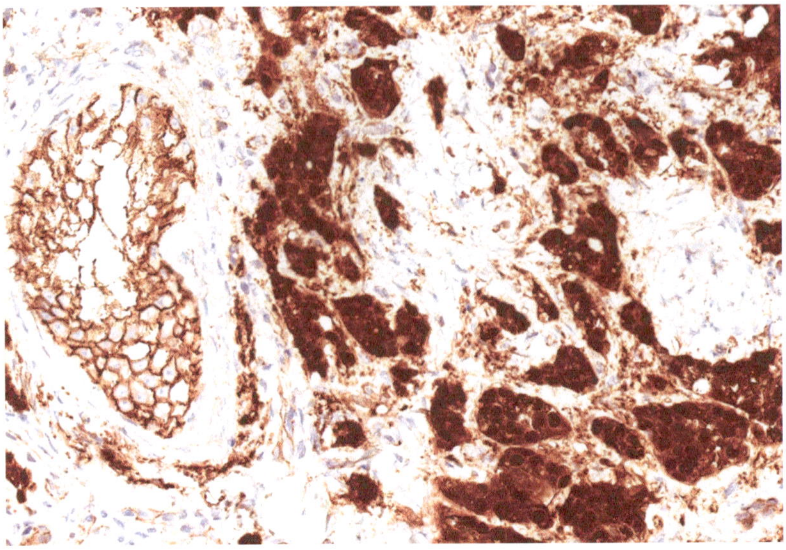

Fig. 6.62 Sertoli cell tumor. Immunoreactivity with β-catenin antibody. The nuclear and cytoplasmic reaction is diffuse in the tumor cells

different from that of the benign variant, but the mitotic activity is brisk (4–14/HPF) compared with the benign counterpart in which mitoses are lacking . Thus, metastases are the only true evidence of malignancy.

Immunohistochemically these tumors behave like the other SCTs. Cytogenetic investigations do not exist.

Differential Diagnosis

Even though the tumor cells microscopically resemble Leydig cells, the lack of a capsule, calcifications, and intratubular growth are features not found in LCT. Moreover, the gross morphology is completely different.

Clinical Features

Painless testicular swelling is the only symptom in sporadic, nonsyndromic cases. Forty percent of cases in adolescent or young men are, however, associated with Carney's complex, which is an autosomal dominant condition. The main symptoms are spotty skin pigmentation, lentigines, and cardiac myxomas, which may lead to embolic stroke and heart failure and even to sudden death [107]. Myxomas may also occur outside the heart, usually in the skin and breast. Endocrine tumors may manifest as disorders such as Cushing's syndrome. The most common endocrine gland manifestation is an ACTH-independent Cushing's syndrome due to primary pigmented adrenocortical microadenomas. STH-producing pituitary microadenoma with acromegaly has also been reported [108].

Table 6.15 Main clinical differences between benign and malignant large-cell calcifying Sertoli cell tumor

Features	Benign LCCSCT	Malignant LCCSCT
Age	Average 17 (range 2–38)	Average 39 (range 28–73)
Location	28 % bilateral and multifocal	Unilateral and unifocal
Association with Carney complex or other endocrine disease	36 %	Almost never

Granulosa Cell Tumor

Granulosa cell tumors of the testis are macro- and microscopically equal to those arising in the ovaries. Because of the different morphology and clinical behavior, two types are distinguished: an adult and a juvenile type.

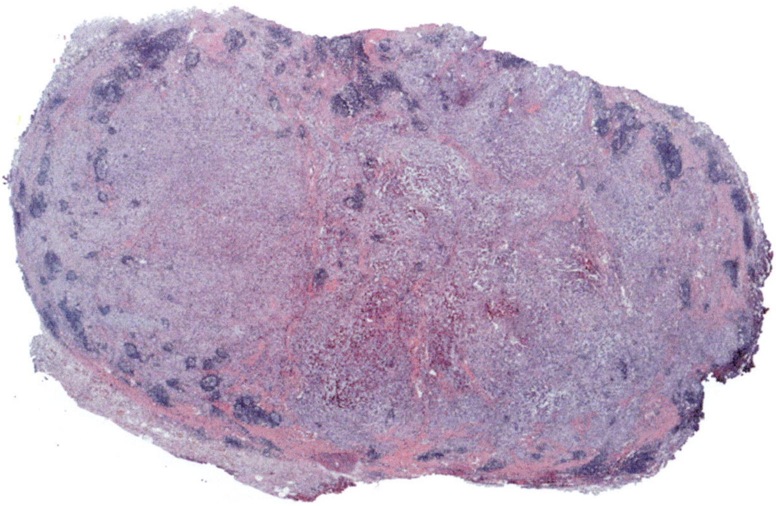

Fig. 6.63 Overview of a large-cell calcifying Sertoli cell tumor which replaces the entire testicular parenchyma. Irregular calcifications are easily visible in the center. The blue areas randomly dispersed in the tumor are lymphocytic infiltrations

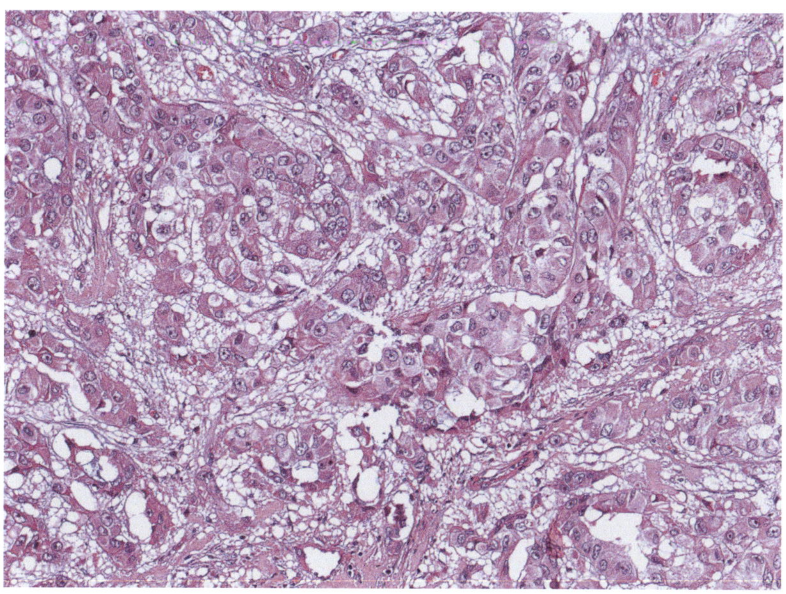

Fig. 6.64 Large-cell calcifying Sertoli cell tumor. The tumor cells have abundant eosinophilic cytoplasm (Published with kind permission of ©Maurizio Colecchia 2015. All Rights Reserved)

Adult Type Granulosa Cell Tumor

Epidemiology

Adult type granulosa cell tumor is believed to be one of the most infrequent testicular tumors. In a recent publication [109], 43 cases were reviewed, but two additional cases were reported shortly after [110, 111]. The tumor arises predominantly between the ages of 40 and 60 (median, 45 years; range, 12–83 years), and only one case has occurred in an adolescent. About 10 % of the reported cases had a malignant course [109].

Morphology

The cut surface has a lobulated appearance; its color is yellow and small cysts can be present.

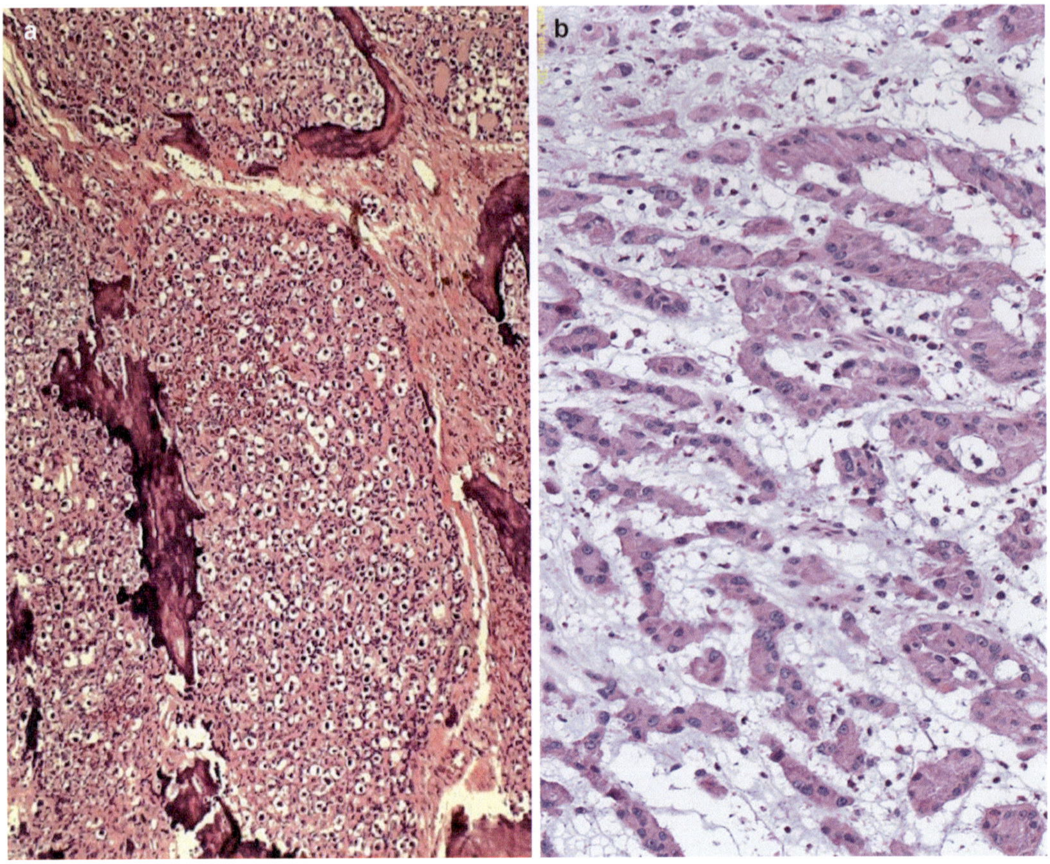

Fig. 6.65 Large-cell calcifying Sertoli cell tumor with irregularly shaped calcifications (**a**) and tumor cells resembling Leydig cells more than Sertoli cells (**b**) embedded in a mucoid stroma

The tumor diameter ranges from 0.7 to 13 cm. Microscopically, the cells have scant cytoplasm, and the nuclei are typically grooved like coffee beans (Fig. 6.66). Many microscopic patterns have been recognized including trabecular, insular, gyriform, macrofollicular, and microfollicular patterns. Call-Exner bodies are usually present though not always. A sarcomatous "heterologous" pattern was observed in one case [109]. Mitoses are rare and there are no microscopically identifiable indicators of malignancy.

Immunohistochemistry

The best immunohistochemical markers of granulosa cell tumor are β-catenin and FOXL2, which are reactive in 100 % of cases (Table 6.14). Other antibodies used in stromal tumors are positive in 50 % of cases at the most [90].

DNA Ploidy and Cytogenetic Analysis

Cytogenetic studies have been performed only in ovarian granulosa cell tumor. The few pertinent studies do not show uniform results. Eighty percent of these tumors are diploid [112]. The main chromosomal aberrations are trisomy 12, monosomy 22 and X, and loss of chromosome 22 [112]. A somatic mutation of the *FOXL2* gene has been reported in virtually all adult type granulosa cell tumors in women. In men the mutation has been found in a smaller proportion than in women [109, 113].

Clinical Features

Apart from testicular swelling, 25 % of men with adult type granulosa cell tumors suffer from gynecomastia. Serum inhibin and anti-müllerian hormone (AMH) are elevated. About 10 % of reported cases were malignant. Reliable morphologic features predictive of malignancy do not exist; hence, the histopathology report should be signed off with the comment that malignancy cannot be excluded. Many of these tumors have been observed to metastasize after years.

Juvenile Type Granulosa Cell Tumor

Epidemiology

Juvenile type granulosa cell tumor is the most common testicular tumor in the perinatal period; it is typically detected before the sixth month of life [114]. It may develop in the gonad of a patient with an abnormal karyotype and ambiguous genitalia and also in infants with true hermaphroditism [115, 116].

Morphology

Given the age of the patients, juvenile type granulosa cell tumors are mostly small and do not exceed a diameter of 2 cm. The cut surface is yellow and shows small cysts. Microscopically, the cysts are lined with cells resembling granulosa cells (Figs. 6.67 and 6.68). Among the cysts, tubules with proliferated Sertoli cells form bizarre structures. The high mitotic count can erroneously suggest malignancy.

Immunohistochemistry

The epithelium lining the cysts stains with different CK antibodies (CK8, CK18, CK19, CAM5.2), α-inhibin, vimentin, and very strongly with AMH [114, 117]. A positive reaction with S100 protein, smooth muscle actin (SMA), and desmin has been observed occasionally.

DNA Ploidy and Cytogenetic Analysis

The number of cytogenetic studies is very limited. In one report, the tumor cells had an aneuploid DNA stem line in the majority of cases. Aneuploid tumors manifested polysomy 12 and monosomy X [118].

Differential Diagnosis

Because of the age of the patients and to a lesser degree the presence of certain similarities, this tumor may be confused with YST, which can be a tragic mistake inasmuch as juvenile type granulosa cell tumor is totally benign and does not require any treatment other than simple surgical enucleation. Compared to YST, the morphology of juvenile granulosa cell tumor is very monotonous. Furthermore, YSTs do not have follicular structures and are positive for AFP. Mistaking a juvenile granulosa cell tumor for a teratoma is less harmful because the therapeutic approach is the same for both tumors.

Clinical Features

Unilateral swelling, predominantly of the left testis, is the only symptom. As already mentioned, these tumors tend to arise in cryptorchid testes (30 %) and in children with dysgenetic gonads and ambiguous genital organs. If possible, simple enucleation of the tumor is the preferred treatment [119].

Thecoma-Fibroma-Type Tumors

The 25 cases known so far [4, 120] were observed in men in their fourth to fifth decade. These tumors are firm, white, and well circumscribed.

Morphology and Immunohistochemistry

The solid, encapsulated, grayish-white testicular mass displays the characteristics of testicular fibroma. The tumor is composed of cellular collagenized plaques and hypercellular areas of fibroblastic spindle cells (Fig. 6.69). Immunohistochemically, the neoplastic cells are reactive to vimentin and SMA.

Differential Diagnosis

Similar tumors arising in the testicular tunics or spermatic cord can invade the testis. Macroscopic inspection will reveal the true location.

Clinical Features

A painful palpable lump is the main symptom of these innocuous tumors.

Mixed Forms and Incompletely Differentiated Gonadal Stromal Tumors

These tumors are composed of randomly mixed Leydig, Sertoli, and granulosa cells as well as

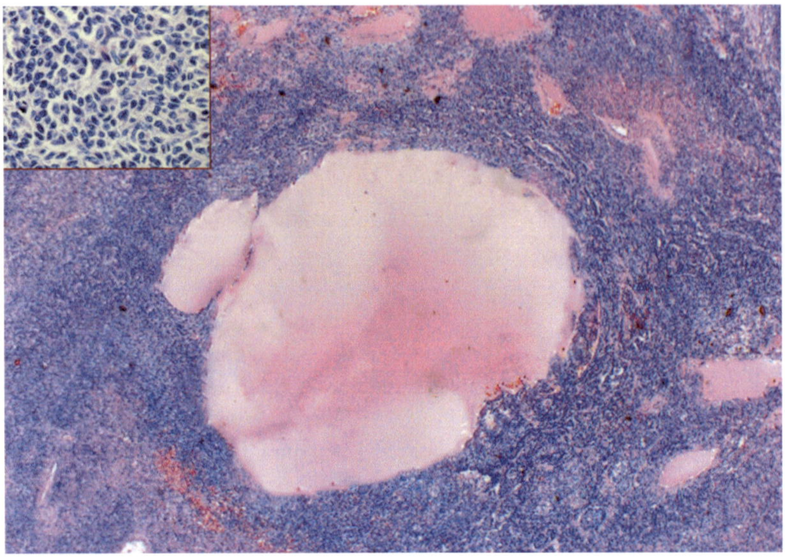

Fig. 6.66 Adult type granulosa cell tumor, with colloid-filled cyst simulating ovarian follicles. Insert: Tumor cells with typical grooved, coffee-bean-like nuclei

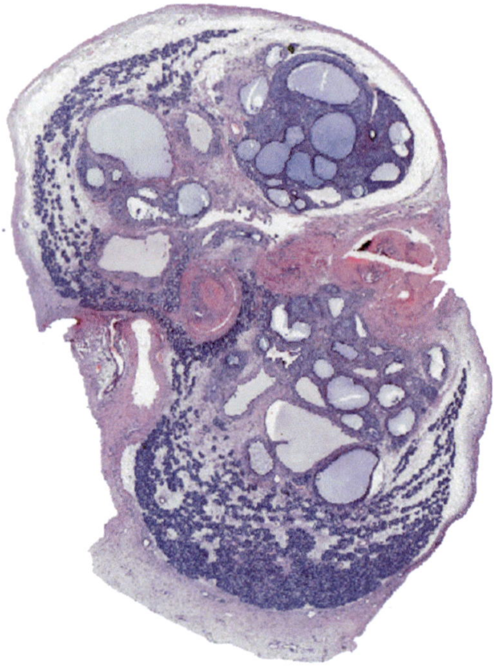

Fig. 6.67 Overview of a juvenile type granulosa cell tumor. Multiple cyst resembling ovarian follicles are the morphological hallmark of the tumor (Copyright Springer Damjanov and Mikuz [149])

less differentiated or undifferentiated cells in which, however, some recognizable cells of specialized gonadal stroma can be detected (Fig. 6.70). Although these tumors are listed separately in the WHO 2004 classification [4], many experts argue that they can hardly be distinguished from each other.

Morphology

Macroscopically, the tumors are nodular and yellow. Microscopically, they usually contain well-differentiated Leydig cells and less differentiated Sertoli cells, but combinations with granulosa cells also occur. The incompletely differentiated cells consist of spindled or more epithelioid cells and may contain differentiated elements. The sarcomatous tumors show brisk mitotic activity, necrotic areas, vascular invasion, and spread to the surrounding structures. Although no cytopathologic hallmarks of malignancy have been identified even in metastasizing cases, large tumor size seems to be an important indicator of malignancy.

Immunohistochemistry and Cytogenetic Analysis

The differentiated cells react with the known antibodies (Table 6.14), while the undifferentiated cells are reactive for S100 protein, SMA, and rarely desmin [121]. In the only cytogenetically analyzed case, gain of many chromosomes was observed (+3, +7, +9, +12, +13, +18, +19, +20) [122].

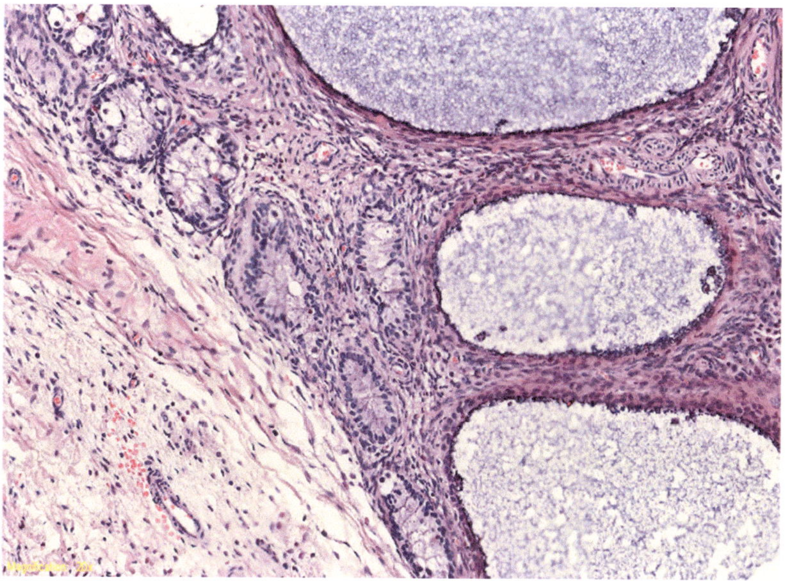

Fig. 6.68 Juvenile type granulosa cell tumor, with follicle-like cysts lined with cuboidal or flattened cylindrical epithelium

Differential Diagnosis

It is very difficult to distinguish between poorly differentiated and undifferentiated tumors. Some authors take the view that when tubular structures can be detected, the tumor should be classified as SCT [123].

Clinical Features

Patient age ranges from 6 months to 60 years. A few cases have presented with gynecomastia. In childhood the tumors are perfectly benign, whereas one-quarter of tumors in adults metastasize to the retroperitoneal lymph nodes and/or abdominal organs. In adults the histopathology report should be signed off with the comment that, although malignancy is unlikely, it cannot be ruled out.

Myoid Gonadal Stromal Tumor

The recently described myoid gonadal stromal tumor is a small (<4 cm) firm nodule composed of spindle cells arranged in fascicles. The nuclei are elongated and the nucleoli scanty. The tumor is strongly positive for SMA, S100 protein, SF1, and FOXL2, focally positive for α-inhibin and calponin, and negative for h-caldesmon, calretinin, and SOX9 [124].

Mixed Germ Cell/Sex Cord/Stromal Tumors

Gonadoblastoma

Gonadoblastoma was first described by Scully [125, 126] and affects only dysgenetic gonads.

Epidemiology

Gonadoblastoma arises more commonly in individuals who are phenotypically female (80 %) than in those who are phenotypically male [127]. The tumor is rare before the age of 12. More than 90 % of these tumors are diagnosed in the first 3 decades of life. Involvement of both gonads is common (30–40 %) [4].

Morphology

Macroscopically, the gonadal surface is lobulated and yellow brown, but in a fair number of cases (25 %), the tumors are only microscopically visible (Fig. 6.71). Prominent calcifications may be present focally. Microscopically, the tumor shows a nesting pattern. Small nests of seminoma cells (and rarely EC cells) are surrounded by Sertoli or granulosa cells in a wreath-like manner (Fig. 6.72), whereas Leydig cells are rather

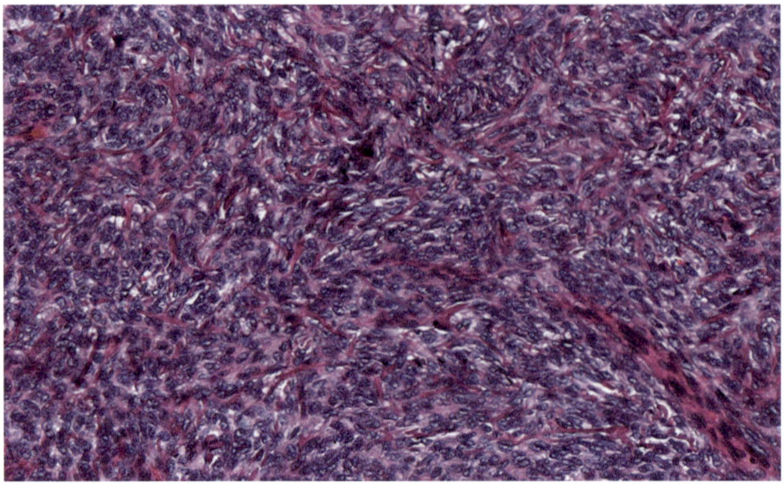

Fig. 6.69 Fibroma-thecoma type of sex cord/stromal tumor composed of fibroblasts-like tumor cells (Published with kind permission of ©Maurizio Colecchia 2015. All Rights Reserved)

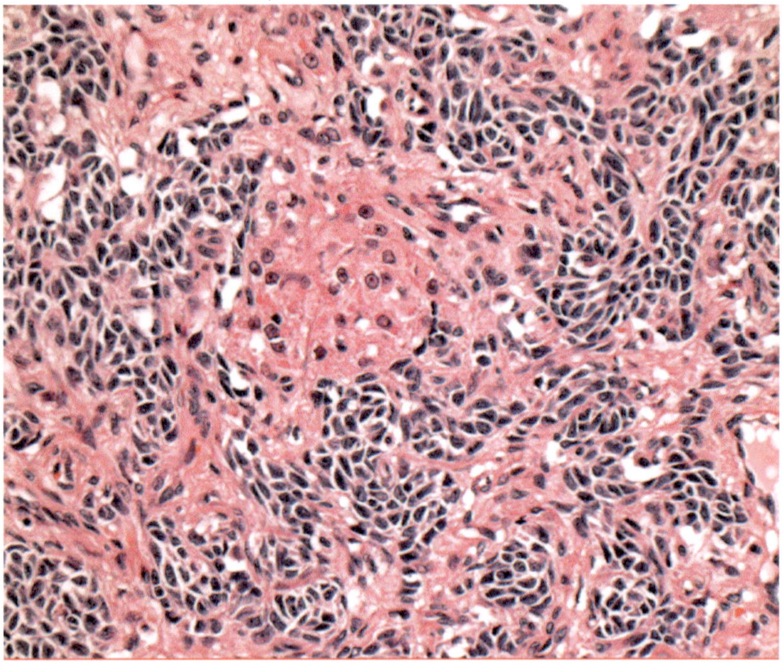

Fig. 6.70 Mixed sex cord/stromal tumor with well-differentiated large Leydig cells with eosinophilic cytoplasm and less differentiated, spindle-shaped Sertoli cells

uncommon. In the center of the nests, the basement membranes are condensed to hyaline nodules, which can calcify to psammoma bodies. If the tumor is not removed early, the germ cells overgrow the stromal cells and in most cases a pure seminoma develops. The development of NSGCT is rather rare (8 %) [4].

Immunohistochemistry

The germ cell component is reactive for PLAP and CD117 (c-kit) as well as for a protein encoded by the Y chromosome (TSPY) [128]. Sertoli or granulosa cells stain clearly with the specific antibodies including AMH. The hyaline nodules react positively with laminin.

DNA Ploidy and Cytogenetic Analysis

Using the FISH technique, a Y chromosome or part of it can be detected in all gonadoblastomas. On the Y chromosome, the candidate gene *TSPY* is responsible for the origin of gonadoblastoma [127, 128]. The germ cell component is aneuploid.

Differential Diagnosis

Sertoli cell nodules show some similarities to gonadoblastoma, but patients with Sertoli cell nodules do not have dysgenetic gonads.

Clinical Features

Patients with dysgenetic gonads often show a chromosomal 45,X/46,XY mosaicism. Patients affected by partial androgen insensitivity syndrome with nonscrotal testes and those with Fraiser and Denys-Drash syndrome also belong to the high-risk group for developing malignancy. These syndromes are characterized by gonadal dysgenesis and glomerular diseases of the kidney because of mutations of the WT1 (Wilms'tumor) suppressor gene. Due to the lack of AMH, the internal genital organs are feminine. In case the neoplastic germ cells have already overgrown the gonadal stroma components, therapy follows the standard protocols for GCTs.

Germ Cell Sex Cord/Gonadal Stromal Tumor, Unclassified

This is the name in the 2004 WHO classification [4] for mixed germ cell and gonadal stromal tumors arising in genotypically and phenotypically normal adult men. Since only a few cases in the testis and in the ovary have been reported to date [129], our knowledge is limited. The tumors consist of germ cells with clear cytoplasm, which are dissimilar from those of seminomas or ECs. The cells are arranged in small clusters surrounded by the predominant stromal component with inhibin-positive, small, often spindled cells (Fig. 6.73). The germ cells do not react with the classical markers PLAP and c-kit and also do not contain i(12p). For this reason, this tumor has been questioned by some authors, who considered the germ cells to be entrapped in a stromal tumor and not be a genuine part of it [130].

Miscellaneous Tumors

Tumors having neither a germ cell nor sex cord/stromal origin are listed in the 2004 WHO classification [4] under this heading.

Malignant Lymphoma and Plasmocytoma

Primary malignant non-Hodgkin lymphomas (NHL) of the testis are defined as isolated manifestations of lymphatic malignancies in the testis without generalized nodal manifestation.

Epidemiology

In different series, 1–7 % of testicular tumors are NHL; nevertheless, they are the most frequent tumors after the age of 50 and also the most frequent bilateral tumors (20–30 %). Testicular NHL accounts for 1–2 % of all lymphomas and has an incidence of 0.26/100,000 [131]. Patients are mostly older than 60 years; in children NHL is less frequent [131].

Solitary extramedullary plasmocytoma of the testis is, with some 60 reported cases, much less frequent than other testicular NHL. The age at diagnosis ranges from 26 to 83 years, although the mean age at diagnosis is 60 years (Fig. 6.74) [132, 133].

In several large case series (Armed Forces Institute of Pathology, British Testicular Tumor Registry, Extranodal Lymphoma Study Group), not a single case of Hodgkin's lymphoma was observed [1, 4, 74, 131].

Morphology

Macroscopically the entire organ is mostly involved. The parenchyma is replaced by a sometimes nodular, cream-pink, or yellowish-brown fish-flesh tumor. Necrosis and hemorrhagic areas are occasionally present. Plasmocytomas are softer, reddish in color, and hemorrhagic.

Microscopically, lymphoma cells diffusely infiltrate the interstitium, narrowing and rarely

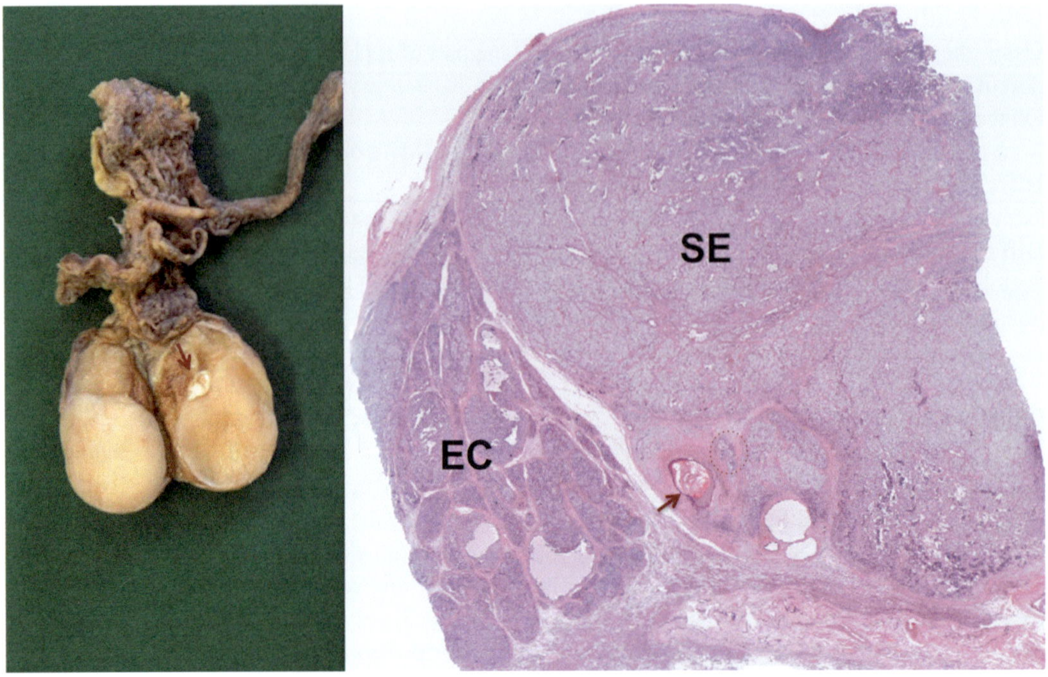

Fig. 6.71 Gonadoblastoma overgrown by a mixed germ cell tumor. Gross morphology (*left*) shows a seminoma-like cut surface with a small teratoma cyst (*arrow*). In the microscopic overview (*right*), only the small encircled area corresponds to the gonadoblastoma. *SE* seminoma, *EC* embryonal carcinoma, *arrow* teratoma cyst lined with squamous epithelium

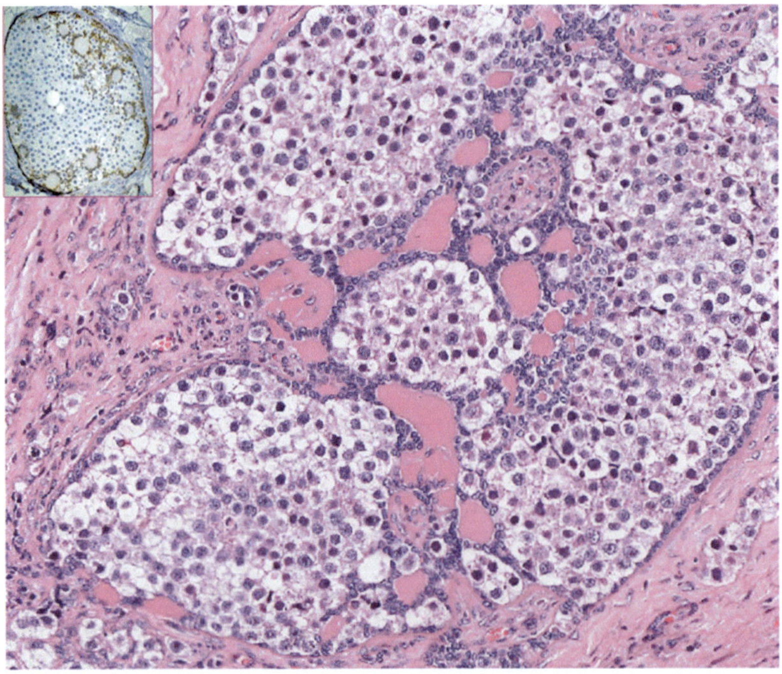

Fig. 6.72 The unique morphology of gonadoblastoma composed of seminoma cells that are surrounded by Sertoli cells in a wreath-like manner. Insert: α-inhibin positive Sertoli cells (With permission of the editor from Gregor Mikuz, Peter Mazal "Hoden und Infertilität beim Mann" Springer-Verlag Berlin Heidelberg, 2016)

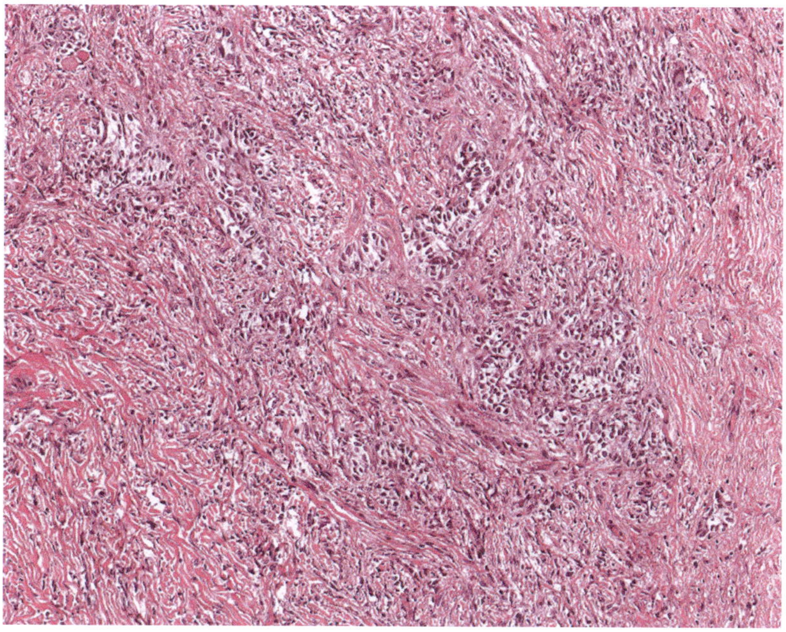

Fig. 6.73 Sex cord/stromal tumor, unclassified. Small foci of sex cord cells are admixed with a more prominent stromal proliferation (Published with kind permission of ©Maurizio Colecchia 2015. All Rights Reserved)

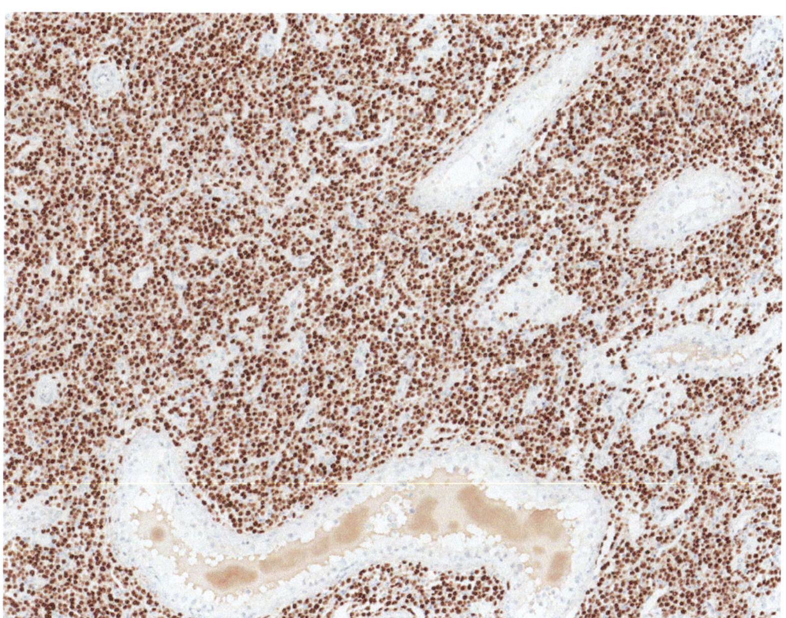

Fig. 6.74 Plasmacytoma of testis. The plasmacytoid nature of the tumor cells is highlighted by the MUM-1 positive reaction (Published with kind permission of ©Maurizio Colecchia 2015. All Rights Reserved)

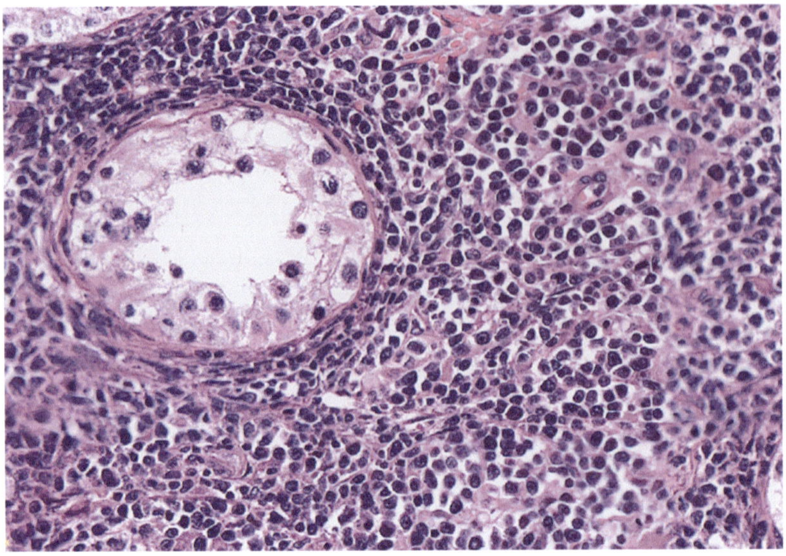

Fig. 6.75 Intratubular infiltration by diffuse large B-cell lymphoma

involving the seminiferous tubules (Fig. 6.75), but intratubular spread may be observed. Interstitial sclerosis, vascular invasion, and spread to the epididymis are frequent.

Plasmocytomas show a similar histologic pattern, but intratubular growth is more frequent than in other NHLs.

Eighty to ninety percent of primary testicular NHLs are large-cell diffuse B-cell lymphomas with or without sclerosis. Other observed lymphomas are mantle cell lymphoma, Burkitt lymphoma, and single cases of T-cell lymphomas [131].

Differential Diagnosis

Seminomas and even more often STs are mistaken for NHL or vice versa. Lymphoma patients are significantly older than GCT patients. Testicular GCTs only rarely invade the epididymis or other paratesticular structures. The use of lymphoma immunohistochemistry (CD45) is helpful, because PLAP is negative not only in lymphomas but also in ST.

Anaplastic large-cell lymphoma can also mimic an EC, but the epithelial nature of the EC cells is unmistakable. Immunohistochemistry (CD45, CAM5.2) can solve the diagnostic dilemma.

Clinical Features

Unilateral or bilateral testicular swelling without B symptoms is the main feature of testicular NHL. In accordance with the definition of testicular NHL, patients are initially at Ann Arbor stage I. Later on the disease generalizes and has a predilection for the CNS: even after therapy, 15 % of recurrences affect the brain. The standard therapy is orchiectomy followed by chemotherapy and/or radiotherapy. In spite of this aggressive regime, the prognosis is poor: the median relapse-free time is 4 years and the survival time 5 years [131]. The prognosis of testicular plasmocytoma is even worse [131].

Leukemia

In postmortem studies, 64 % of patients with acute leukemia and 22 % of those with chronic leukemia showed involvement of the testes [134]. Clinically this was mostly symptomless, because only 5 % of patients had swollen testicles. Best known is testicular involvement in children with acute myelocytic or lymphatic leukemia. Since recurrences were found to develop in the testis in 36 % of cases, it was common practice in the past to carry out testicular biopsies for diagnosis of relapse [135, 136]. However, given that an early diagnosis does not improve the prognosis, testicular biopsy is no longer recommended [137]. All these diseases tend to rapidly generalize and recur and therefore have a poor prognosis.

Recently also extramedullary testicular involvement in myelodysplastic and myeloproliferative diseases has been described [138, 139]. Among these diseases, myelosarcomas (granulocytic sarcoma, chloroma) seem to be the most frequent.

Macroscopically and microscopically, it is difficult to distinguish leukemia from lymphomas. The presence of eosinophilic granulocytes is highly suggestive of a myeloid tumor. A diagnosis can only be reached with the naphthol AS-D chloroacetate esterase reaction or with immunohistochemical proof of lysozymes or myeloperoxidases.

Primary Testicular Carcinoid and Nephroblastoma (Wilms' Tumor)

Usually these tumors arise in teratomas as a somatic-type malignancy. However, some of the reported cases did not originate in such a tumor. The histogenesis of primary carcinoids is mysterious, because the normal testicular parenchyma does not harbor neuroendocrine cells, which in contrast are abundant in teratomas [71]. One may argue that so-called primary testicular carcinoids also arise from neuroendocrine cells in teratoma, which slowly overgrow the other tissue components.

Carcinoids account for 0.2–1 % of all tumors of the testis in various statistics. Patients' age ranged from 19 to 83 years. Sixty-one of the 80 (76 %) well-documented cases of testicular carcinoids were not associated with teratoma [140]. Obviously, for a correct diagnosis, a metastasis of a carcinoid located in the gut or elsewhere must be clinically ruled out. After surgery the prognosis is excellent. The few patients with metastatic disease died of their tumors.

Primary nephroblastomas (Wilms'tumor) can arise in heterotopic renal anlage. Clinically they behave like kidney tumors and require the same treatment.

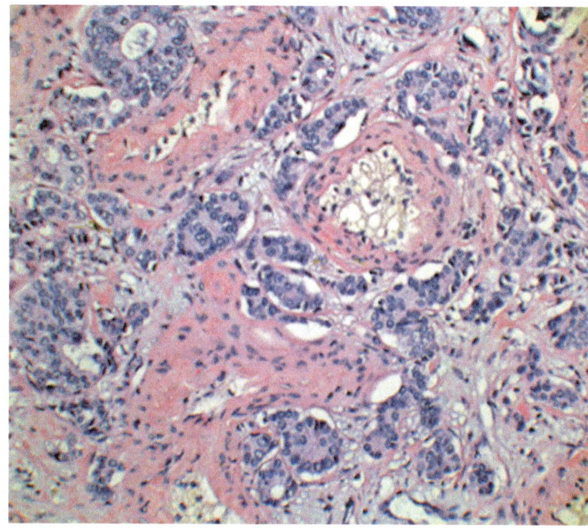

Fig. 6.76 Testicular metastasis. Intratubular spread of prostate cancer glands

Metastases

Metastases of solid neoplasia are surprisingly very rare in the testis. In postmortem studies, their incidence oscillates between 0 and 3.6 % [141–143]. Patients with secondary testicular neoplasms are generally older than those with GCTs. The tumors most commonly reported to metastasize to the testis are in decreasing order of frequency: prostate (Fig. 6.76), lung, melanoma, colon, kidney, stomach, and pancreas carcinoma. Neuroblastoma, retinoblastoma, carcinoid tumor (Fig. 6.77), Merkel carcinoma (Fig. 6.78), and cancers of the bile duct, ureter, bladder, salivary gland, and thyroid have also involved the testis secondarily (Table 6.16).

Macroscopically, metastases are recognizable as small, single, or multiple nodules. Histologically, the presence of extensive lymphatic and vascular invasion and an interstitial pattern in which the seminiferous tubules are spared is typical. Although metastases can easily be distinguished from testicular GCTs, confusion of melanoma metastases with seminoma has been reported [144].

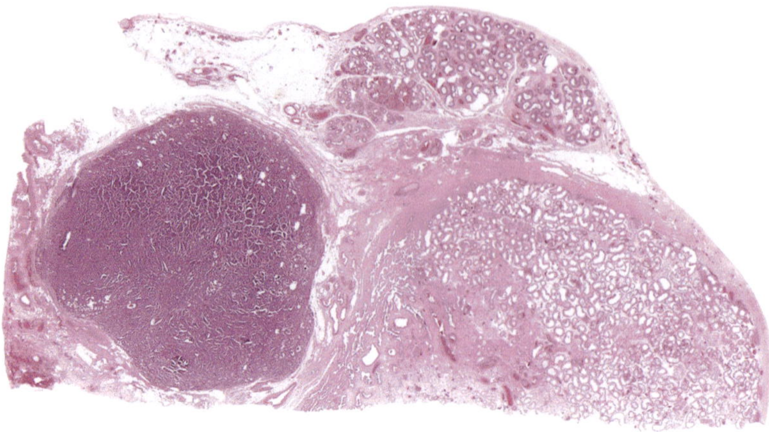

Fig. 6.77 Neuroendocrine carcinoma metastatic to fat tissue adjacent to the testicular parenchyma

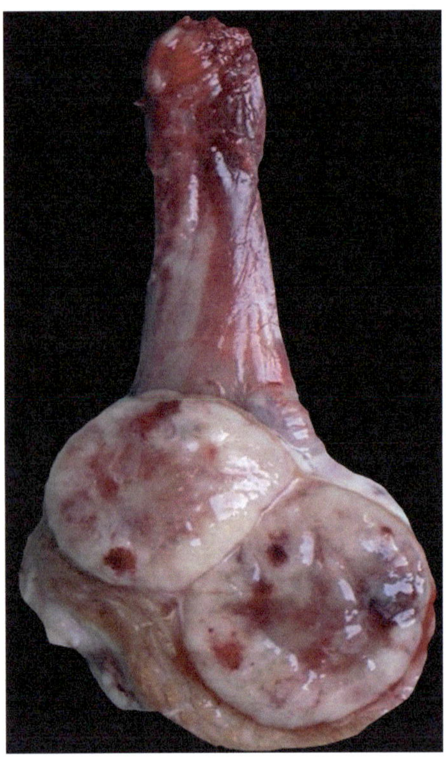

Fig. 6.78 Unusual presentation of Merkel cell carcinoma metastatic to the testis (Published with kind permission of ©Maurizio Colecchia 2015. All Rights Reserved)

Tumorlike Lesions

Some nonneoplastic lesions can cause a mass in the scrotum or a testicular swelling and have mainly the gross appearance of tumors. Most of such lesions are located in the testicular appendages or tunics and only few in the testis.

Table 6.16 Most frequent sites of primary tumors metastasizing to the testis (range from different studies)

Prostate	35–60 %
Lung	5–15 %
Melanoma	9–15 %
Colon	5–9 %
Kidney	5–9 %
Stomach	4 %
Miscellaneous	1–10 %

Testotoxicosis is an active Leydig cell differentiation associated with premature onset of spermatogenesis in children in the absence of pituitary gonadotropin stimulation. The testis enlargement is due to diffuse or nodular proliferation of mature Leydig cells [145].

The granulomatous forms of orchitis with slow onset, like syphilis or leprosy, which lead to fibrosis and induration of the gonad, might be mistaken for neoplasia. In particular the so-called idiopathic or pseudogranulomatous orchitis is clinically indistinguishable from a testicular tumor. It affects men in the fifth and sixth decades with a history of urinary tract infection. The testicular parenchyma is replaced by a tan-yellow mass resembling a seminoma (Fig. 6.79). Microscopically, the more or less destroyed tubules are filled with macrophages, which give the lesion the appearance of a granuloma [146].

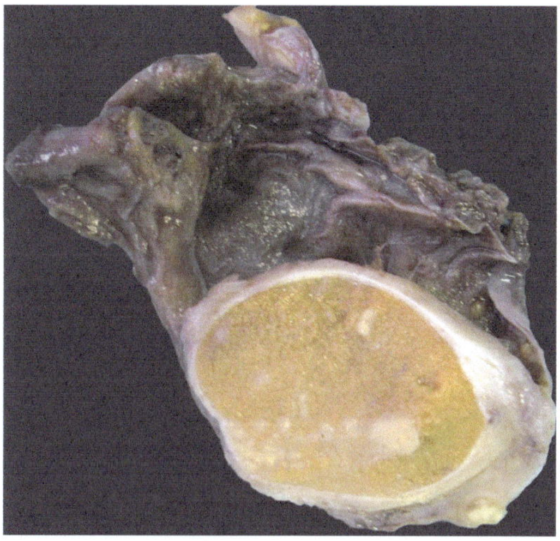

Fig. 6.79 Multiple white nodules involve the testicular parenchyma resembling a germ cell tumor (Published with kind permission of ©Maurizio Colecchia 2015. All Rights Reserved)

A special form is malacoplakia, which is grossly not very different from pseudogranulomatous orchitis. Microscopically, the tissue is replaced by large epithelioid cells with eosinophilic cytoplasm sometimes containing targetoid basophilic inclusions called Michaelis-Gutmann bodies.

Infarcts and hemorrhage can lead to sudden testicular swelling. Hemorrhagic infarction in young men is commonly caused by testicular torsion. Hematomas are the result of trauma or vasculitis, which is either localized or a manifestation of generalized disease. The most common type of vasculitis in the testis is due to Henoch-Schönlein purpura [147]. Less frequent are polyarteritis nodosa and Wegener's granulomatosis.

Testicular lipomatosis in Cowden syndrome is histologically characterized by multiple foci of fat tissue in the testicular interstitium. On ultrasound imaging, these areas appear as diffuse bilateral hyperechoic lesions. Cowden syndrome is a rare autosomal dominant disorder characterized by multiple tumorlike growths called hamartomas and an increased risk of certain forms of cancer. The *PTEN/MMAC1/TEP1* tumor suppressor gene on chromosome 10q23.3 has proven to contain a germline mutation predisposing to uncontrolled cell growth [148].

References

1. Pugh RCB, editor. Pathology of the testis. Oxford/London/Edinburgh/Melbourne: Blackwell Scientific Publications; 1976.
2. Mostofi FK, Sobin LH. Histological typing of tumors of the testis, International histological classification of tumors, vol. 16. Geneva: WHO; 1977.
3. Skakkebaek NE. Possible carcinoma in situ of the testis. Lancet. 1972;2:516–7.
4. Eble JN, Sauter G, Epstein JI, Sesterhenn IA, editors. Pathology & genetics. Tumors of the urinary system and male genital organs, WHO classification of tumors. Lyon: IARC Press; 2004. p. 218–9.
5. Moch H, Humprey PA, Ulbright TM, Reuter VE. WHO Classification of Tumours of the Urinary System and Male Genital Organs. Fourth edition IARC Lyon, 2016. chapter 4; p.185–258.
6. Hochstetter AR, Hedinger CE. The differential diagnosis of testicular germ cell tumors in theory and practice. A critical analysis of two major systems of classification and review of 389 cases. Virchows Arch A Pathol Anat Histol. 1982;396:247–77.
7. Stiens R. Testikuläre Keimzelltumoren: Histologie, Klassifikation, Pathologie und Häufigkeit. In: Weißbach L, Hildenbrand G, editors. Register und Verbundstudie fur Hodentumoren–Bonn, Ergebnisse einer prospektiven Untersuchung. Munchen: W Zuckschwerdt Verlag; 1982. p. 27–50.
8. Jacobsen KG, Barlebo H, Olsen J, Schultz HP, Starklint H, Søgaard H, Vaeth M. Testicular germ cell tumors in Denmark 1976 1980. Pathology of 1058 consecutive cases. Acta Radiol Oncol. 1984;23:239–47.
9. Horwich A, Shipley J, Huddart R. Testicular germ-cell cancer. Lancet. 2006;367:754–65.
10. Dieckmann KP, Loy V, Buttner P. Prevalence of bilateral testicular germ cell tumours and early detection based on contralateral intra-epithelial neoplasia. Br J Urol. 1993;71:340–5.
11. Cools M, van Aerde K, Kersemaekers AM, Boter M, Drop SL, Wolffenbuttel KP, Steyerberg EW, Oosterhuis JW, Looijenga LH. Morphological and immunohistochemical differences between gonadal maturation delay and early germ cell neoplasia in patients with undervirilization syndromes. J Clin Endocrinol Metab. 2005;90:5295–303.
12. Loy V, Dieckmann KP. Prevalence of contralateral testicular intraepithelial neoplasia (carcinoma in situ) in patients with testicular germ cell tumour. Results of the German multicentre study. Eur Urol. 1993;23:120–2.
13. Mostofi FK, Sesterhenn IA. Histological typing of testis tumours. 2nd ed. Berlin Heidelberg: Springer; 1998.
14. Hailelemariam S, Engler DS, Bannwart F, Amin MB. Primary mediastinal germ cell tumor with intratubular germ cell neoplasia of the testis- further support for germ cell origin of these tumors: a case report. Cancer. 1997;79:1031–6.

15. Emerson RE, Ulbright TM. Intratubular germ cell neoplasia of the testis and its associated cancers: the use of novel biomarkers. Pathology. 2010;42: 344–55.
16. Ulbright TM, Tickoo SK, Berney DM, Srigley JR, Members of the ISUP Immunohistochemistry in Diagnostic Urologic Pathology Group. Best practices recommendations in the application of immunohistochemistry in testicular tumors: report from the International Society of Urological Pathology consensus conference. Am J Surg Pathol. 2014;38:e50–9.
17. Nielsen JE, Kristensen DM, Almstrup K, Jørgensen A, Olesen IA, Jacobsen GK, Horn T, Skakkebaek NE, Leffers H, Rajpert-De Meyts E. A novel double staining strategy for improved detection of testicular carcinoma in situ cells in human semen samples. Andrologia. 2012;44:78–85.
18. El-Naggar AK, Ro JY, McLemore D, Ayala AG, Batsakis JG. DNA ploidy in testicular germ cell neoplasms. Histogenetic and clinical implications. Am J Surg Pathol. 1992;16:611–8.
19. Looijenga LH, Rosenberg C, van Gurp RJ, Geelen E, van Echten-Arends J, de Jong B, Mostert M, Wolter Oosterhuis J. Comparative genomic hybridization of microdissected samples from different stages in the development of a seminoma and a non-seminoma. J Pathol. 2000;191:187–92.
20. Rosenberg C, Van Gurp RJ, Geelen E, Oosterhuis JW, Looijenga LH. Overrepresentation of the short arm of chromosome 12 is related to invasive growth of human testicular seminomas and nonseminomas. Oncogene. 2000;19:5858–62.
21. Dieckmann KP, Skakkebaek NE. Carcinoma in situ of the testis: review of biological and clinical features. Int J Cancer. 1999;83:815–22.
22. Grigor KM, Rorth M. Should the contralateral testis be biopsied? Round table discussion. Eur Urol. 1993;23:129–35.
23. Dieckmann KP, Classen J, Loy V. Diagnosis and management of testicular intraepithelial neoplasia (carcinoma in situ) – surgical aspects. APMIS. 2003;111:64–8.
24. Christensen TB, Daugaard G, Geertsen PF, von der Maase H. Effect of chemotherapy on carcinoma in situ of the testis. Ann Oncol. 1998;9:657–60.
25. Herr HW, Sheinfeld J. Is biopsy of the contralateral testis necessary in patients with germ cell tumors? J Urol. 1997;158:1331–4.
26. McGlynn KA, Devesa SS, Sigurdson AJ, Brown LM, Tsao L, Tarone RE. Trends in the incidence of testicular germ cell tumors in the United States. Cancer. 2003;97:63–70.
27. Kay R. Prepubertal testicular tumor registry. J Urol. 1993;150:671–4.
28. Bols B, Jensen L, Jensen A, Brændstrup O. Immunopathology of *in situ* seminoma. Int J Exp Pathol. 2000;81:211–7.
29. Mostofi FK, Sesterhenn IA. Pathology of germ cell tumors of testes. Prog Clin Biol Res. 1985;203:1–34.
30. Ye H, Ulbright TM. Difficult differential diagnoses in testicular pathology. Arch Pathol Lab Med. 2012;136:435–46.
31. Idrees M, Saxena R, Cheng L, Ulbright TM, Badve S. Podoplanin, a novel marker for seminoma: a comparison study evaluating immunohistochemical expression of podoplanin and OCT3/4. Ann Diagn Pathol. 2010;14:331–6.
32. Hittmair A, Rogatsch H, Hobisch A, Mikuz G, Feichtinger H. CD30 expression in seminoma. Hum Pathol. 1996;27:1166–71.
33. Hittmair A, Rogatsch H, Feichtinger H, Hobisch A, Mikuz G. Testicular seminomas are aneuploid tumors. Lab Invest. 1995;72:70–4.
34. Mikuz G. Update on the pathology of testicular tumors. Anal Quant Cytopathol Histpathol. 2015;37: 75–85.
35. van Echten J, Osterhuis JW, Looijenga LH, van de Pol M, Wiersema J, te Meerman GJ, Schraffordt Koops H, Sleijfer DT, de Jong B. No recurrent structural abnormalities apart from i(12p) in primary germcell tumors of the adult testis. Genes Chromosomes Cancer. 1995;14:133–44.
36. Cao D, Li J, Guo CC, Allan RW, Humphrey PW. SALL4 is a novel diagnostic marker for testicular germ cell tumor. Am J Surg Pathol. 2009;33:1065–77.
37. Warde P, Specht L, Horwich A, Oliver T, Panzarella T, Gospodarowicz M, von der Maase H. Prognostic factors for relapse in stage I seminoma managed by surveillance: a pooled analysis. J Clin Oncol. 2002;20:4448–52.
38. Chung P, Daugaard G, Tyldesley S, Atenafu EG, Panzarella T, Kollmannsberger C, Warde P. Evaluation of a prognostic model for risk of relapse in stage I seminoma surveillance. Cancer Med. 2015;4:155–60.
39. Cohn-Cedermark G, Stahl O, Tandstad T; SWENOTECA. Surveillance vs. adjuvant therapy of clinical stage I testicular tumors – a review and the SWENOTECA experience. Andrology. 2015;3: 102–10.
40. Masson P. Etude sur le séminome. Rev Can Biol. 1946;5:361–87.
41. Lim J, Goriely A, Turner GD, Ewen KA, Jacobsen GK, Graem N, Wilkie AO, Rajpert-De Meyts E. OCT2, SSX and SAGE1 reveal the phenotypic heterogeneity of spermatocytic seminoma reflecting distinct subpopulations of spermatogonia. J Pathol. 2011;224:473–83.
42. Mikuz G. Spermatocytic seminoma-a tumor with many faces. Pathologe. 2014;35:232–7.
43. Carrière P, Baade P, Fritschi L. Population based incidence and age distribution of spermatocytic seminoma. J Urol. 2007;178:125–8.
44. Rosai J, Khodadoust K, Silber I. Spermatocytic seminoma. II. Ultra- structural study. Cancer. 1969;24:103–16.
45. Lombardi M, Valli M, Brisigotti M, Rosai J. Spermatocytic seminoma: review of the literature

and description of a new case of the anaplastic variant. Int J Surg Pathol. 2012;19:5–10.
46. Albores-Saavedra J, Huffman H, Alvarado-Cabrero I, Ayala AG. Anaplastic variant of spermatocytic seminoma. Hum Pathol. 1996;27:650–5.
47. Mikuz G, Böhm GW, Behrend M, Schäfer G, Colecchia M, Verdorfer I. Therapy-resistant metastasizing anaplastic spermatocytic seminoma – a cytogenetical hybrid. Anal Quant Cytol Histol. 2014;39:382–5.
48. Kao CS, Badve SS, Ulbright TM. The utility of immunostaining for NUT, GAGE7 and NY-ESO-1 in the diagnosis of spermatocytic seminoma. Histopathology. 2014;65:35–44.
49. Talerman A, Fu YS, Okagaki T. Spermatocytic seminoma. Ultrastructural and microspectrometric observations. Lab Invest. 1984;51:343–9.
50. Takahashi H. Cytometric analysis of testicular seminoma and spermatocytic seminoma. Acta Pathol Jpn. 1993;43:121–9.
51. Verdorfer I, Rogatsch H, Tzankov A, Steiner H, Mikuz G. Molecular cytogenetic analysis of human spermatocytic seminomas. J Pathol. 2004;204: 277–81.
52. Jacobsen GK. Alpha-fetoprotein (AFP) and human chorionic gonadotropin (HCG) in testicular germ cell tumours. A comparison of histologic and serologic occurrence of tumour markers. APMIS. 1983;91:183–90.
53. Giannatempo P, Paolini B, Miceli R, Raggi D, Nicolai N, Farè E, Catanzaro M, Biasoni D, Torelli T, Stagni S, Piva L, Mariani L, Salvioni R, Colecchia M, Gianni AM, Necchi A. Persistent CD30 expression by embryonal carcinoma in the treatment time course: prognostic significance of a worthwhile target for personalized treatment. J Urol. 2013; 190:1919–24.
54. Delozier-Blanchet CD, Walt H, Engel E, Vuagnat P. Cytogenetic studies of human testicular germ cell tumours. Int J Androl. 1987;10:69–77.
55. Williams SD, Einhorn LH. Neoplasms of the testis. In: Calabresi P, Schein PS, Rosenberg SA, editors. Medical oncology: basic principles and clinical management of cancer. New York: Macmillan; 1985. p. 1077–88.
56. Teilum G. Endodermal sinus tumors of the ovary and testis. Comparative morphogenesis of the so-called mesoephroma ovarii (Schiller) and extraembryonic (yolk sac-allantoic) structures of the rat's placenta. Cancer. 1959;12:1092–105.
57. Ross JH, Kay R. Prepubertal testis tumors. Rev Urol. 2004;6:11–8.
58. Baik K, Kang M, Park K, Choi H. Prepubertal testicular tumors in Korea: a single surgeon's experience of more than 20 years. Korean J Urol. 2013;54:399–403.
59. Brown LM, Pottern LM, Hoover RN, Devesa SS, Aselton P, Flannery JT. Testicular cancer in the United States: trends in incidence and mortality. Int J Epidemiol. 1986;15:164–70.
60. Kao CS, Idrees MT, Young RH, Ulbright TM. Solid pattern yolk sac tumor: a morphologic and immunohistochemical study of 52 cases. Am J Surg Pathol. 2012;36:360–7.
61. Silver SA, Wiley JM, Perlman EJ. DNA ploidy analysis of pediatric germ cell tumors. Mod Pathol. 1994;7:951–6.
62. Perlman EJ, Cushing B, Hawkins E, Griffin CA. Cytogenetic analysis of childhood endodermal sinus tumor: a Pediatric Oncology Group study. Pediatr Pathol. 1994;14:695–708.
63. Ulbright TM, Young RH, Scully RE. Trophoblastic tumors of the testis other than classic choriocarcinoma: "monophasic" choriocarcinoma and placental site trophoblastic tumor: a report of two cases. Am J Surg Pathol. 1997;21:282–8.
64. McCluggage WG, Ashe P, McBride H, Maxwell P, Sloan JM. Localization of the cellular expression of inhibin in trophoblastic tissue. Histopathology. 1998;32:252–6.
65. Niehans GA, Manivel JC, Copland GT, Scheithauer BW, Wick MR. Immunohistochemistry of germ cell and trophoblastic neoplasms. Cancer. 1988;62:1113–23.
66. Manivel JC, Niehans G, Wick MR, Dehner LP. Intermediate trophoblast in germ cell neoplasm. Am J Surg Pathol. 1987;11:693–701.
67. Rabes HM. Proliferation of human testicular tumours. Int J Androl. 1987;10:127–37.
68. Bosl GJ, Dmitrovsky E, Reuter VE, Samaniego F, Rodriguez E, Geller NL, Chaganti RS. Isochromosome of the short arm of chromosome 12: clinically useful markers for male germ cell tumors. J Natl Cancer Inst. 1989;81:1874–8.
69. Logothetis CJ, Samuels ML, Selig DE, Ogden S, Dexeus F, Swanson D, Johnson D, von Eschenbach A. Cyclic chemotherapy with cyclophosphamide, doxorubicin, and cisplatin plus vinblastine and bleomycin in advanced germinal tumors. Am J Med. 1986;81:219–28.
70. Virchow R. Die krankhaften Geschwülste. Hirschwald/Berlin: Verlag A; 1863.
71. Pichmann S, Mikuz G, Schmid KW. Chromogranins A and B in nonseminomatous testicular tumors. J Urol Pathol. 1993;1:43–54.
72. Shah KH, Maxted WC, Chun B. Epidermoid cyst of the testis: a report of three cases and analysis of 141 cases from the world literature. Cancer. 1981;47: 577–82.
73. Mikuz G, Colecchia M. Teratoma with somatic-type malignant components of the testis. A review and an update. Virchows Arch. 2012;461:27–32.
74. Ulbright TM, Amin MB, Young RH. Tumors of the testis, adnexa, spermatic cord, and scrotum. AFIP Atlas of tumor pathology, 3rd series, Fascicle 25. Washington, DC: Armed Forces Institute of Pathology; 1999.
75. Molenaar WM, Oosterhuis JW, Meiring A, Sleyfer DT, Schraffordt Koops H, Cornelisse CJ. Histology and DNA contents of a secondary malignancy

arising in a mature residual lesion six years after chemotherapy for a disseminated nonseminomatous testicular tumor. Cancer. 1986;58:264–8.
76. Motzer RJ, Amsterdam A, Prieto V, Sheinfeld J, Murty VV, Mazumdar M, Bosl GJ, Chaganti RS, Reuter VE. Teratoma with malignant transformation: diverse malignant histologies arising in men with germ cell tumors. J Urol. 1998;159:133–8.
77. Shukla AR, Woodard C, Carr MC, Huff DS, Canning DA, Zderic SA, Kolon TF, Snyder 3rd HM. Experience with testis sparing surgery for testicular teratoma. J Urol. 2004;171:161–3.
78. Colecchia M, Necchi A, Paolini B, Nicolai N, Salvioni R. Teratoma with somatic-type malignant components in germ cell tumors of the testis: a clinicopathologic analysis of 40 cases with outcome correlation. Int J Surg Pathol. 2011;19:321–7.
79. Mosharafa AA, Foster RS, Leibovich BC, Ulbright TM, Bihrle R, Einhorn LH, Donohue JP. Histology in mixed germ cell tumors. Is there a favourite pairing? J Urol. 2004;171:1471–3.
80. Heidenreich A, Sesterhenn IA, Mostofi FK, Moul JW. Prognostic risk factors that identify patients with clinical stage I nonseminomatous germ cell tumors at low risk and high risk for metastasis. Cancer. 1998;83:1002–11.
81. Fung CY, Kalish LA, Brodsky GL, Richie JP, Garnick MB. Stage I nonseminomatous germ cell testicular tumor: prediction of metastatic potential by primary histopatology. J Clin Oncol. 1988;6:1467–73.
82. Azzopardi JG, Mostofi FK, Theiss EA. Lesions of testes observed in certain patients with widespread choriocarcinoma and related tumors. Am J Pathol. 1961;38:207–25.
83. Daugaard G, von der Maase H, Olsen J, Rorth M, Skakkebaek NE. Carcinoma in situ testis in patients with assumed extragonadal germ-cell tumours. Lancet. 1987;2:528–30.
84. Balzer BL, Ulbright TM. Spontaneous regression of testicular germ cell tumors: an analysis of 42 cases. Am J Surg Pathol. 2006;30:858–65.
85. Teilum G. Special tumors of ovary and testis. Copenhagen: Munksgaard; 1971.
86. Kim I, Young RH, Scully RE. Leydig cell tumors of the testis: a clinico-pathological analysis of 40 cases and review of the literature. Am J Surg Pathol. 1985;9:177–92.
87. Sogge MR, McDonald SD, Cofold PB. The malignant potential of the dysgenetic germ cell in Klinefelter's syndrome. Am J Med. 1979;66: 515–8.
88. Ulbright TM, Srigley JR, Hatzianastassiou DK, Young RH. Leydig cell tumors of the testis with unusual features: adipose differentiation, calcification with ossification, and spindle-shaped tumor cells. Am J Surg Pathol. 2002;26:1424–33.
89. Cheville JC, Sebo TJ, Lager DJ, Bostwick DG, Farrow GM. Leydig cell tumor of the testis: a clinicopathologic, DNA content and MIB-1 comparison of nonmetastasizing and metastasizing tumors. Am J Surg Pathol. 1998;22:1361–7.
90. Divatia M, Smith S, Colecchia M, Aron M, Amin M, Shen SS, Hansel D, Tamboli P, Paner GP, de Peralta-Venturina M, Herrera Hernandez L, Gowen AM. Diagnostic utility of comprehensive immunohistochemical (IHC) panel for testicular sex cord stromal tumors (TSCST): a study of 76 cases. USCAP 2015. Abstractbook: Abstract 860. p. 216A.
91. Joensuu H, Klemi PJ. DNA aneuploidy in adenomas of endocrine organs. Am J Pathol. 1988;132: 145–51.
92. Verdorfer I, Horst D, Höllrigl A, Susani M, Hartmann A, Rogatsch H, Mikuz G. Leydig cell tumors of the testis: a molecular-cytogenetic study based on a large series of patients. Oncol Rep. 2007;17:585–9.
93. Canto P, Soderlund D, Ramon G, Nishimura E, Mendez JP. Mutational analysis of the luteinizing hormone receptor gene in two individuals with Leydig cell tumors. Am J Med Genet. 2002;8:148–52.
94. Wang Z, Yang S, Shi H, Du H, Xue L, Wang L, Dong Y, Han A. Histopathological and immunophenotypic features of testicular tumour of the adrenogenital syndrome. Histopathology. 2011;58:1013–8.
95. Datta MW, Young RH. Malignant melanoma metastatic to the testis: a report of three cases with clinically significant manifestations. Int J Surg Pathol. 2000;8:49–57.
96. Grem JL, Robins I, Wilson KS, Gilchrist K, Trump DK. Metastatic Leydig cell tumor of the testis. Report of three cases and review of the literature. Cancer. 1986;58:2116–9.
97. Gilcrease MZ, Delgado R, Albores-Saavedra J. Testicular Sertoli cell tumor with a heterologous sarcomatous component: immunohistochemical assessment of Sertoli cell differentiation. Arch Pathol Lab Med. 1998;122:907–11.
98. Zuckerberg LR, Young RH, Scully RE. Sclerosing Sertoli cell tumor of the testis: a report of 10 cases. Am J Surg Pathol. 1991;15:829–64.
99. Verdorfer I, Höllrigl A, Susani M, Hartmann A, Rogatsch H, Mikuz G. Molecular cytogenetic characterisation of sex cord-stromal tumors: CHG analysis in Sertoli cell tumours of the testis. Virchows Arch. 2007;450:425–31.
100. Perrone F, Bertolotti A, Montemurro G, Paolini B, Pierotti MA, Colecchia M. Frequent mutation and nuclear localization of β-catenin in sertoli cell tumors of the testis. Am J Surg Pathol. 2014;38:66–71.
101. Lawrence WD, Young RH, Scully RE. Sex cord-stromal tumors. In: Talerman A, Roth LM, editors. Pathology of the testis and its adnexa. New York/ Edinburgh/London/Melbourne: Churchill Livingstone; 1986. p. 67–92.
102. Young RH, Koelliker DD, Scully RE. Sertoli cell tumors of the testis, not otherwise specified. A clinicopathologic analysis of 60 cases. Am J Surg Pathol. 1998;22:709–21.

103. Carney JA. Carney complex: the complex of myxomas, spotty pigmentation, endocrine overactivity, and schwannomas. Semin Dermatol. 1995;14:90–8.
104. Kratzer SS, Ulbright TM, Talerman A, Srigley JR, Roth LM, Wahle GR, Moussa M, Stephens JK, Millos A, Young RH. Large cell calcifying Sertoli cell tumor of the testis: contrasting features of six malignant and six benign tumors and a review of the literature. Am J Surg Pathol. 1997;21:1271–80.
105. Bufo P, Pennella A, Serio G, Mastropasqua MG, Cenacchi G, Rogatsch H, Mikuz G. Malignant large cell calcifying Sertoli cell tumor of the testis (LCCSCTT). Report of a case in an elderly man and review of the literature. Pathologica. 1999;91: 107–14.
106. Proppe KH, Dickersin GR. Large-cell calcifying Sertoli cell tumor of the testis: light microscopic and ultrastructural study. Hum Pathol. 1982;13:1109–14.
107. Rothschild JA, Kreso M, Slodzinski M. Sudden death in a patient with Carney's complex. Anesth Pain Med. 2013;2:182–5.
108. Birla S, Aggarwal S, Sharma A, Tandon N. Rare association of acromegaly with left atrial myxoma in Carney's complex due to novel PRKAR1A mutation. Endocrinol Diabetes Metab Case Rep. 2014; 2014:140023.
109. Schubert TE, Stoehr R, Hartmann A, Schöne S, Löbelenz M, Mikuz G. Adult type granulosa cell tumor of the testis with a heterologous sarcomatous component: case report and review of the literature. Diagn Pathol. 2014;9:107.
110. Rane SU, Menon S, Desai S, Bakshi G, Joshi A. Granulosa cell tumor of testis: clinicopathological correlation of a rare tumor. Indian J Pathol Microbiol. 2014;57:564–73.
111. Giulianelli R, Mirabile G, Vincenti G, Pellegrino F, Soda G. A very rare case of adult-type granulosa cell tumor. Arch Ital Urol Androl. 2015;87:98–9.
112. Mayr D, Kaltz-Wittmer C, Arbogast S, Amann G, Aust DE, Diebold J. Characteristic pattern of genetic aberrations in ovarian granulosa cell tumors. Mod Pathol. 2002;15:951–7.
113. Lima JF, Jin L, de Araujo AR, Erikson-Johnson MR, Oliveira AM, Sebo TJ, Keeney GL, Medeiros F. FOXL2 mutations in granulosa cell tumors occurring in males. Arch Pathol Lab Med. 2012;136: 825–8.
114. Harms D, Kock LR. Testicular juvenile granulosa cell and Sertoli cell tumours: a clinicopathological study of 29 cases from the Kiel Paediatric Tumour Registry. Virchows Arch. 1997;430:301–9.
115. Young RH, Lawrence WD, Scully RE. Juvenile granulosa cell tumor–another neoplasm associated with abnormal chromosomes and ambiguous genitalia. A report of three cases. Am J Surg Pathol. 1985;19:737–43.
116. Tanaka Y, Sasaki Y, Tachibana K, Suwa S, Terashima K, Nakatani Y. Testicular juvenile granulosa cell tumor in an infant with X/XY mosaicism clinically diagnosed as true hermaphroditism. Am J Surg Pathol. 1994;18:316–22.
117. Rey R, Sabourin JC, Venara M, Long WQ, Jaubert F, Zeller WP, Duvillard P, Chemes H, Bidart JM. Anti-Müllerian hormone is a specific marker of Sertoli and granulosa – cell origin in gonadal tumors. Hum Pathol. 2000;31:1202–8.
118. Kemp B, Silva E, Elnaggar A. Juvenile granulosa-cell tumor of the ovary – interphase cytogenetics for chromosome-12 and chromosome-x and flow cytometric DNA-ploidy study. Int J Oncol. 1995;7:661–5.
119. Shukla AR, Huff DS, Canning DA, Filmer RB, Snyder 3rd HM, Carpintieri D, Carr MC. Juvenile granulosa cell tumor of the testis: contemporary clinical management and pathological diagnosis. J Urol. 2004;171:1900–2.
120. Deveci MS, Deveci G, Ongürü O, Kilciler M, Celasun B. Testicular gonadal stromal fibroma: case report and review of the literature. Pathol Int. 2002;52:326–30.
121. Renshaw AA, Gordon M, Corless CL. Immunohistochemistry of unclassified sex cord–stromal tumors of the testis with a predominance of spindle cells. Mod Pathol. 1997;10:693–700.
122. Yang DT, Lowichik A, Chen J, Snow BW, Ulbright TM, Chen Z. Cytogenetics of a pediatric unclassified sex cord-stromal tumor of the testis: a case report. Cancer Genet Cytogenet. 2005;156:80–2.
123. Young RH, Talerman A. Testicular tumors other than germ cell tumors. Semin Diagn Pathol. 1987;4:342–60.
124. Kao CS, Ulbright TM. Myoid gonadal stromal tumor: a clinicopathologic study of three cases of a distinctive testicular tumor. Am J Clin Pathol. 2014;142:675–82.
125. Scully RE. Gonadoblastoma. A gonadal tumor related to the dysgerminoma (seminoma) and capable of sex hormone production. Cancer. 1953;6: 445–63.
126. Scully RE. Gonadoblastoma. A review of 74 cases. Cancer. 1970;25:1340–56.
127. Delbridge ML, Longepied G, Depetris D, Mattei MG, Disteche CM, Marshall Graves JA, Mitchell MJ. TSPY, the candidate gonadoblastoma gene on the human Y chromosome, has a widely expressed homologue on the X – implications for Y chromosome evolution. Chromosome Res. 2004;12:345–56.
128. Lau Y, Chou P, Iezzoni J, Alonzo J, Komuves L. Expression of a candidate gene for the gonadoblastoma locus in gonadoblastoma and testicular seminoma. Cytogenet Cell Genet. 2000;91: 160–4.
129. Michal M, Vanecek T, Sima R, Mukensnabl P, Hes O, Kazakov DV, Matoska J, Zuntova A, Dvorak V, Talerman A. Mixed germ cell sex cord-stromal tumors of the testis and ovary. Morphological, immunohistochemical and molecular genetic study of seven cases. Virchows Arch. 2006;448:612–22.

130. Ulbright TM, Srigley JR, Reuter VE, Wojno K, Roth LM, Young RH. Sex cord–stromal tumors of the testis with entrapped germ cells: a lesion mimicking unclassified mixed germ cell sex cord-stromal tumors. Am J Surg Pathol. 2000;24:535–42.
131. Zucca E, Conconi A, Mughal TI, Sarris AH, Seymour JF, Vitolo U, Klasa R, Ozsahin M, Mead GM, Gianni MA, Cortelazzo S, Ferreri AJ, Ambrosetti A, Martelli M, Thieblemont C, Moreno HG, Pinotti G, Martinelli G, Mozzana R, Grisanti S, Provencio M, Balzarotti M, Laveder F, Oltean G, Callea V, Roy P, Cavalli F, Gospodarowicz MK, International Extranodal Lymphoma Study Group. Patterns of outcome and prognostic factors in primary large-cell lymphoma of the testis in a survey by the International Extranodal Lymphoma Study Group. J Clin Oncol. 2003;21:20–7.
132. Finn LS, Viswanatha DS, Belasco JB, Snyder H, Huebner D, Sorbara L, Raffeld M, Jaffe ES, Salhany KE. Primary follicular lymphoma of the testis in childhood. Cancer. 1999;85:1626–35.
133. Anghel G, Petti N, Remotti D, Ruscio C, Blandino F, Majolino I. Testicular plasmacytoma: report of a case and review of the literature. Am J Hematol. 2002;71:98–104.
134. Givler RL. Testicular involvement in leukaemia and lymphoma. Cancer. 1969;23:1290–5.
135. Quaranta BP, Halperin EC, Kurtzberg J, Clough R, Martin PL. The incidence of testicular recurrence in boys with acute leukemia treated with total body and testicular irradiation and stem cell transplantation. Cancer. 2004;101:845–50.
136. Miller DR, Leikin S, Albo VC, Palmer NF, Sather HN, Hammond GD. The prognostic value of testicular biopsy in childhood acute lymphoblastic leukemia: a report from the Childrens Cancer Study Group. J Clin Oncol. 1990;8:57–66.
137. Trigg ME, Steinherz PG, Chappell R, Johnstone HS, Gaynon PS, Kersey JH, Cherlow JM, Grossman NJ, Sather HN, Hammond GD. Early testicular biopsy in males with acute lymphoblastic leukemia: lack of impact on subsequent event-free survival. J Pediatr Hematol Oncol. 2000;22:27–33.
138. McIlwain L, Sokol L, Moscinski LC, Saba HI. Acute myeloid leukemia mimicking primary testicular neoplasm. Presentation of a case with review of literature. Eur J Haematol. 2003;70:242–5.
139. Constantinou J, Nitkunan T, Al-Izzi M, McNicholas TA. Testicular granulocytic sarcoma, a source of diagnostic confusion. Urology. 2004;64:807–9.
140. Kato N, Motoyama T, Kameda N, Hiruta N, Emura I, Hasegawa G, Murata T, Kimura M, Tsuda H, Ishihara T. Primary carcinoid tumor of the testis: immunohistochemical, ultrastructural and FISH analysis with review of the literature. Pathol Int. 2003;53:680–5.
141. Pienkos JE, Jablokow VR. Secondary testicular tumors. Cancer. 1972;30:481–5.
142. Haupt HM, Mann RB, Trump DL, Abeloff MD. Metastatic carcinoma involving the testis. Clinical and pathologic distinction from primary testicular neoplasms. Cancer. 1984;54:709–14.
143. Patel SR, Richardson RL, Kvols L. Metastatic cancer to the testes: a report of 20 cases and review of the literature. J Urol. 1989;142:1003–5.
144. Richardson PG, Millward MJ, Shrimankar JJ, Cantwell BM. Metastatic melanoma to the testis simulating primary seminoma. Br J Urol. 1992; 69:663–5.
145. Gondos B, Egli CA, Rosenthal SM, Grumbach MM. Testicular changes in gonadotropin-independent familial male sexual precocity. Familial testotoxicosis. Arch Pathol Lab Med. 1985;109:990–5.
146. Mikuz G, Damjanov I. Inflammation of the testis, epididymis, peritesticular membranes, and scrotum. Pathol Annu. 1982;17:101–28.
147. Mikuz G, Hofstadter F, Hager J. Testis involvement in Schönlein–Henoch purpura. Pathol Res Pract. 1979;165:323–9.
148. Woodhouse JB, Delahunt B, English SF, Fraser HH, Ferguson MM. Testicular lipomatosis in Cowden's syndrome. Mod Pathol. 2005;18:1151–6.
149. Damjanov I, Mikuz G. Tumors of the testis and epididymis. In: Jezek D, editor. Atlas on human testis. Normal morphology and pathology. London: Springer; 2013.

7 Prognostic and Predictive Factors in Pathology of the Testis

Nicola Nicolai

Introduction

Testis tumors encompass germ cell tumors (GCTs), which represent about 95 % of cases, and sex cord stromal tumors (SCSTs), which account for the remaining 5 %. GCTs are characterized by a very favorable prognosis even when metastatic spread is proven. SCSTs are frequently benign, although about 10 % display a clinically unfavorable course.

GCT

Outcome Predictors

Stage I GCT

A significant proportion of GCT patients present with nonmetastatic disease. Current figures indicate that the incidence and age at onset of GCT are increasing and that seminoma tends to be more frequent than nonseminoma. Moreover, about 70 % of nonseminoma and 90 % of seminoma patients are diagnosed with no disease beyond the testis (clinical stage I) [1, 2]. Only a proportion of these patients will progress, but the prognosis remains excellent, with a cure rate very close to 100 %. Micrometastases are present in about 15–20 % of seminomas and about 30 % of nonseminomas at stage I. So far, postorchiectomy treatment in this setting has been prophylactic, and many patients will not benefit from therapy but may suffer from its side effects. Since the 1970s, clinical researchers have tried to identify clinical and pathologic parameters that may predict metastases, in order to tailor postorchiectomy treatment according to different risks of progression.

As radiation therapy was a consolidated, effective, and supposedly safe strategy for seminoma up to the 1990s, the issue mainly concerned nonseminoma, where the introduction of effective cisplatin-based chemotherapy could permit the delay of treatment until the appearance of metastases, without compromising the favorable outcome.

Thanks to the Medical Research Council trials, predictive parameters of metastatic spread were identified and then validated by two prospective studies. Lymphatic invasion, venous invasion, absence of yolk sac tumor (YST), and undifferentiated cancer (embryonal carcinoma [EC]) were distinguished as independent predictors of metastatic disease in clinical stage I nonseminoma [3, 4]. Since then, lymphatic invasion and venous invasion have been considered as a single feature (i.e., vascular invasion), given that only 10 % of cases with lymphatic invasion did not display venous invasion as well.

N. Nicolai
Testis Surgery Unit, Fondazione IRCCS Istituto Nazionale dei Tumori di Milano, Milan, Italy
e-mail: nicola.nicolai@istitutotumori.mi.it

M. Colecchia (ed.), *Pathology of Testicular and Penile Neoplasms*,
DOI 10.1007/978-3-319-27617-5_7

A clear limitation in many histology reports is the unavailability of information on vascular invasion. Orchiectomy is usually performed in peripheral primary care hospitals, following which most patients are referred to tertiary academic or research centers. This implies that the first pathologic examination will not include information about the vascular invasion status, as was documented in only 6 % of cases at Indiana University [5] but as many as 50 % of cases seen at Istituto Nazionale dei Tumori, Milan, Italy [6]. This induced some researchers to explore other factors that would be easy to evaluate or reevaluate. Albers et al. first reported on Ki67 staining by MIB-1 expression and found that MIB-1 expression greater than 80 % was predictive of micrometastases [7].

The proportion of EC in the primary tumor has been considered a predictive factor of occult metastases. This parameter was associated with a higher risk of metastases in clinical series from medical and surgical experiences [8–10]. Nonetheless, the proportion of EC associated with a higher risk of metastases varied across series. It was as high as 90 % in patients undergoing observation only [8], while only the prevalence of this histologic type was significant in a surgical series [9, 10]. The proportion of EC in the primary tumor as a definitive and reproducible cutoff was never defined.

Other studies evaluated the role of predictive factors in stage I nonseminoma patients undergoing primary retroperitoneal lymph node dissection (RPLND). In the early 1990s, Klepp et al., on behalf of the SWENOTECA group, reported on a series of 279 patients undergoing RPLND and found that the presence of vascular invasion, a normal alpha-fetoprotein (AFP) level prior to orchiectomy, or, after excluding AFP, the absence of teratoma and YST in the primary tumor was associated with an increased risk of nodal or distant metastases [11]. In a further series of 250 patients from the same group, vascular invasion only was confirmed, while AFP was no longer identified as a risk factor [12]. Studies addressing the sole risk of nodal metastases at RPLND were carried out at Indiana University and Istituto Nazionale dei Tumori, Milan. At Indiana, a complex model including the volume of EC (threshold 2 mL), a short axis of retroperitoneal lymph nodes at cross-sectional CT imaging, and MIB-1 staining (thresholds of 80 or 90 % according to EC volume) was proposed to identify patients with a low risk of bearing nodal metastases at RPLND [13]. However, no further studies using this complicated algorithm have been published. An Italian study reported a simple model to predict nodal metastases at RPLND based on the presence of vascular invasion and the percent of EC (threshold 90 %). Patients with at least 1 factor had a risk of nodal metastases as high as 35 %, whereas in patients with no risk factors, the risk was 10 % [14].

From a practical point of view, vascular invasion became the most reliable and applicable parameter. A meta-analysis by Vergouwe et al. [15] including more than 5,000 clinical stage I patients from the literature confirmed that vascular invasion was the strongest predictive parameter of occult metastases, with an odds ratio (OR) greater than 5, higher than the ORs of other factors. Vascular invasion is currently recommended as the sole informative parameter in stage I nonseminoma by the most important international guidelines [16, 17].

Parameters associated with the risk of metastases in stage I seminoma have been explored more recently, following experiences with active surveillance. Warde et al. [18] reported that a tumor size greater than 4 cm and the presence of rete testis invasion might have predictive value. The presence of one or both factors was associated with an about 30 % rate of nodal metastases, whereas the absence of these factors implied a no greater than 10 % rate of metastases in a series of 638 patients. Although these factors were not fully validated by a subsequent dataset of 687 patients recruited by mostly the same centers [19], Spanish researchers started studies that provided observation only for patients with no risk factors and adjuvant chemotherapy with carboplatin for those with 1 or 2 risk factors. These studies strongly underscored that patients with no risk factors in the modern era have a risk of recurrence not exceeding 6–10 %, thus calling particular attention to the recommendation of no treatment for patients without unfavorable features [20, 21].

An important study by the SWENOTECA group did not find significant prognostic factors of recurrence among 514 patients undergoing surveillance only. More recently, a multicenter dataset of clinical stage I seminoma patients showed that the probability of recurrence increases as the size of the primary tumor increases and that vascular invasion or invasion of the epididymis had prognostic significance in a series of as many as 1,954 patients with stage I seminoma [22]. Studies to confirm these data will not be easy to conduct because of the difficulty to recruit a sufficient number of cases.

Metastatic Disease

Metastatic GCTs can still have a generally favorable prognosis following cisplatin-based chemotherapy. Pathologic parameters are not in use to determine different gradients of curability. International datasets have been analyzed to offer clinicians reproducible means to distinguish different prognostic profiles.

In 1996, the IGCCCG classification study, based on more than 6,000 cases of metastatic disease, identified good-prognosis, intermediate-prognosis, and poor-prognosis categories with a 5-year overall survival of more than 90 %, about 75 %, and 48 %, respectively (Table 7.1) [23]. This classification was essentially based on clinical features. The only pathologic parameter was the distinction between nonseminoma and seminoma, but a poor-prognosis category for the latter could not be defined.

Further studies showed that the prognosis of these categories improved. Interestingly, the survival rate of poor-prognosis patients improved in some cases to a 5-year survival of 70 %. The cause of this gain may be the introduction of more effective salvage strategies, including high-dose chemotherapy and more effective and timely postchemotherapy surgery, rather than a simple stage migration effect due to the improved efficacy of staging devices [24]. More recently, the proportion of patients in the intermediate-prognosis category seems to decrease and the prognosis of these patients to approximate that of good-prognosis patients [25, 26]. The reasons for this are not clear.

In 2010, another international effort permitted to identify as many as five different prognostic profiles among patients who relapsed or were not cured following first-line chemotherapy (Table 7.2) [27]. Also this classification, commonly known as the IGCCCG-2 score, is based on clinical parameters, and the only pathologic piece of information is the diagnosis of seminoma. The best prognostic category includes this histology and a minimal nodal metastatic burden. It is debated how different therapy schedules (essentially standard-dose versus high-dose chemotherapy) may impact prognosis [28]. Although the retrospective results of this dataset show a trend in favor of high-dose regimens, the lack of prospective trials does not permit a conclusive assessment.

Molecular Factors

In recent years many efforts have been made to identify molecular parameters that could help to individualize prognosis and treatment. Interestingly, gene expression profiling including 140 different genes has been carried out in a training set and a validation set of patients with pretreated GCTs. Specific gene expression signatures accurately predicted outcome in terms of 5-year survival, and some gene signatures could therefore be considered predictive of poor outcome or chemoresistance [29].

An Italian study addressing retained expression of CD30 in viable EC cells following chemotherapy showed that persistent CD30 positivity was a significant prognostic factor for progression-free survival and overall survival in a small cohort of patients and could represent a target for treatment [30].

Sex Cord Stromal Tumors

These tumors are rare but usually have a favorable prognosis. Nonetheless, unfavorable outcomes have been reported in about 10 % of cases. Kim et al. [31] first reported on different prognostic

Table 7.1 IGCCCG prognostic classification

Good-prognosis group	
Nonseminoma (56 % of cases)	All of the following criteria:
5-year PFS 89 %	Testis/retroperitoneal primary
5-year survival 92 %	No nonpulmonary visceral metastases
	AFP <1,000 ng/mL
	hCG <5,000 IU/L (1,000 ng/mL)
	LDH <1.5 × ULN
Seminoma (90 % of cases)	All of the following criteria:
5-year PFS 82 %	Any primary site
5-year survival 86 %	No nonpulmonary visceral metastases
	Normal AFP
	Any hCG
	Any LDH
Intermediate-prognosis group	
Nonseminoma (28 % of cases)	All of the following criteria:
5-year PFS 75 %	Testis/retroperitoneal primary
5-year survival 80 %	No nonpulmonary visceral metastases
	AFP 1,000–10,000 ng/mL or
	hCG 5,000–50,000 IU/L or
	LDH 1.5–10 × ULN
Seminoma (10 % of cases)	All of the following criteria:
5-year PFS 67 %	Any primary site
5-year survival 72 %	Nonpulmonary visceral metastases
	Normal AFP
	Any hCG
	Any LDH
Poor-prognosis group	
Nonseminoma (16 % of cases)	Any of the following criteria:
5-year PFS 41 %	Mediastinal primary
5-year survival 48 %	Nonpulmonary visceral metastases
	AFP >10,000 ng/mL or
	hCG >50,000 IU/L (10,000 ng/mL) or
	LDH >10 × ULN
Seminoma	No patients classified as poor prognosis

Modified from International Germ Cell Cancer Collaborative Group [23]
PFS progression-free survival, *AFP* alpha-fetoprotein, *hCG* human chorionic gonadotropin, *LDH* lactate dehydrogenase, *ULN* upper limit of normal

factors associated with a worse prognosis in Leydig cell tumors. These factors include infiltrative growth, presence of mitoses, high proliferation index, presence of necrosis and vascular invasion, and a size greater than 5 cm. These factors have been subsequently extended to other stromal tumors [32]. The presence of at least 2 unfavorable factors is considered an unfavorable condition prompting strict follow-up [16] or, according to some schools of thought, prophylactic RPLND. In patients with nodal involvement, RPLND can be an effective treatment, as it cures a proportion of patients with small nodal metastases. However, there is not sufficient evidence to recommend prophylactic RPLND for clinical stage I patients with unfavorable features [33–35].

The size of a SCST may represent a key marker of aggressive behavior, and small tumors (<5 cm) usually do not display other unfavorable features and therefore allow safe testis-conserving surgery [35]. Patients with no risk factors may be spared continuative and intensive follow-up [14, 33].

Table 7.2 IGCCCG-2 prognostic classification

Points	−1 (very low)	0 (low)	1 (intermediate)	2 (high)	3 (very high)
Variable					
Histology	Seminoma	Nonseminoma			
Primary site		Gonadal	Retroperitoneal		Mediastinal
Response		CR/PRm-	PRm ± SD	PD	
PFI		>3 months	≤3 months		
AFP salvage		Normal	<1,000	1,000	
hCG salvage		<1,000	1,000		
LBB		No	Yes		
2-year PFS (%)	75.1	52.6	42.8	26.4	11.5
3-year OS (%)	77.0	69.0	57.3	31.7	14.7

Modified from Lorch et al. [27]

CR complete remission; *PR* partial remission; *SD* stable disease; *PD* progressive disease; *m−* no evidence of metastasis; *m+* evidence of metastasis; *PFI* progression-free interval (time to relapse); *AFP* alpha-fetoprotein; *hCG* human chorionic gonadotropin; *LBB* liver, brain, or bone metastases; *PFS* progression-free survival; *OS* overall survival

References

1. Verhoeven RH, Karim-Kos HE, Coebergh JW, Brink M, Horenblas S, de Wit R, Kiemeney BA. Markedly increased incidence and improved survival of testicular cancer in the Netherlands. Acta Oncol. 2014;53:342–50.
2. Ruf CG, Isbarn H, Wagner W, Fisch M, Matthies C, Dieckmann KP. Changes in epidemiologic features of testicular germ cell cancer: age at diagnosis and relative frequency of seminoma are constantly and significantly increasing. Urol Oncol. 2014;32:33.e1–6.
3. Freedman LS, Parkinson MC, Jones WG, Oliver RT, Peckham MJ, Read G, Newlands ES, Williams CJ. Histopathology in the prediction of relapse of patients with stage I testicular teratoma treated by orchidectomy alone. Lancet. 1987;2:294–8.
4. Read G, Stenning SP, Cullen MH, Parkinson MC, Horwich A, Kaye SB, Cook PA. Medical Research Council prospective study of surveillance for stage I testicular teratoma. Medical Research Council Testicular Tumors Working Party. J Clin Oncol. 1992;10:1762–8.
5. Sesterhenn IA, Weiss RB, Mostofi FK, Stablein DM, Rowland RG, Falkson G, Rivkind SE, Vogelzang NJ. Prognosis and other clinical correlates of pathologic review in stage I and II testicular carcinoma: a report from the Testicular Cancer Intergroup Study. J Clin Oncol. 1992;10:69–78.
6. Nicolai N, Colecchia M, Biasoni D, Catanzaro M, Stagni S, Torelli T, Necchi A, Piva L, Milani A, Salvioni R. Concordance and prediction ability of original and reviewed vascular invasion and other prognostic parameters of clinical stage I nonseminomatous germ cell testicular tumors after retroperitoneal lymph node dissection. J Urol. 2011; 186:1298–302.
7. Albers P, Ulbright TM, Albers J, Miller GA, Orazi A, Crabtree WN, Baniel J, Reister T, Sidner RA, Foster RS, Donohue JP. Tumor proliferative activity is predictive of pathological stage in clinical stage A nonseminomatous testicular germ cell tumors. J Urol. 1996;155:579–86.
8. Nicolai N, Pizzocaro G. A surveillance study of clinical stage I nonseminomatous germ cell tumors of the testis: 10-year followup. J Urol. 1995;154:1045–9.
9. Sweeney CJ, Hermans BP, Heilman DK, et al. Results and outcome of retroperitoneal lymph node dissection for clinical stage I embryonal carcinoma—predominant testis cancer. J Clin Oncol. 2000;18:358–62.
10. Stephenson AJ, Bosl GJ, Bajorin DF, Stasi J, Motzer RJ, Sheinfeld J. Retroperitoneal lymph node dissection in patients with low stage testicular cancer with embryonal carcinoma predominance and/or lymphovascular invasion. J Urol. 2005;174:557–60.
11. Klepp O, Olsson AM, Henrikson H, Aass N, Dahl O, Stenwig AE, Persson BE, Cavallin-Ståhl E, Fosså SD, Wahlqvist L. Prognostic factors in clinical stage I nonseminomatous germ cell tumors of the testis: multivariate analysis of a prospective multicenter study. Swedish-Norwegian Testicular Cancer Group. J Clin Oncol. 1990;8:509–18.
12. Klepp O, Dahl O, Flodgren P, Stierner U, Olsson AM, Oldbring J, Nilsson S, Daehlin L, Tørnblom M, Småland R, Starkhammar H, Abramsson L, Wist E, Raabe N, Edekling T, Cavallin-Ståhl E. Risk-adapted treatment of clinical stage 1 non-seminoma testis cancer. Eur J Cancer. 1997;33:1038–44.
13. Leibovitch I, Foster RS, Kopecky KK, Albers P, Ulbright TM, Donohue JP. Identification of clinical stage A nonseminomatous testis cancer patients at extremely low risk for metastatic disease: a combined

approach using quantitive immunohistochemical, histopathologic, and radiologic assessment. J Clin Oncol. 1998;16:261–8.
14. Nicolai N, Miceli R, Artusi R, Piva L, Pizzocaro G, Salvioni R. A simple model for predicting nodal metastasis in patients with clinical stage I nonseminomatous germ cell testicular tumors undergoing retroperitoneal lymph node dissection only. J Urol. 2004;171:172–6.
15. Vergouwe Y, Steyerberg EW, Eijkemans MJ, Albers P, Habbema JD. Predictors of occult metastasis in clinical stage I nonseminoma: a systematic review. J Clin Oncol. 2003;21:4092–9.
16. European Association of Urology. Guidelines on testicular cancer. 2015. www.uroweb.org
17. NCCN Clinical Practice Guidelines in Oncology. Testicular Cancer. Version 1.2015. At URL: www.nccn.org. Accessed on 19 Nov 2014.
18. Warde P, Specht L, Horwich A, Oliver T, Panzarella T, Gospodarowicz M, von der Maase H. Prognostic factors for relapse in stage I seminoma managed by surveillance: a pooled analysis. J Clin Oncol. 2002;20:4448–52.
19. Chung PW, Daugaard G, Tyldesley S, Panzarella T, Kollmannsberger CK, Gospodarowicz MK, Warde PR. Prognostic factors for relapse in stage I seminoma managed with surveillance: a validation study. J Clin Oncol. 2010;28:Abstract 4535
20. Aparicio J, Germà JR, García del Muro X, Maroto P, Arranz JA, Sáenz A, Barnadas A, Dorca J, Gumà J, Olmos D, Bastús R, Carles J, Almenar D, Sánchez M, Paz-Ares L, Satrústegui JJ, Mellado B, Balil A, López-Brea M, Sánchez A, Second Spanish Germ Cell Cancer Cooperative Group. Risk-adapted management for patients with clinical stage I seminoma: the Second Spanish Germ Cell Cancer Cooperative Group study. J Clin Oncol. 2005;23:8717–23.
21. Aparicio J, Maroto P, del Muro XG, Gumà J, Sánchez-Muñoz A, Margelí M, Doménech M, Bastús R, Fernández A, López-Brea M, Terrassa J, Meana A, del Prado PM, Sastre J, Satrústegui JJ, Gironés R, Robert L, Germà JR. Risk-adapted treatment in clinical stage I testicular seminoma: the third Spanish Germ Cell Cancer Group study. J Clin Oncol. 2011;29:4677–81.
22. Tandstad T, Smaaland R, Solberg A, Bremnes RM, Langberg CW, Laurell A, Stierner UK, Ståhl O, Cavallin-Ståhl EK, Klepp OH, Dahl O, Cohn-Cedermark G. Management of seminomatous testicular cancer: a binational prospective population-based study from the Swedish norwegian testicular cancer study group. J Clin Oncol. 2011;29:719–25.
23. International Germ Cell Consensus Classification: a prognostic factor-based staging system for metastatic germ cell cancers. International Germ Cell Cancer Collaborative Group. J Clin Oncol. 1997;15:594–603
24. van Dijk MR, Steyerberg EW, Habbema JD. Survival of non-seminomatous germ cell cancer patients according to the IGCC classification: an update based on meta-analysis. Eur J Cancer. 2006;42:820–6.
25. Albany C, Satpute SR, Brames MJ, Suleiman Y, Al-Nasrallah N, Perkins SM, Hanna NH, Einhorn LH. A retrospective analysis of patients with intermediate-risk germ cell tumor (IRGCT) treated at Indiana University from 2000 to 2010. J Clin Oncol. 2012;30:Abstract 4534
26. Raggi D, Mariani L, Giannatempo P, Lo Vullo S, Giardiello D, Nicolai N, Piva L, Biasoni D, Catanzaro M, Torelli T, Stagni S, Maffezzini M, Calareso G, Magni M, Di Nicola M, Verzoni E, Grassi P, Procopio G, De Braud F, Pizzocaro G, Salvioni R, Necchi A. Prognostic reclassification of patients with intermediate-risk metastatic germ cell tumors: implications for clinical practice, trial design, and molecular interrogation. Urol Oncol. 2015;33:332.e19–24.
27. Lorch A, Beyer J, Bascoul-Mollevi C, Kramar A, Einhorn LH, Necchi A, Massard C, De Giorgi U, Fléchon A, Margolin KA, Lotz JP, Germa Lluch JR, Powles T, Kollmannsberger CK. Prognostic factors in patients with metastatic germ cell tumors who experienced treatment failure with cisplatin-based first-line chemotherapy. J Clin Oncol. 2010;28:4906–11.
28. Lorch A, Bascoul-Mollevi C, Kramar A, Einhorn L, Necchi A, Massard C, De Giorgi U, Fléchon A, Margolin K, Lotz JP, Germà-Lluch JR, Powles T, Kollmannsberger C, Beyer J. Conventional-dose versus high-dose chemotherapy as first salvage treatment in male patients with metastatic germ cell tumors: evidence from a large international database. J Clin Oncol. 2011;29:2178–84.
29. Korkola JE, Houldsworth J, Feldman DR, Olshen AB, Qin LX, Patil S, Reuter VE, Bosl GJ, Chaganti RS. Identification and validation of a gene expression signature that predicts outcome in adult men with germ cell tumors. J Clin Oncol. 2009;27:5240–7.
30. Giannatempo P, Paolini B, Miceli R, Raggi D, Nicolai N, Farè E, Catanzaro M, Biasoni D, Torelli T, Stagni S, Piva L, Mariani L, Salvioni R, Colecchia M, Gianni AM, Necchi A. Persistent CD30 expression by embryonal carcinoma in the treatment time course: prognostic significance of a worthwhile target for personalized treatment. J Urol. 2013;190:1919–24.
31. Kim I, Young RH, Scully RE. Leydig cell tumors of the testis. A clinicopathological analysis of 40 cases and review of the literature. Am J Surg Pathol. 1985;9:177–92.
32. Young RH, Koelliker DD, Scully RE. Sertoli cell tumors of the testis, not otherwise specified: a clinicopathologic analysis of 60 cases. Am J Surg Pathol. 1998;22:709–21.
33. Mosharafa AA, Foster RS, Bihrle R, Koch MO, Ulbright TM, Einhorn LH, Donohue JP. Does retroperitoneal lymph node dissection have a curative role for patients with sex cord-stromal testicular tumors? Cancer. 2003;98:753–7.
34. Silberstein JL, Bazzi WM, Vertosick E, Carver BS, Bosl GJ, Feldman DR, Bajorin DF, Motzer RJ, Al-Ahmadie H, Reuter VE, Sheinfeld J. Clinical outcomes of local and metastatic testicular sex cord-stromal tumors. J Urol. 2014;192:415–9.
35. Nicolai N, Necchi A, Raggi D, Biasoni D, Catanzaro M, Piva L, Stagni S, Maffezzini M, Torelli T, Faré E, Giannatempo P, Pizzocaro G, Colecchia M, Salvioni R. Clinical outcome in testicular sex cord stromal tumors: testis sparing vs radical orchiectomy and management of advanced disease. Urology. 2015;85:402–6.

Handling of the Surgical Specimen and Pathology Reporting of Malignant Germ Cell and Sex Cord-Stromal Tumors of the Testis

8

Marina Scarpelli, Roberta Mazzucchelli, Matteo Santoni, Valeria Sotte, Alessandro Conti, Antonio Lopez-Beltran, Liang Cheng, and Rodolfo Montironi

Introduction

This chapter discusses handling of the partial orchiectomy or radical orchiectomy specimens and focuses on pathology reporting of malignant germ cell. A similar approach can be adopted for sex cord-stromal tumors. Clinical information is critical for the pathological assessment of orchiectomy specimens.

M. Scarpelli (✉) • R. Mazzucchelli • R. Montironi
Pathological Anatomy, Polytechnic University of the Marche Region, School of Medicine, United Hospitals, Ancona, Italy
e-mail: m.scarpelli@univpm.it; r.mazzucchelli@univpm.it; r.montironi@univpm.it

M. Santoni • V. Sotte
Medical Oncology, Polytechnic University of the Marche Region, School of Medicine, United Hospitals, Ancona, Italy
e-mail: mattymo@alice.it; valeria.sotte@gmail.it

A. Conti
Department of Odontostomatologic and Specialized Clinical Sciences, Section of Urology, Polytechnic University of the Marche Region, School of Medicine, United Hospitals, Ancona, Italy
e-mail: alessandro.conti@hotmail.com

A. Lopez-Beltran
Department of Pathology and Surgery, Faculty of Medicine, University of Cordoba, Cordoba, Spain
e-mail: em1lobea@uco.es

L. Cheng
Department of Pathology and Laboratory Medicine, Indiana University School of Medicine, Indianapolis, IN, USA
e-mail: lcheng@iupui.edu

Handling of the Surgical Specimen

Testis specimen should be handled in such manner to allow gathering of comprehensive and accurate pathological information [1–3].

Measurements of the three dimensions of the orchiectomy specimen must be reported together with the length of spermatic cord. The following macroscopic data must be recorded [1, 2]:

- Length, width, and thickness of the neoplasm
- Heterogeneity in color and consistency
- Necrotic and/or hemorrhagic areas
- Zones that appear different from the remaining tumor (e.g., cysts or bone)
- Multiple neoplastic nodules
- Relation of the neoplasm with tunica vaginalis, testis hilum, epididymis, and spermatic cord
- Pathological findings of the testicular tissue uninvolved by the neoplasm, such as fibrosis

M. Colecchia (ed.), *Pathology of Testicular and Penile Neoplasms*, DOI 10.1007/978-3-319-27617-5_8

Sampling should include [1, 2]:

- Neoplasm and its interface with nontumorous testis.
- Any macroscopic different looking areas of the neoplasm. Any area showing necrosis or hemorrhage must be sampled. A hemorrhagic area has to be included entirely, since tumors such as choriocarcinoma can be extensively hemorrhagic leaving just little viable cancer.
- Testis hilum and mediastinum, epididymis.
- Testicular tissue not involved by the neoplasm, including the tunica vaginalis and tunica albuginea. Every abnormality of tunica vaginalis and albuginea must be sampled.
- Spermatic cord, including its margin. It is important to assess and incise spermatic cord before sectioning the orchiectomy specimen in order to avoid the so-called tumor smearing, i.e., the blade used to incise testis transfers neoplastic cells, relocating them in successive sections, including in the vascular lumen, thus giving the impression of lymphovascular invasion.
- Any other lesion (or lesions) identified.

Since patient management depends on the identification of different tumor types within the same specimen, cancer sampling should be adequate to allow the identification of different tumor types and patterns, including the presence of lymphovascular invasion and intratubular germ cell neoplasia unclassified (IGCNU) [1]. If the blocks needed to sample the tumor are equal or less than 10, the whole testis neoplasm can be included. In case of neoplasms larger than 10 cm, it is preferable to take one block for each centimeter of the maximum length [2]. It is important to block tumor interface with uninvolved testicular tissue and tunica albuginea, also at a distance from neoplastic cells. Indeed, it is known that lymphovascular invasion is better evaluated in peri-tumoral parenchyma.

Pathology Reporting

Germ Cell and Sex Cord-Stromal Tumors of the Testis: Histologic Type

Histologic type must be recorded [1–5]. The new WHO classification is listed in Chap. 6. TGCTs (testicular germ cell tumours) include pure and mixed forms. In mixed forms, the percentage of the distinct tumor types must be assessed and reported [6, 7]. Syncytiotrophoblast may be found in TGCTs, with the syncytiotrophoblast presenting as single cells or very small groups, with no cytotrophoblast to indicate associated choriocarcinoma. This finding should be reported.

Necrosis

Complete necrosis is a rare event. Tumors with complete necrosis should be reported as TGCTs without further classification. Necrotic tumors must be distinguished from testicular infarction, where the normal architecture in the background is still preserved [1, 2].

Scar

Testicular scarring, particularly in metastatic patients without clinically apparent testicular primary lesions, may represent regressed testicular TGCTs (i.e., *regressed* (*burnt-out*) *TGCTs*) [4, 5]. Among features that favor such diagnosis, the reporting pathologist should consider [1, 2, 8, 9]:

- Residual TGCT
- Associated intratubular calcifications
- IGCNU or differentiated type
- Lymphoplasmacytic inflammatory infiltrate
- Hemosiderin-containing macrophages
- Seminiferous tubule hyalinization/atrophy
- Serum GCT marker elevation
- Extratesticular TGCT

Scars with residual invasive cancer should be considered as a partial regression of the tumor. In pure seminoma forms, testicular scarring may derive from the partial regression of a nonseminomatous TGCT component, and this should be taken into account to guide treatment decisions.

TNM Staging

The TNM staging system is currently accepted worldwide [10]. The year of publication or the edition of the cancer staging system employed must be indicated in the pathologic report. Its revision should be available by the end of 2015. The T parameter is assigned to not previously treated primary tumors. The prefix "p" indicates a pathological classification, whereas "c" stands for a clinical definition of the extent of the disease [10]. Pathological classification is based on histological evidence: pT requires either the excision of the primary neoplasm or a biopsy suitable for determining the pT class (Table 8.1; Fig. 8.1). pN implies the resection of lymph nodes adequate to identify metastases (Table 8.2), whereas pM involves the evaluation of distant secondary metastatic sites (Table 8.3). Pathologic staging is commonly performed after surgery and depends on the pathologic evaluation of the extent of disease.

Tumor invasion of the rete testis consists in the direct invasion of the stroma and does not include pagetoid spread of IGCN into the tubules of the rete. Invasion of rete testis or epididymis is not recorded as a higher stage, while the invasion of the tunica vaginalis (perforating the mesothelial lining) is assigned as pT2. The presence of rete testis invasion, as well as a tumor size >4 cm, has been associated with a higher risk of metastatic spread in patients with stage I seminomas. Tumor invasion of hilar soft tissue is the predominant pathway of extratesticular extension for testicular neoplasms. However, the issue of hilar soft tissue invasion and its clinical significance has not been completely studied [2].

Table 8.1 Primary tumor (pT)

pTX:	Cannot be assessed
pT0:	No evidence of primary tumor (includes scar)
pTis:	Intratubular germ cell neoplasia (carcinoma in situ)
pT1:	Tumor limited to the testis and epididymis without vascular/lymphatic invasion; tumor may invade tunica albuginea but not tunica vaginalis
pT2:	Tumor limited to the testis and epididymis with vascular/lymphatic invasion or tumor extending through the tunica albuginea with involvement of the tunica vaginalis
pT3:	Tumor invades the spermatic cord with or without vascular/lymphatic invasion
pT4:	Tumor invades the scrotum with or without vascular/lymphatic invasion

Edge et al. [10]

Lymphovascular Invasion

The presence of lymphovascular invasion has been associated with a higher risk of developing distant metastases. This situation is particularly important in clinical stage I disease, i.e., without serum and/or imaging evidence of spread outside the testis [11–14]. Some clinicians manage patients with clinical stage I disease without lymphovascular invasion in their orchiectomy specimens and other favorable prognostic elements (including a small amounts of embryonal carcinoma) by close follow-up rather than adjuvant chemotherapy. The AJCC TNM staging system does not specifically takes into account the vascular invasion in the spermatic cord [10]. While the invasion of the cord is indicated as a pT3 stage, it would be logical to report vascular invasion in the cord as pT2 stage, unless the tumor penetrates through the vessel wall into the perivascular soft tissues of the cord.

Intratubular Germ Cell Neoplasia Unclassified (IGCNU)

The presence or absence of IGCNU (*synonyms: carcinoma in situ testis (CIS), testicular intraepithelial neoplasia (TIN), and gonocytoma in situ*) must be specified [1–5]. IGCNU is defined by gonocyte-like germ cells with abundant clear cytoplasm and large (10–11 μm) nuclei with coarse chromatin, located within the seminiferous

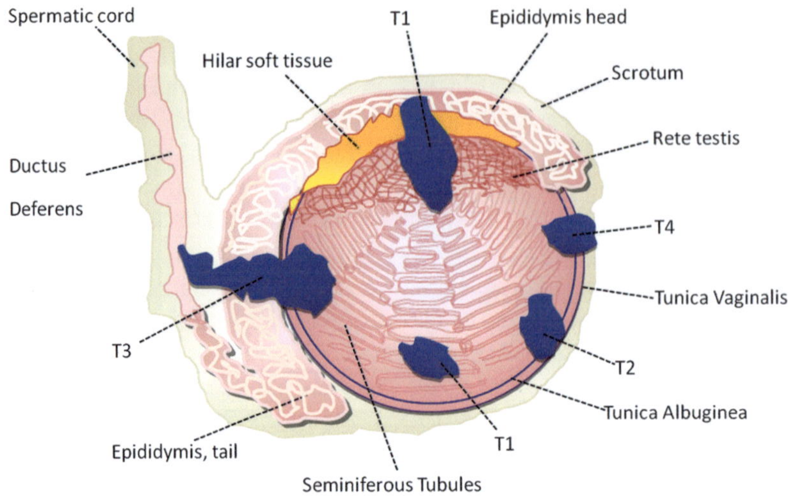

Fig. 8.1 Staging of testicular neoplasms. Diagrammatic representation

Table 8.2 Regional lymph nodes (pN)

pNX:	Cannot be assessed
pN0:	No regional lymph node metastasis
pN1:	Metastasis with a lymph node mass 2 cm or less in greatest dimension and less than or equal to 5 nodes positive, none more than 2 cm in greatest dimension
pN2:	Metastasis with a lymph node mass more than 2 cm but not more than 5 cm in greatest dimension or more than 5 nodes positive, none more than 5 cm, or evidence of extranodal extension of tumor
pN3:	Metastasis with a lymph node mass more than 5 cm in greatest dimension

Edge et al. [10]

Table 8.3 Distant metastasis (pM)

pM1:	Distant metastasis present
pM1a:	Nonregional nodal or pulmonary metastasis
pM1b:	Distant metastasis other than to nonregional lymph nodes and lung

Edge et al. [10]

tubules and expressing embryonic germ cell markers [15]. IGCNU should be differentiated from intratubular seminoma, intratubular non-seminoma, spermatogenic arrest at the stage of spermatogonia, pre-IGCNU cells, and maturation-delayed gonocytes persisting outside the fetal/infantile period.

IGCNU is the most recognized intratubular proliferation associated with the development of testicular TGCTs. However, other tumor types are also occasionally identified, nearly always in association with IGCNU and invasive TGCTs [16, 17]. It is unclear if these additional types are preinvasive neoplastic lesions or represent the growth of an existing invasive TGCT into tubules.

Additional Findings

The list of additional relevant findings that should be evaluated and included in the pathology report include [1, 2]:

- Leydig cell hyperplasia
- Scarring
- The presence of macrophages containing hemosiderin in their cytoplasm
- Intratubular calcifications, which may be interpreted as tumor regression
- Abnormal development of the testis, such as androgen-insensitivity syndrome and dysgenesis and testicular atrophy

Ancillary Studies

The use of ancillary studies may provide additional information on lineage, clonality, or disease classification [4]. Furthermore, they can provide prognostic and predictive biomarkers of tumor response to targeted therapies [4]. The majority of testicular tumors can be identified by histological examination. However, the differentiation among some types (i.e., the identification of trophoblast) may result as difficult. In this context, the employ of immunohistochemistry may provide useful information that should be reported in the pathology reports [4, 5].

Serum Markers

The serum tumor marker category includes alpha-fetoprotein (AFP), human chorionic gonadotropin (hCG), and lactate dehydrogenase (LDH). Serum marker status and trend should be monitored in TGCT inasmuch as they guide pathological specimen management (Table 8.4). High concentrations of beta-human chorionic gonadotropin (b-hCG) or alpha-fetoprotein (AFP) without a pathological equivalent in the preliminary morphological examination of the specimens might suggest the necessity of supplementary sampling of the specimen. Pre-orchiectomy serum levels of lactate dehydrogenase (LDH), AFP, and b-hCG are required to define the "S" parameter of TGCT staging [1, 2, 10]. Oncologic markers should be transcribed in the pathology report.

Metastatic Tumor

The distinction of metastatic residual teratoma from non-teratomatous types of TGCT is fundamental in those patients who present with metastatic testicular germ cell neoplasms following chemotherapy. The differentiation between these tumor types allows to distinguish patients with pure teratomatous metastasis, who usually undergo surgical excision alone, from patients with residual TGCT, who are treated with additional chemotherapy [1, 2, 4].

Table 8.4 Serum tumor markers (S)

SX:	Serum marker studies not available or performed			
S0:	Serum marker study levels within normal limits			
	LDH		*HCG (mIU/mL)*		*AFP (ng/mL)*
S1:	<1.5×N[a]	and	<5,000	and	<1,000
S2:	1.5–10×N	or	5,000–50,000	or	1,000–10,000
S3:	>10×N	or	>50,000	or	>10,000

Edge et al. [10]

[a]*N* indicates the upper limit of normal for the LDKH assay

Conclusions

Macroscopic and microscopic items included in a pathology report have prognostic implications. Clinical information is critical for the pathological assessment of orchiectomy specimens. It is recommended to include in the pathology report anamnestic data such as cryptorchidism and previous TGCT, along with acknowledged risk factors (e.g., positive family history for testicle germ cell neoplasm). Serum marker status and trend should be monitored in TGCT inasmuch as they guide pathological specimen management.

References

1. Royal College of Pathologists of Australasia (RCPA). Functional requirements for laboratory information systems to support structured pathology reporting of cancer protocols. 2011. Available from: http://www.rcpa.edu.au/Publications/StructuredReporting/LISFunctionalRequirements.htm.
2. Tickoo SK, Reuter VE, Amin MB, Chang SS, Humphrey PA, McKiernan J, Srigley JR, Ulbright TM, Zhou M. Protocol for the examination of specimens from patients with malignant germ cell and sex cord-stromal tumors of the testis. 2011. Available from: http://www.cap.org/apps/cap.portal.
3. Berney DM, Algaba F, Amin M, Delahunt B, Compérat E, Epstein JI, Humphrey P, Idrees M, Lopez-Beltran A, Magi-Galluzzi C, Mikuz G, Montironi R, Oliva E, Srigley J, Reuter VE, Trpkov K, Ulbright TM, Varma M, Verrill C, Young RH, Zhou M, Egevad L. Handling and reporting of orchidectomy specimens with testicular cancer: areas of consensus and variation among 25 experts and 225 European pathologists. Histopathology. 2015;67:313–24.
4. Eble JN, Sauter G, Epstein JI, Sesterhenn IA editors. World Health Organization classification of tumours. pathology and genetics: tumours of the urinary system and male genital organ. In: Tumours of the testis and paratesticular tissue. Lyon: IARC Press; 2004. pp. 216–78

5. Ulbright TM, Young HY. Tumors of the testis and adjacent structures. In: Silverberg SG, editor. AFIP atlas of tumor pathology. Series 4, vol. 18. Silver Spring: ARP; 2013.
6. Moul JW, McCarthy WF, Fernandez EB, Sesterhenn IA. Percentage of embryonal carcinoma and of vascular invasion predicts pathological stage in clinical stage I nonseminomatous testicular cancer. Cancer Res. 1994;54:362–4.
7. Daugaard G, Gundgaard MG, Mortensen MS, Agerbæk M, Holm NV, Rørth M, von der Maase H, Christensen IJ, Lauritsen J. Surveillance for stage I nonseminoma testicular cancer: outcomes and long-term follow-up in a population-based cohort. J Clin Oncol. 2014;32:3817–23.
8. Balzer BL, Ulbright TM. Spontaneous regression of testicular germ cell tumors: an analysis of 42 cases. Am J Surg Pathol. 2006;30:858–65.
9. Angulo JC, González J, Rodríguez N, Hernández E, Núñez C, Rodríguez-Barbero JM, Santana A, López JI. Clinicopathological study of regressed testicular tumors (apparent extragonadal germ cell neoplasms). J Urol. 2009;182:2303–10.
10. Edge SE, Byrd DR, Compton CC, Fritz AG, Greene FL, Trotti A editors. Cancer staging handbook. In: AJCC Cancer Staging Manual. 7th ed. New York: Springer; 2010. pp. 539–46
11. Fung CY, Kalish LA, Brodsky GL, Richie JP, Garnick MB. Stage I nonseminomatous germ cell testicular tumor: prediction of metastatic potential by primary histopathology. J Clin Oncol. 1988;6:1467–73.
12. Heidenreich A, Sesterhenn IA, Mostofi FK, Moul JW. Prognostic risk factors that identify patients with clinical stage I nonseminomatous germ cell tumors at low risk and high risk for metastasis. Cancer. 1998;83:1002–11.
13. Albers P, Siener R, Kliesch S, Weissbach L, Krege S, Sparwasser C, Schulze H, Heidenreich A, de Riese W, Loy V, Bierhoff E, Wittekind C, Fimmers R, Hartmann M, German Testicular Cancer Study Group. Risk factors for relapse in clinical stage I nonseminomatous testicular germ cell tumors: results of the German Testicular Cancer Study Group Trial. J Clin Oncol. 2003;21:1505–12.
14. Yilmaz A, Cheng T, Zhang J, Trpkov K. Testicular hilum and vascular invasion predict advanced clinical stage in nonseminomatous germ cell tumors. Modern Pathol. 2013;26:579–86.
15. Skakkebaek NE. Possible carcinoma-in-situ of the testis. Lancet. 1972;2:516–7.
16. Jacobsen GK, Henriksen OB, von der Maase H. Carcinoma in situ of testicular tissue adjacent to malignant germ-cell tumors: a study of 105 cases. Cancer. 1981;47:2660–2.
17. Oosterhuis JW, Kersemaekers AM, Jacobsen GK, Timmer A, Steyerberg EW, Molier M, Van Weeren PC, Stoop H, Looijenga LH. Morphology of testicular parenchyma adjacent to germ cell tumours. An interim report. APMIS. 2003;111:32–42.

Cysts and Epithelial Proliferations of the Testicular Collecting System

9

Antonio Lopez-Beltran, Rita Canas-Marques, Maria R. Raspollini, Rodolfo Montironi, Marina Scarpelli, and Liang Cheng

Introduction

Paratesticular tumors are uncommon, accounting for less than 10 % of intrascrotal neoplasms; most are benign and morphologically similar to their counterparts in other organs. In the presence of a paratesticular mass, the differential diagnosis must consider both tumorlike lesions and primary neoplasms. Not infrequently, metastases to the paratesticular region count as an additional diagnostic challenge in uropathology practice. This chapter provides a pathological synopsis of epithelial neoplasms and pseudotumors arising in the paratesticular region.

A. Lopez-Beltran (✉)
Department of Pathology and Surgery, Faculty of Medicine, University of Cordoba, Cordoba, Spain
e-mail: em1lobea@uco.es

R. Canas-Marques
Champalimaud Foudation, Lisbon, Portugal
e-mail: rita.marques@fundacaochampalimaud.pt

M.R. Raspollini
Division of Histology and Molecular Diagnostics, University Hospital Careggi, University of Florence, Florence, Italy
e-mail: mariarosaria.raspollini@unifi.it

R. Montironi • M. Scarpelli
Pathological Anatomy, Polytechnic University of the Marche Region, School of Medicine, United Hospitals, Ancona, Italy
e-mail: r.montironi@univpm.it; m.scarpelli@univpm.it

L. Cheng
Department of Pathology and Laboratory Medicine, Indiana University School of Medicine, Indianapolis, IN, USA
e-mail: lcheng@iupui.edu

Basic Anatomy

The paratesticular region is a rich anatomic structure that comprises the intratesticular duct system, the excretory genital duct, the spermatic cord, and the tunics of the testis [1–5]. Here we summarize the main anatomical features of the paratestis to introduce the malformations and tumors occurring in this region. The rete testis consists of a complex network of channels covered by flat or cuboidal cells (Fig. 9.1), which receives the content of the seminiferous tubules and their twisted loops at the testicular hilum. Up to twenty efferent ductules arise from the extratesticular portion of the rete testis, which merge into the epididymis. The epididymis is composed of a head, a body, and a tail consisting of a long duct that goes on in the ductus deferens, a 30–40-cm tubular structure which merges with the seminal vesicles in the ejaculatory duct [6]. The head and tail of the epididymis occasionally have a cribriform architecture with some lipochrome pigment (Fig. 9.2a–c). The spermatic cord is filled with a loose connective tissue matrix with scattered bundles of smooth muscle fibers; it is covered by spermatic and

M. Colecchia (ed.), *Pathology of Testicular and Penile Neoplasms*,
DOI 10.1007/978-3-319-27617-5_9

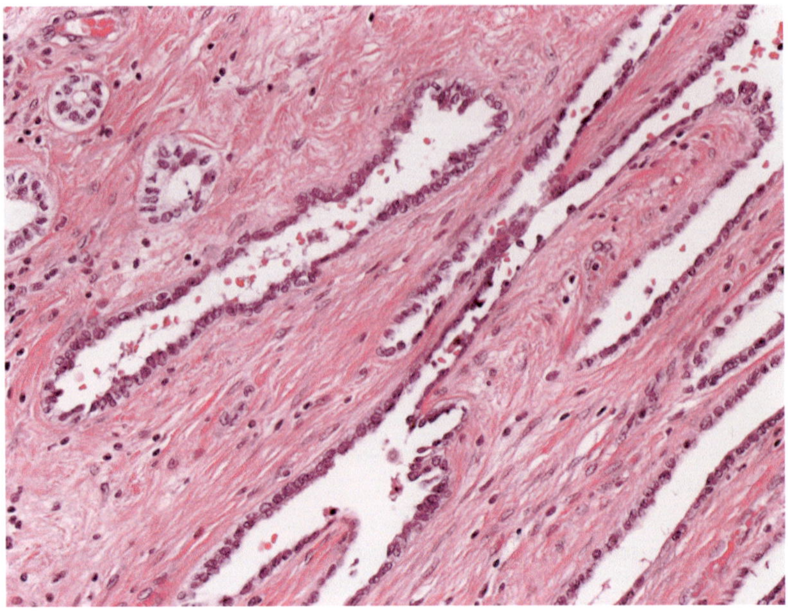

Fig. 9.1 Anastomosing channels of rete testis covered by flat to cuboidal epithelium

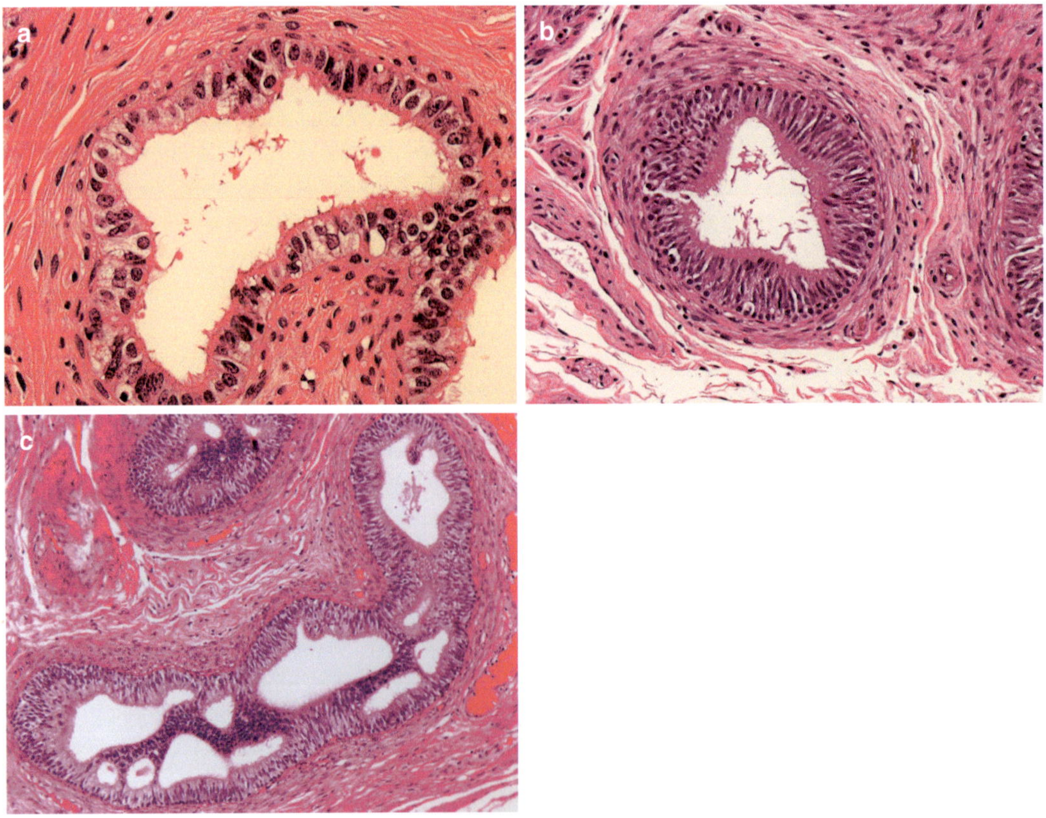

Fig. 9.2 Head (**a**) and tail (**b**) of the epididymis, which may occasionally present a cribriform architecture (**c**)

cremasteric fasciae, which are also constitutive layers of the scrotal wall. The testis is covered by numerous structures including the inner (visceral) portion of the tunica vaginalis, its external counterpart (parietal tunica vaginalis), the internal spermatic fascia, the cremasteric muscle, the external spermatic fascia, and the external structures of the scrotal skin. The tunica vaginalis consists of thick fibrous tissue containing elastic and smooth muscle fibers covered by mesothelium (Fig. 9.3). The tunica vaginalis surrounds all of the testis except the testicular hilum.

Cysts of the Testicular Collecting System

Most cysts with a tumorlike presentation are paratesticular but may occasionally occur in the testis, where they can be confused with neoplasms arising in the tunica albuginea [7, 8].

Congenital Cysts

Cystic change in the rete testis may be associated with cryptorchidism or may occur as cystic dysplasia of the rete testis (associated with renal agenesis or cystic dysplasia of the kidney). Epididymal cysts may affect patients with von Hippel-Lindau disease. Congenital hydrocele may also occur, generally before the age of 2 years.

Cystic Transformation of the Rete Testis

Cystic transformation of the rete testis (CTRT), or giant cystic degeneration of the rete testis, is the result of a partial or complete obstruction of the head of the epididymis (Fig. 9.4). CTRT is frequently associated with vascular alterations of testicular or epididymal arteries, while occasional bilateral efferent duct atrophy has been reported. CTRT has been found in 1.1 % of autopsy and 3.5 % of surgical series. Other etiologic aspects include mechanical factors (compression of the epididymis by an epididymal spermatic cord tumor or as a result of long-standing epididymitis or traumatic hematocele), hormones (in cirrhotic patients), ischemia, and malformation (cryptorchidism). CTRT was related to ipsilateral renal agenesis in two cases. Ectasia of the rete testis is sometimes associated with columnar transformation of the epithelium,

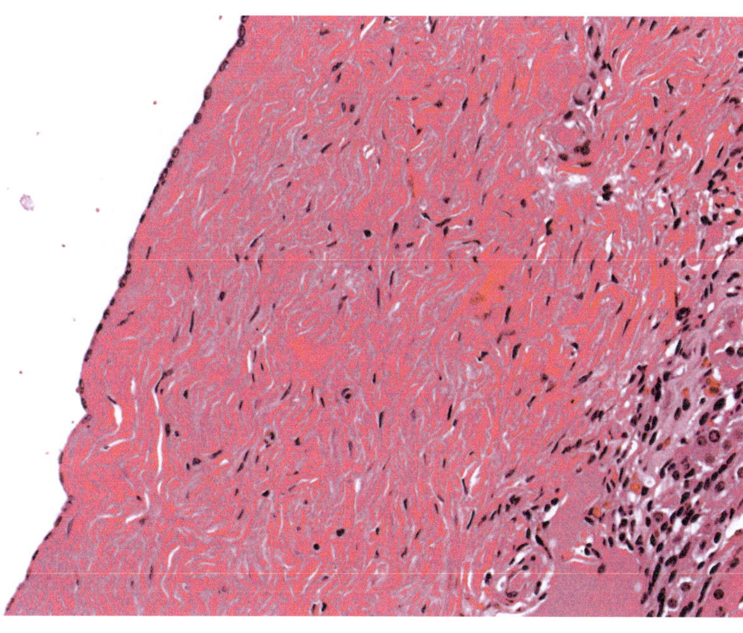

Fig. 9.3 Tunica albuginea covered by the mesothelial tunica vaginalis testis (*right*)

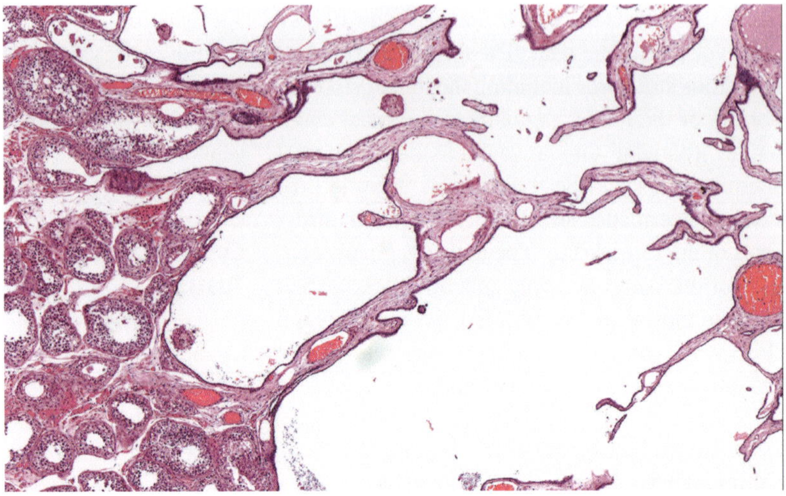

Fig. 9.4 Cystic transformation of the rete testis

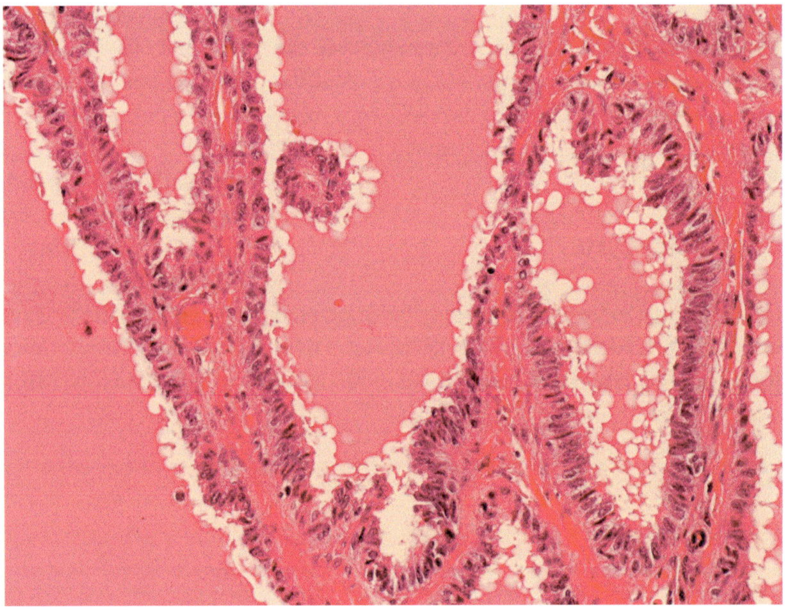

Fig. 9.5 Acquired cysts of rete testis with columnar transformation seen in a patient with varicocele

leading to nodular proliferation with or without calcification of the connective tissue [9–16]. Malformations in cryptorchidism with testis and epididymis dissociation (derived from the sex cords and mesonephric ducts, respectively) may result in CTRT [17].

Acquired Cysts of the Rete Testis

Acquired cysts of the rete testis are related to obstruction of the epididymis or the intratesticular excretory ducts due to varicocele (Fig. 9.5) or can be secondary to hemodialysis in patients with renal failure [14, 18]. The rete testis is composed of dilated channels lined with high columnar or pseudostratified epithelium with occasional papillary proliferations; the ductuli efferentes epithelium may show intracytoplasmic eosinophilic granules. In both structures, the lumen usually contains spermatozoa, proteinaceous material, and calcium oxalate crystals with occasionally multinucleated giant cells [14, 18].

Tubular Ectasia of the Rete Testis

Tubular ectasia of the rete testis is an uncommon entity that is usually discovered incidentally during ultrasound evaluation of epididymal abnormalities, in most cases a spermatocele. This cystic lesion is usually located in the mediastinum testes, where there is dilatation of the tubules of the rete testis often associated with some degree of obstruction at the epididymal level, either post-traumatic or post-infectious in nature. Bilaterality is a common finding. When severe, it may show complete testicular parenchyma substitution. Bilateral cases may be associated with azoospermia [19, 20].

Multicystic Mass of Probable Wolffian Origin

Multicystic mass of probable Wolffian origin (Wolffian hamartoma) is a benign tumor believed to arise from Wolffian duct remnants at supraepididymal, paravasal locations suggesting its origin in the paradidymis. It is very rare in men and more common in women. It occurs as a unilocular or multicystic mass lined with a single layer of cuboidal to tall columnar epithelium with apical cilia surrounded by fibromuscular tissue [21]. The nuclei are usually bland with rare mitoses. Secretions are commonly observed on the apical aspect of cells and in the lumen but without sperm in the lumen as is seen in spermatocele (Fig. 9.6a, b).

Epididymal Cyst and Spermatocele

Epididymal cysts and spermatoceles are common lesions resulting from inflammatory processes that are often included in the differential diagnosis with other cystic lesions.

Epididymal cysts are usually small and benign, with a diameter of up to 2 cm. They mostly occur in the head of the epididymis and arise from the efferent ductules. Painful torsion of these cysts may occur. The prevalence is high in patients with von Hippel-Lindau disease, polycystic kidney disease, early-onset renal cell carcinoma, and in sons of diethylstilbestrol-treated mothers. The cysts are usually translucent, unilocular, or multilocular and covered by a single layer of flat to cuboidal cells with variable numbers of cilia. There is no evidence of cellular atypia. Small papillary structures containing connective tissue cores lined with a single layer of non-atypical epithelium may protrude into the cysts. The cyst wall is thin and composed of fibromuscular tissue. Epididymal cysts may be associated with chronic inflammation, foreign-body giant cell reaction, cholesterol clefts, and occasionally calcification. The lumen contains proteinaceous material, and if spermatozoa are also present, these cysts are called spermatoceles (Fig. 9.7). Shedding of rete testis cells has been related to associated hydrocele, sometimes with signs of inflammation and scrotal swelling. This finding is a potential diagnostic pitfall, as it may lead to confusion with metastatic small cell

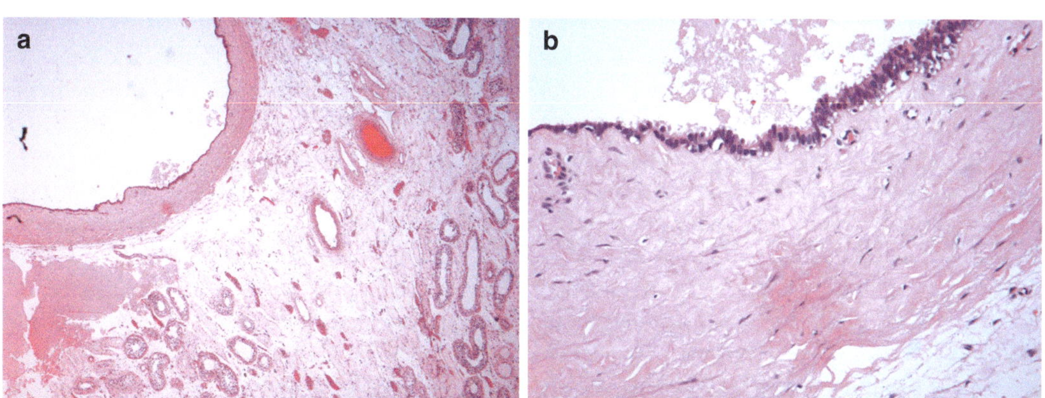

Fig. 9.6 Cystic lesion of probable Wolffian origin at low- (**a**) and medium-power (**b**) magnification

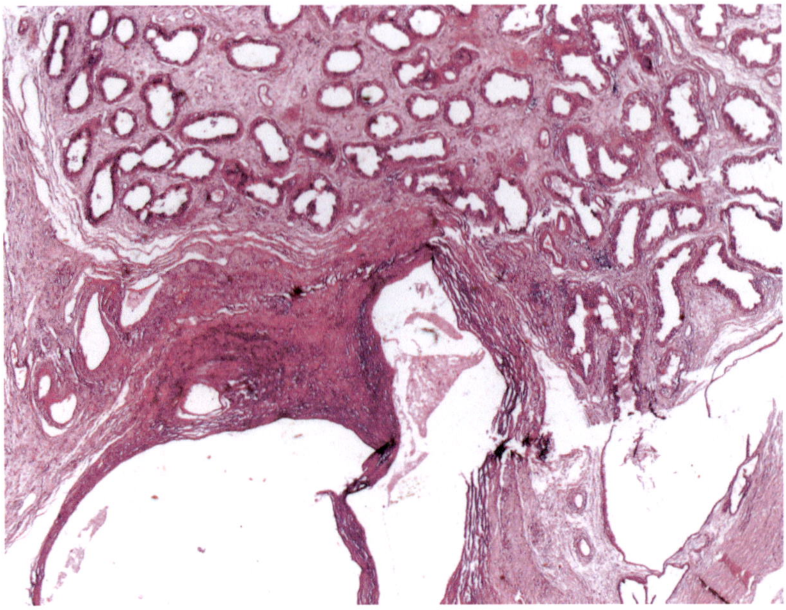

Fig. 9.7 Spermatocele associated with epididymitis

carcinoma: even in the presence of bland nuclear morphology, the high nuclear-to-cytoplasmic ratio along with nuclear hyperchromatism is a misleading feature. Synaptophysin and chromogranin negativity and a low Ki67 index attest to the benign nature of the cells [22–25].

Acquired Hydrocele and Hematocele

Hydrocele consists of serous fluid accumulation between the parietal and visceral tunica vaginalis of the testis. It usually presents as a painless scrotal swelling. Hydroceles can be congenital (prevalence of 6 % at birth and 1 % in adulthood) or acquired; the acquired form may be either idiopathic or secondary to inguinal hernia, scrotal trauma, epididymo-orchitis, or cancer. A single layer of cuboidal or flattened mesothelial cells, sometimes with prominent atypia, and underlying connective tissue stroma line the hydrocele. Mesothelial papillary hyperplasia and/or subepithelial chronic inflammation and fibrosis may be present in some cases. The luminal fluid is usually clear and serous unless the hydrocele is complicated by infection or hemorrhage. The surface is often covered with fibrinous adhesions and inflammatory cells [26].

Hematocele (hematoma) is a collection of blood in the space between the parietal and visceral tunica vaginalis, with causative factors similar to those of hydrocele. Patients with hematocele usually present with a scrotal mass and pain. Long-standing hematocele may become calcified and fibrotic, showing hemosiderin-laden macrophages.

Spermatic Cord Cysts

The majority of these cysts do not cause any diagnostic difficulties, but occasionally an epidermoid cyst can mimic neoplasia. Epidermoid cysts represent about 1 % of the tumor masses of the testis and are less commonly found in the paratesticular region and in the epididymis (Fig. 9.8). They consist of a lining of benign mature keratinizing squamous epithelium and a wall composed of fibrous connective tissue, often with inflammation or, occasionally, a granulomatous reaction. Recent genetic studies have shown that there is no chromosome 12p abnormality, thus supporting its distinction from true teratoma [27]. Suggested origins include squamous metaplasia of Wolffian duct structures, squamous metaplasia of mesothelial cyst,

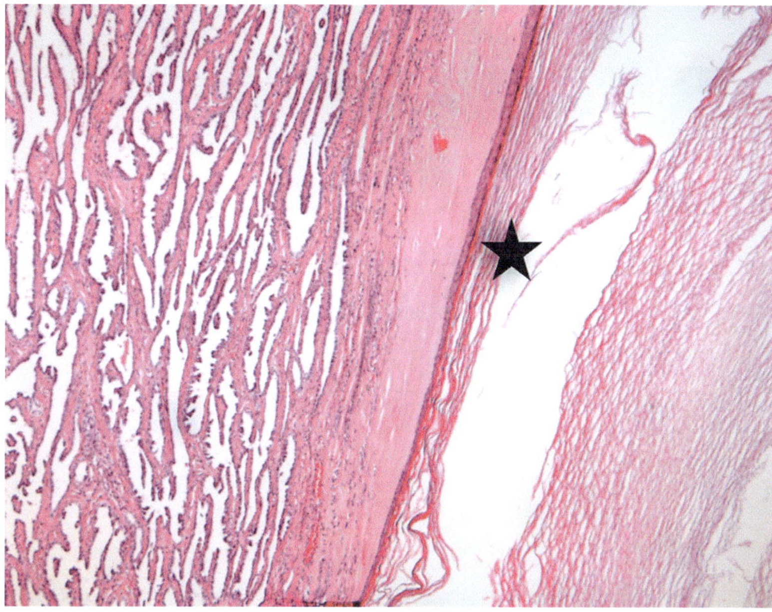

Fig. 9.8 Epidermoid cyst (*star*) extending to the rete testis (left)

displacement of squamous epithelium from the scrotal skin to paratesticular structures during embryogenesis, and monomorphic epidermal development of a teratoma. Epidermoid cysts in the paratesticular area do not recur after surgical excision [28–33].

Mesothelial cysts can arise within the tunica vaginalis, tunica albuginea (usually located anteriorly and laterally to the testis), and, less frequently, epididymis and spermatic cord. Those originating from the tunica vaginalis or albuginea may represent an embryonic remnant or an inclusion of mesothelium after trauma, inflammation, or cancer, while spermatic cord cysts probably arise from embryonic mesothelial remnants (processus vaginalis). These cysts can be unilocular or multilocular, and their diameter can be up to 4 cm. They are lined with a single layer of uniform cuboidal to flattened mesothelial cells and are filled with clear or blood-tinged serous fluid. Multilocular cysts must be distinguished from the exceptionally rare cystadenoma of putative müllerian origin. Nodular or diffuse proliferation of mesothelial cells, sometimes with squamous metaplasia, is seen in some cases [34, 35].

Epithelial Tumors

Tumors of Ovarian (Müllerian) Epithelial Type

Most types of ovarian epithelial tumors described in the testis originate from the appendix testis (müllerian rest) (Fig. 9.9a–d) or from müllerian metaplasia of the tunica vaginalis. Serous tumors are more common than mucinous tumors but both types are rare. Serous tumors typically occur in men with an average age of 55 years, while the reported age range for mucinous tumors is 11–70 years [36].

Benign and borderline tumors are cystic, while carcinomas are non-cystic, firm masses. Depending on the lining epithelium, the cysts contain either serous fluid or gelatinous material. In serous tumors, small papillae lining the cysts protrude into the lumen. Serous cystadenomas and cystadenocarcinomas are lined with columnar, frequently ciliated epithelium that is bland in benign tumors and more atypical with a variable amount of mitotic figs. in borderline lesions. Papillae and psammoma bodies are characteristic of serous differentiation.

Mucinous cystadenomas are lined with columnar cells having basally located nuclei. Borderline

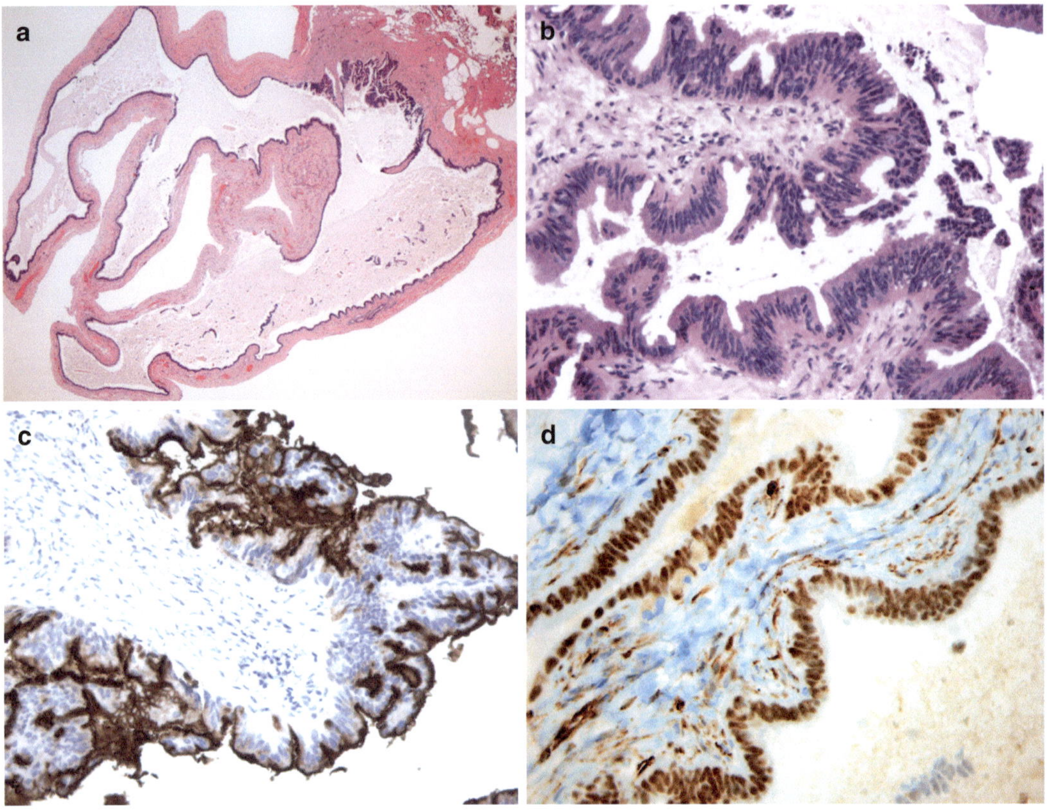

Fig. 9.9 Low- (**a**) and high-power (**b**) view and CA125 (**c**) and WT1 (**d**) expression in a case of paratesticular ovarian-type tumor originating from the appendix testis

tumors and mucinous cystadenocarcinomas are lined with intestinal-type cells that produce large amounts of mucin. Extravasated mucin and dystrophic calcifications are further hallmarks of borderline or malignant cases. Rarely, endometrioid carcinoma, clear cell carcinoma, squamous cell carcinoma, and Brenner tumors may arise in this location [37]. Müllerian tumors are not easy to distinguish from mesothelioma of the testicular tunics.

The epithelium of serous tumors is immunoreactive for CA125, WT1, and CD117 (Fig. 9.9c, d). Mucinous tumors are positive for CEA and CK20. The mesothelium reacts with cytokeratin antibodies but not with CEA or CD117. Other common immunohistochemical findings in mesothelioma are positivity for WT1, calretinin, CK7, and podoplanin and negativity for CK20, LeuM1, and D2-40.

Tumors of the Collecting Ducts and Rete Testis

The deeper part of the rete testis – the tubuli recti – connects the 2 ends of the seminiferous tubule loops to the rete testis, whose channels lead to the efferent ductules in the head of the epididymis. These channels are covered by ciliated columnar epithelium. The anatomy is the clue to the diagnosis of tumors of the collecting ducts; therefore they must have an anatomic relationship to this area. The main categories are described in the following paragraphs.

Adenoma

Rare cases of cystadenoma, papillary cystadenoma, adenofibroma, and adenoma have been reported in the literature. Mean age at presentation is 25 years. Hyperplasia of the rete testis encountered in cryptorchid testes and other diseases can mimic an adenoma; the lesion, however, shows clear continuity with the rete. Microscopic examination shows cystic, sometimes papillary lesions lined with cuboidal cells without atypia or mitotic figures. One case of adenofibroma and a few cases of sertoliform cystadenoma have been reported in the rete testis. Immunohistochemistry is positive for inhibin in both sertoliform cystadenoma and Sertoli cell tumors and is therefore not helpful in the differential diagnosis. The anatomic location and the absence of a coexisting Sertoli cell tumor in the testis point to a primary rete testis tumor.

Adenocarcinoma of the Rete Testis

Rete testis carcinoma is rare and aggressive. Age at presentation ranges between 17 and 91 years; the mean age is 54 years and there is an incidence peak around age 70. Tumors are never bilateral. The prognosis is poor, with an overall 5-year survival rate of 12 %. A significant prognostic factor is tumor size: about 75 % of patients with tumors smaller than 5 cm survive at least 5 years.

The diameter of the tumors ranges from 1 to 12 cm; many are multifocal and/or extending to the tunica and the spermatic cord. Pathologic reporting supports two main types of adenocarcinoma of the rete testis: solid and cystic. Solid lesions tend to be firm and rubbery, usually have a whitish cut surface, and characteristically penetrate the testis and surrounding structures (Fig. 9.10). Cystic lesions recall papillary serous cystadenocarcinomas arising in the ovary and peritoneum, and they may be multiloculated.

The morphologic criteria required for diagnosis include (i) involvement of the testicular mediastinum, (ii) transition from normal rete testis epithelium to neoplasia, (iii) intact parietal tunica vaginalis, and (iv) absence of any other primary tumor.

Immunohistochemistry is not specific for adenocarcinoma of the rete testis but may help to exclude other tumors such as mesothelioma or papillary serous carcinoma.

Adenocarcinomas of the rete are diffusely positive for cytokeratin, CD10, and EMA and negative for β-hCG, S100, AFP, LeuM1, PLAP, and PSA. Malignant mesotheliomas are positive for calretinin, CK5/6, and WT1 and negative for CEA, LeuM1, and CD30. Serous carcinoma is positive for CA125 and WT1.

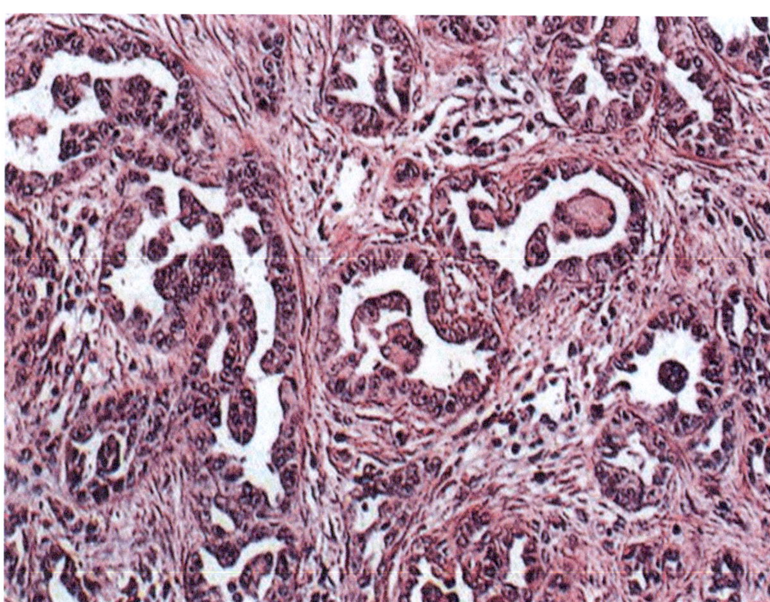

Fig. 9.10 Microscopic features of adenocarcinoma of the rete testis

Papillary Cystadenoma of the Epididymis

Papillary cystadenoma is a cystic tumor measuring up to 5 cm in diameter, lined with columnar cells having water-clear, glycogen-rich cytoplasm. The cells form papillae protruding into the lumen of the cyst filled with a colloid-like fluid. No malignancy-associated features including mitotic figures, nuclear pleomorphism, or necrosis should be present (Fig. 9.11).

Affected men seek help because of sterility and therefore these tumors are often incidental findings. Papillary cystadenoma is rather common (18 %) in men with von Hippel-Lindau disease and is then frequently bilateral. Sporadic cases are extremely rare. Mutations of the VHL gene (chromosome 3p25) are present in some cases. Immunohistochemistry is unnecessary in these tumors. A solid variant of papillary cystadenoma of the epididymis has been described [38].

Differential diagnosis with metastatic clear cell renal cell carcinoma should be considered in selected cases. Immunohistochemistry is of limited help in this differential since staining with CK7 (positive), RCC marker (negative), PAX8 (positive), carbonic anhydrase IX (positive), and AMACR (negative) overlaps [39]. Only CD10 staining can be helpful, because it is negative in papillary cystadenoma of the epididymis and positive in metastatic clear cell renal cell carcinoma [38, 39].

Adenocarcinoma of the Epididymis

Primary adenocarcinoma arising in the epididymis is one of the rarest malignancies, with fewer than 15 cases reported in the literature. Patients' age ranges between 25 and 82 years (mean age 67 years). Tumor size ranges between 1 and 15 cm, and the tumor is usually centrally located in the epididymis with or without infiltration of the adjacent tissues. Histologically, adenocarcinoma of the epididymis has a tubulopapillary structure and clear cells like adenoma, but there are evident features of malignancy. It is not associated with von Hippel-Lindau disease. Immunohistochemistry shows positivity for cytokeratin and EMA with no other specific features.

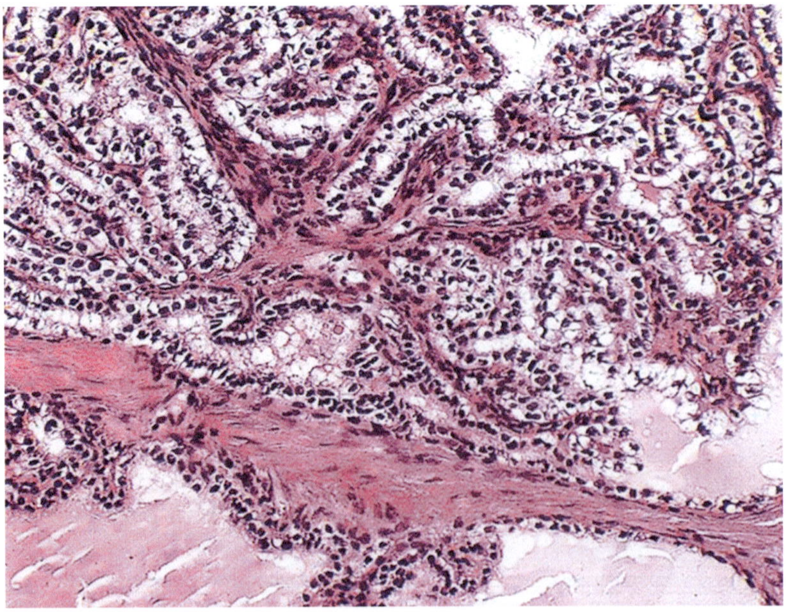

Fig. 9.11 Microscopic appearance of papillary cystadenoma of the rete testis

Mesothelial Tumors

Adenomatoid Tumor (Benign Mesothelioma of the Genital Tract)

Adenomatoid tumor is a benign proliferation of mesothelial origin that accounts for 30 % of all paratesticular neoplasms and is the second most common tumor after lipoma in this location [40]. Most reported cases originated in the epididymis, but these tumors may also arise in the testicular tunica, spermatic cord, ejaculatory ducts, prostate, and suprarenal recess. In rare cases the tumor has an intratesticular location. Adenomatoid tumors occur in both sexes; in women, they may develop in the uterus, fallopian tubes, and, less frequently, ovary.

Adenomatoid tumors of the paratesticular region occur in men of a wide range of ages and with a peak incidence between 20 and 50 years. The tumors are firm and whitish-yellow in color; they are frequently spherical and the size varies from a few millimeters to 5 cm (Fig. 9.12). The cuboidal tumor cells with intracytoplasmic vacuoles grow in solid cords or form pseudoglandular structures, which can be mistaken for a hemangioma or even a Sertoli cell tumor. Like all mesothelial cells, the tumor cells are immunoreactive for all types of cytokeratin antibodies, calretinin, WT1, and vimentin.

Mesothelioma of the Tunica Vaginalis Testis

Mesothelioma derives from mesothelium, the lining of the serous cavities. Irrespective of the primary location, there is a well-documented association with asbestos exposure and poor outcome. Mesothelioma of the tunica vaginalis testis is an extremely rare tumor [41].

The current WHO classification of mesotheliomas of the tunica vaginalis testis distinguishes between benign and malignant types; the benign form is further subdivided into papillary and cys tic types, but a clear distinction and prediction of the biological behavior is not always possible.

Malignant mesothelioma of the tunica vaginalis testis can arise at any age and has been reported to occur in males between 7 and 87 years of age. There is also a form of mesothelioma of uncertain malignant potential. Most mesotheliomas of the tunica vaginalis present as a papillary exophytic lesion growing in the lumen of a hydrocele sac or show only more or less pronounced thickening of the tunica vaginalis with formation of small nodules.

There are three general types of mesothelioma: the epithelial type (Fig. 9.13a, b), the fibrous or sarcomatous type, and a mixture of these two

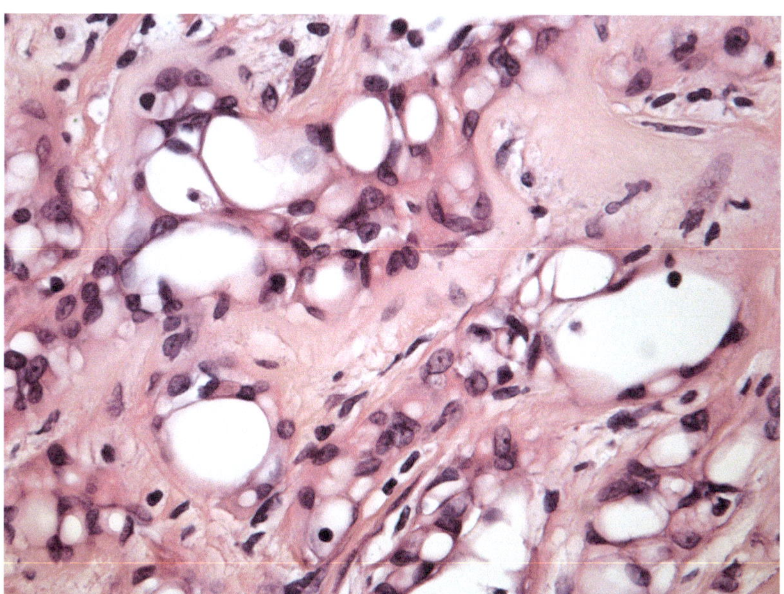

Fig. 9.12 Microscopic appearance of an adenomatoid tumor of the epididymis

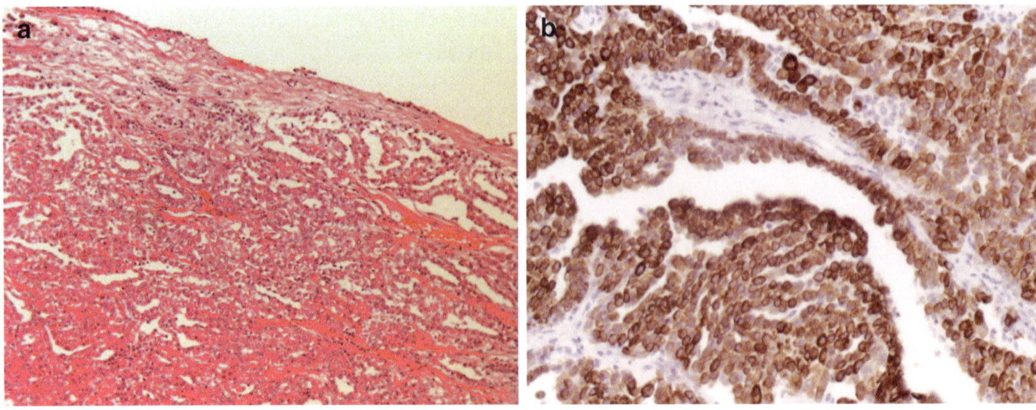

Fig. 9.13 Histologic appearance of an epithelioid mesothelioma (**a**) showing cytokeratin 7 expression (**b**)

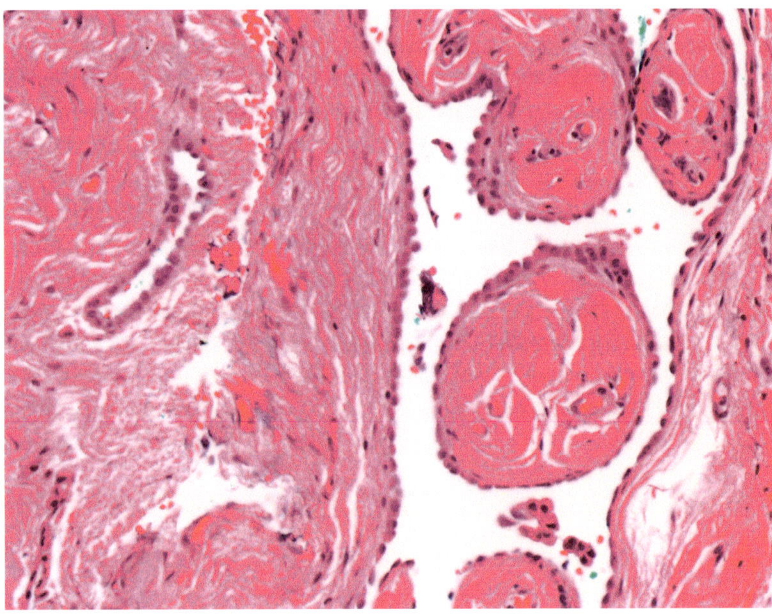

Fig. 9.14 Benign reactive mesothelial proliferation in association with hydrocele

types, the biphasic type. In the tunica vaginalis, the epithelial type accounts for 60 % and the biphasic type for 35 % of mesotheliomas. The sarcomatous type is very rare.

Even so-called benign papillary mesotheliomas show invasion of the wall of the tunica in one-quarter of cases, and another fifth infiltrate to the testis. The only benign mesothelioma is the cystic type, which consists of a multilocular cyst lined with mesothelium.

Benign reactive mesothelial proliferations in hydroceles may look histologically worrisome and are one of the main differential diagnoses (Fig. 9.14). Such proliferations are nonetheless circumscribed, never macroscopically visible, and always microscopically discovered in the wall of a resected hydrocele. Mesotheliomas are always macroscopically visible.

As mentioned earlier, epithelial mesotheliomas can also be mistaken for ovarian-type cystadenomas or carcinomas. However, they have a different immunophenotype, with mesotheliomas being positive for calretinin, CK5/6, WT1, and D2-40 and negative for CEA, LeuM1, and BerEP4 (CD30) [42, 43].

Other Rare Tumors

Rare cases of primary paratesticular germ cell tumors, sex cord-stromal tumors, neuroblastoma, paraganglioma, carcinoid, Wilms' tumor, and one case of squamous cell carcinoma have been reported. Their pathologic characteristics are described in other sections of this book.

Melanotic Neuroectodermal Tumor of Infancy

(Synonyms and old terms: congenital melanocarcinoma, retinal anlage tumor, pigmented congenital epulis, melanotic progonoma.)

Melanotic neuroectodermal tumor of infancy is a rare neoplasm. The lesion most commonly affects the maxilla of infants during the first year of life, but it may also occur in the mandible, skull, brain, epididymis, testis, and other rare locations. Most patients range between 4 months and 18 years of age. The tumor is circumscribed and cream colored with black spots and shows two cell types: small immature neuroblast-like cells and large columnar or cuboidal epithelial-like cells with or without melanin granules. Some cases metastasize to lymph nodes. Immunohistochemical analysis shows positivity for CD57 (Leu7) and NSE in the smaller cells and positivity for cytokeratins, HMB-45, Melan-A, and EMA in pigmented larger cells. Both small and large cells show negative staining for S100 protein.

Desmoplastic Small Round Cell Tumor

Desmoplastic small round cell tumor is a rare intra-abdominal tumor that has a poor outcome. Rare cases may occur in the tunica vaginalis or in the recess between the rete testis and epididymis. Macroscopically, the tumor is tan and firm. Microscopically, it is composed of typical small round blue cells that have a prominent round nucleus with finely dispersed chromatin and a small rim of cytoplasm. Tumor cell nests are surrounded by desmoplastic stroma. There is a distinctive immunophenotype with positivity for keratin, vimentin, desmin, and NSE, as well as a characteristic chromosomal abnormality, the EWS/WT1 fusion transcript t(11, 22)(p13,q12). Tumor metastases occur usually intra-abdominally and in the lung.

Secondary Tumors

Secondary tumors are rarely seen in the testicular tunics, epididymis, and spermatic cord, mostly in men over 50 years of age with disseminated high-grade carcinomas. Stomach cancer is the most frequent primary tumor. Other primary tumor sites include the testis, skin (melanoma), intestine, lung, kidney, bladder, and pancreas [44]. Prostate cancer may spread through the vas deferens.

Other Lesions and Proliferations

Ectopic Adrenocortical Tissue

Ectopic adrenocortical tissue is relatively frequent in the tunica albuginea, rete testis, epididymis, and spermatic cord and occasionally reaches a size that will make it symptomatic. It is made up of mature adrenal cortical tissue of about 5 mm in diameter surrounded by a band of connective tissue [45, 46].

Splenic-Gonadal Fusion

Fusion of the spleen and a gonad is more frequent on the left side. Morphologically, the ectopic splenic tissue can be in close relation to the head of the epididymis or the upper pole of the testis [47].

Testicular Appendages

There are five testicular appendages, but only three are of interest in the context of surgical pathology: the appendix testis or hydatid of Morgagni

(Fig. 9.15), the appendix epididymis, and the paradidymis or organ of Giraldés. Aberrant superior and inferior ductuli (organ of Haller) are usually seen near the head or body of the epididymis (superior) or at the junction of the tail of the epididymis and the vas deferens (inferior) (Fig. 9.16). Some may express CD10. In rare cases of large-sized cysts, they may present as a paratesticular mass. Ectopic epididymal tissue may occasionally be seen in testicular appendages.

Sertoli Cell Hyperplasia (Sertoli Cell Nodule)

Non-encapsulated nodules of Sertoli cells found especially in cryptorchid testes are known as Pick's adenomas. Because of their appearance, the nodules should be distinguished from actual Sertoli cell tumors, which are generally larger. Rare nodules of Sertoli cells may be seen in the paratesticular region,

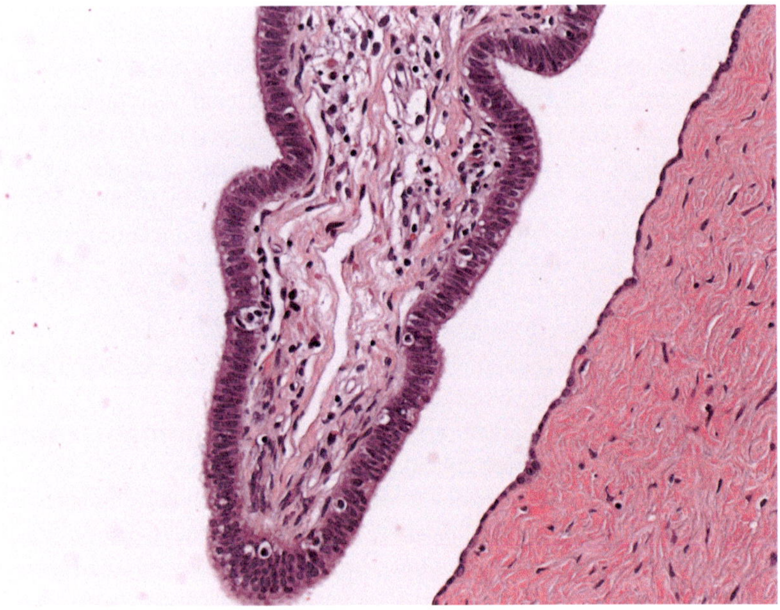

Fig. 9.15 Histologic features of appendix testis

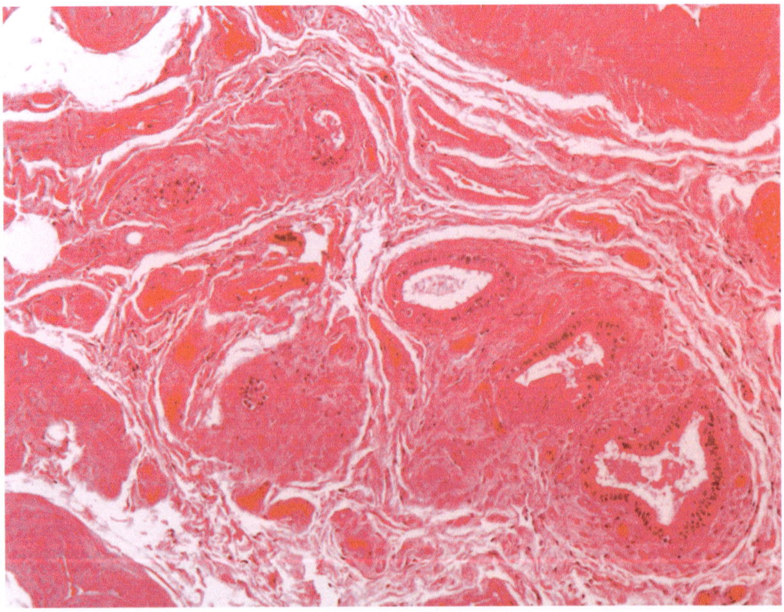

Fig. 9.16 Microscopic view of aberrant ductuli

where they might be large enough to become palpable (Fig. 9.17).

Leydig Cell Hyperplasia

Leydig cell hyperplasia is seen in testicles with marked tubular atrophy, such as in Klinefelter syndrome, but it is also possible to see Leydig cell nodules that must be distinguished from Leydig cell tumors. The interstitial growth pattern without expansion favors hyperplasia. Nodules of eosinophilic cells appearing to be Leydig cells are found in patients with adrenogenital syndrome and Nelson's syndrome. The nodules are usually bilateral and large in size with cellular pleomorphism and pigmentation. Clusters of Leydig cells are frequently seen in the paratesticular region but only rarely form large enough nodules to become palpable.

Hyperplasia of the Rete Testis

In atrophic testes the rete testis sometimes shows a slight prominence with micropapillary growth of a hyperplastic-like appearance. The most common presentation is so-called adenomatous hyperplasia of the rete testis, which maintains its arborizing architecture without any cytologic atypia. There are cystically dilated tubulopapillary channels filled with sperm or proteinaceous secretions (Fig. 9.18), and the presence of intracellular eosinophilic hyaline globules may lead to confusion with yolk sac tumor (Fig. 9.19).

Smooth muscle hyperplasia (stromal hyperplasia; hamartoma) of the rete testis is a rare tumorlike condition observed as an intrascrotal palpable mass in men aged 46–80 years. It most frequently involves the epididymis. Microscopic examination shows a nodular or diffuse increase in periductal, perivascular, or interstitial smooth muscle [48–50].

Cribriform Hyperplasia and Atypical Nuclei in the Epididymis

The simple columnar epithelium of the epididymis may sometimes display a cribriform pattern (usually focal and in rare cases extensive) suggestive of a hyperplastic process (Fig. 9.20). Enlarged, atypical nuclei may also occur in the epididymis as well as in the efferent ductuli and vas deferens [51–53] (Fig. 9.21).

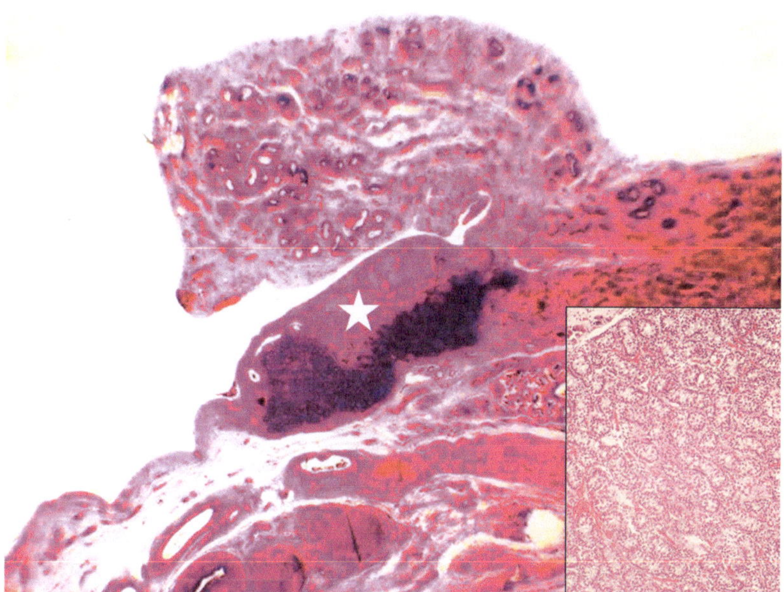

Fig. 9.17 Nonencapsulated extratesticular Sertoli cell nodule (*asterisk*) composed of Sertoli cell-only tubules (*inset*)

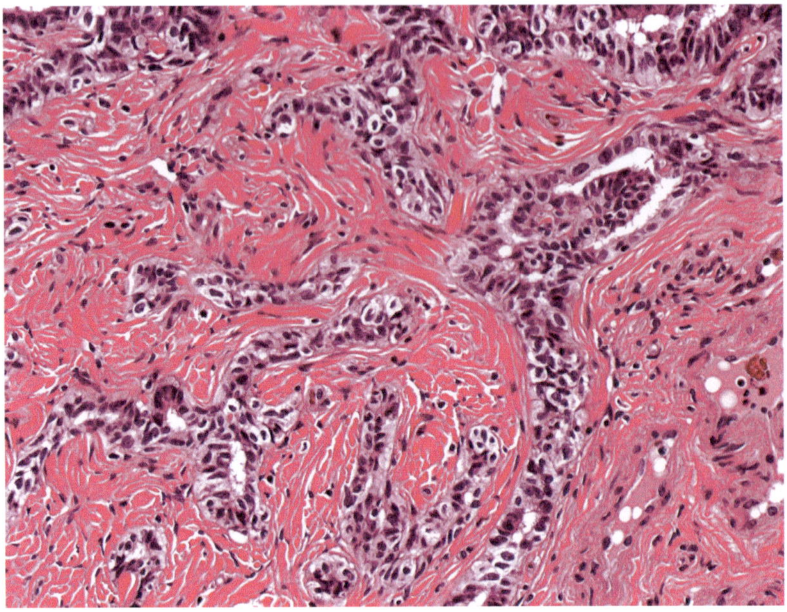

Fig. 9.18 Adenomatous hyperplasia of the rete testis

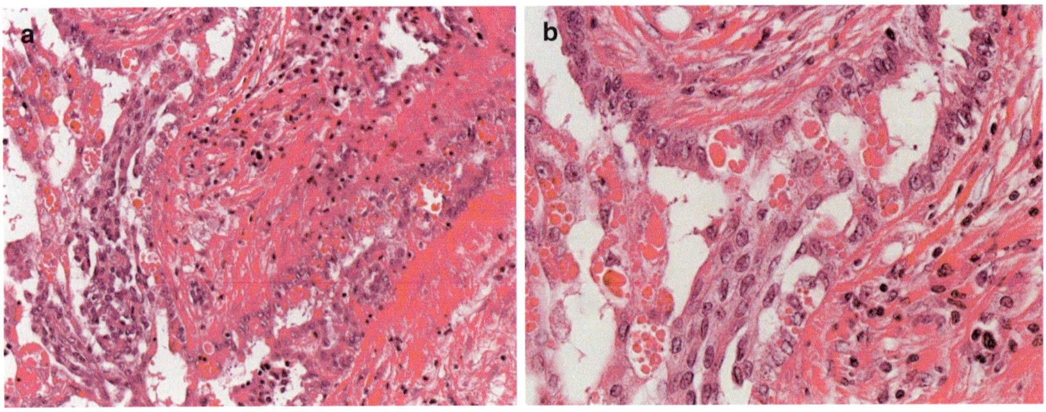

Fig. 9.19 Hyperplasia of the rete testis in association with germ cell tumor (**a**). High-power view highlights hyaline globules, a finding that should not be mistaken for a yolk sac tumor (**b**)

Reactive Mesothelial Hyperplasia and Mesothelial Cysts

Reactive mesothelial hyperplasia is the most important benign mimicker of testicular malignancy and is seen in reactive situations such as hydrocele or hernia. The mesothelial proliferation has an epithelial and occasionally tubular appearance with retraction artifacts and rarely shows spindle cell features.

In the differential diagnosis with mesothelioma, the bland nuclear features, lack of stromal invasion, and associated inflammatory/reactive background are useful. WT1 immunoreactivity confirms the mesothelial nature of the lesion.

Vasitis/Epididymitis Nodosa

Vasitis/epididymitis nodosa consists of a ductular proliferation with a microglandular appearance, mild nuclear atypia, and perineural growth or benign vascular invasion. It generally occurs after vasectomy or trauma and may be clinically mistaken for malignancy. The coincidence with microscopic sperm granulomas and an inflammatory reaction can

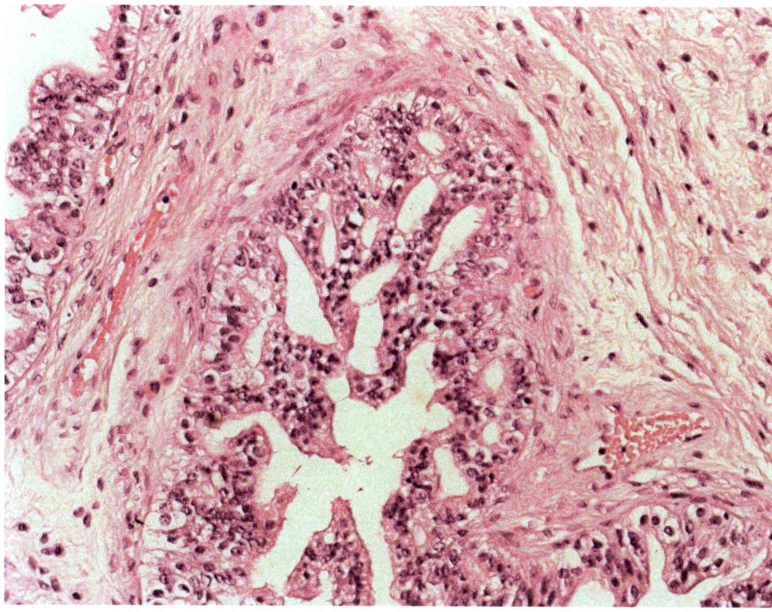

Fig. 9.20 So-called cribriform hyperplasia of the epididymis

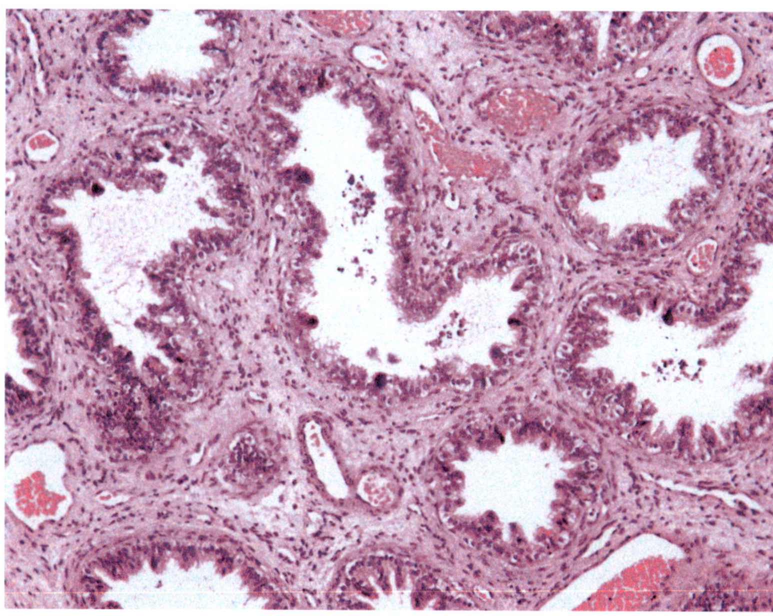

Fig. 9.21 Enlarged and atypical nuclei seen occasionally in the epididymis

help in the correct diagnosis. An epididymal lesion with similar histology may occur [54].

Embryonic Remnants

Rare embryonic remnants such as the presence of seminiferous tubules within the tunica albuginea; Leydig cells in the rete testis, tunica albuginea, and spermatic cord or within sclerotic tubules; prostate gland in the epididymis; muscular rete testis hyperplasia; and ectopic renal tissue can all mimic neoplasia. A rare case of endometriosis after long-term diethylstilbestrol administration has been reported [55, 56].

Ductal or glandular structures similar in morphology to vas-deferens-like (CD10-negative, SMA-positive), müllerian-like (CD10-negative), or epididymis-like (sometimes CD10-positive) structures may be seen in about 7 % of inguinal hernia sacs in young boys and should not be misdiagnosed as transected vas deferens. Ductal/glandular inclusion remnants do not affect reproduction.

References

1. Trainer TD. Testis and excretory duct system. In: Sternberg SS, editor. Histology for pathologists. New York: Raven; 2007. p. 943–62.
2. Srigley JR. The paratesticular region: histoanatomic and general considerations. Semin Diagn Pathol. 2000;17:258–69.
3. Kuo T, Gomez LC. Monstrous epithelial cells in human epididymis and seminal vesicles. A pseudomalignant change. Am J Surg Pathol. 1981;5:483–90.
4. Manely RE. Epididymal structure and function. A historical and critical review. Acta Zool (Stockh). 1959;40:1–21.
5. Madara JL, Haggitt RC, Federman M. Intranuclear inclusions of the human vas deferens. Arch Pathol Lab Med. 1978;102:648–50.
6. Paniagua R, Regadera J, Nistal M, Abaurrea MA. Histological, histochemical and ultrastructural variations along the length of the human vas deferens before and after puberty. Acta Anat (Basel). 1982;111:190–203.
7. Srigley J, Hartwick RW. Tumors and cysts of the paratesticular region. Pathol Annu. 1990;25:51–108.
8. Jones EC, Murray SK, Young RH. Cysts and epithelial proliferations of the testicular collecting system (including rete testis). Semin Diagn Pathol. 2000;17:270–93.
9. Nistal M, Regadera J, Paniagua R. Cystic dysplasia of the testis. Light and electron microscopic study of three cases. Arch Pathol Lab Med. 1984;108:579–83.
10. Cimador M, Rosone G, Castagnetti M, Libri M, Bertozzi M, Lima M, De Grazia E. Cystic dysplasia of rete testis associated with ipsilateral renal agenesis. Case report. Minerva Pediatr. 2003;55:175–9.
11. Wegmann W, Illi O, Kummer-Vago M. Cystic testis dysplasia with ipsilateral kidney agenesis. Schweiz Med Wochenschr. 1984;114:144–8.
12. Nistal M, Mate A, Paniagua R. Cystic transformation of the rete testis. Am J Surg Pathol. 1996;20:1231–9.
13. Busto Martín LA, García DL, Barghouti I, Abal VC, Castañón LB. Giant cystic degeneration of the rete testis. Arch Esp Urol. 2009;62:592–5.
14. Nistal M, Jiménez-Heffernan JA, García-Viera M, Paniagua R. Cystic transformation and calcium oxalate deposits in rete testis and efferent ducts in dialysis patients. Hum Pathol. 1996;27:336–41.
15. Meyer DR, Hüppe T, Lock U, Hodek E, Friedrich M. Pronounced cystic transformation of the Rete testis. MRI appearance. Invest Radiol. 1999;34:600–3.
16. Nistal M, Riestra ML, Paniagua R. Focal orchitis in undescended testes: discussion of pathogenetic mechanisms of tubular atrophy. Arch Pathol Lab Med. 2002;126:64–9.
17. Michael H, Srigley J. Pathology of the paratesticular region. In: Amin MB, Eble J, editors. Urological pathology. Philadelphia: Lippincott Williams & Wilkins; 2014. p. 816–7.
18. Nistal M, Santaaria L, Paniagua R. Acquired cystic transformation of the rete testis secondary to renal failure. Hum Pathol. 1989;20:1065–70.
19. Colangelo SM, Fried K, Hyacinthe LM, Fracchia JA. Tubular ectasia of the rete testis: an ultrasound diagnosis. Urology. 1995;45:532–4.
20. Weingarten BJ, Kellman GM, Middleton WD, Gross ML. Tubular ectasia within the mediastinum testis. J Ultrasound Med. 1992;11:349–53.
21. Schned AR, Seremetis GM, Rous SN. Paratesticular multicystic mass of Wolffian, probably paradidymal, origin. Am J Clin Pathol. 1994;101:543–6.
22. Jassie M, Mahmood P. Torsion of spermatocele: a newly described entity with 2 cases. J Urol. 1985;133:683–4.
23. Engelbrecht K, Bornman M, du Plessis D. Multicystic epididymis and seminal vesicles in a patient with polycystic kidney disease. Br J Urol. 1995;75:554–5.
24. Kroes HY, Sijmons RH, Van Den Berg A, Van Der Hout AH. Early-onset renal cell cancer and bilateral epididymal cysts as presenting symptoms of von Hippel-Lindau disease. Br J Urol. 1998;81:915.
25. Bibbo M, Al-Naqeeb M, Baccarini I, Gill W, Newton M, Sleeper KM, Sonek RN, Wied GL. Follow-up study of male and female offspring of DES-treated mothers a preliminary report. J Reprod Med. 1975;15:29–32.
26. Rinker JR, Allen L. Lymphatic defect in hydrocele. Am Surg. 1951;17:681.
27. Cheng L, Zhang S, MacLennan GT, Poulos CK, Sung MT, Beck SD, Foster RS. Interphase fluorescence in situ hybridization analysis of chromosome 12p abnormalities is useful for distinguishing epidermoid cysts of the testis from pure mature teratoma. Clin Cancer Res. 2006;12:5668–72.
28. Nistal M, Iniguez L, Paniagua R. Histological classification of spermatic cord cysts in relation to their histogenesis. Eur Urol. 1987;13:327–30.
29. Wiesenthal JD, Ettler H, Razvi H. Testicular epidermoid cyst: a case report and review of the clinicopathologic features. Can J Urol. 2004;11:2133–5.
30. Shah KH, Maxted WC, Chun B. Epidermoid cysts of the testis: a report of three cases and analysis of 141 cases from the world literature. Cancer. 1981;47:577–82.
31. Katergiannakis V, Lagoudianakis EE, Markogiannakis H, Manouras A. Huge epidermoid cyst of the spermatic cord in an adult patient. Int J Urol. 2006;13:95–7.
32. Ford Jr J, Singh S. Paratesticular dermoid cyst in a 6-month old infant. J Urol. 1988;139:89–90.
33. Wegner H, Herbst H, Dieckmann KP. Paratesticular epidermoid cyst and ipsilateral spermatic cord dermoid cyst: case report and discussion of pathogenesis, diagnosis and treatment. J Urol. 1994;152: 2101–3.

34. Mancilla-Jiminez R, Matsuda GT. Cysts of the tunica albuginea. Report of 4 cases and review of the literature. J Urol. 1975;114:730–3.
35. Tammela TL, Karttunen TJ, Mattila SI, Mäkäräinen HP, Hellström PA, Kontturi MJ. Cysts of the tunica albuginea – more common testicular masses than previously thought? Br J Urol. 1991;68:280–4.
36. Eble JN, Sauter G, Epstein JI, Sesterhenn IA, editors. WHO Classification of tumors. Pathology & genetics. Tumors of the urinary system and male genital organs. Lyon: IARCPress; 2004. p. 218–19.
37. Brennan MB, Srigley JR. Brenner tumors of testis and paratestis: case report and literature review. J Urol Pathol. 1999;10:219–28.
38. Yang L, Xu WS, Melamed J, Zhou M, Deng FM. Solid variant of papillary cystadenoma of the epididymis. Histopathology. 2015;67:138–41.
39. Cox R, Vang R, Epstein JI. Papillary cystadenoma of the epididymis and broad ligament: morphologic and immunohistochemical overlap with clear cell papillary renal cell carcinoma. Am J Surg Pathol. 2014;38:713–8.
40. Perez-Ordonez B, Srigley JR. Mesothelial lesions of the paratesticular region. Semin Diagn Pathol. 2000;17:294–306.
41. Butnor KJ, Sporn TA, Hammar SP, Roggli VL. Well-differentiated papillary mesothelioma. Am J Surg Pathol. 2001;25:1304–9.
42. Tolhurst SR, Lotan T, Rapp DE, Lyon MB, Orvieto MA, Gerber GS, Sokoloff MH. Well-differentiated papillary mesothelioma occurring in the tunica vaginalis of the testis with contralateral atypical mesothelial hyperplasia. Urol Oncol. 2006;24:36–9.
43. Tyagi G, Munn CS, Kiser LC, Wetzner SM, Tarabulcy E. Malignant mesothelioma of tunica vaginalis testis. Urology. 1989;34:102–4.
44. Manav AN, Kazan E, Ertek MŞ, Amasyalı AS, Culhacı N, Erol H. A rare cause of testicular metastasis: upper tract urothelial carcinoma. Case Rep Urol. 2014;2014:759858.
45. Claahsen-van der Grinten HL, Otten BJ, Takahashi S, Meuleman EJ, Hulsbergen-van de Kaa C, Sweep FC, Hermus AR. Testicular adrenal rest tumors in adult males with congenital adrenal hyperplasia: evaluation of pituitary-gonadal function before and after successful testis-sparing surgery in eight patients. J Clin Endocrinol Metab. 2007;92:612–5.
46. Dahl EV, Bahn RC. Aberrant adrenal cortical tissue near the testis in human infants. Am J Pathol. 1962;40:587–98.
47. Gouw AS, Elema JD, Bink-Boelkens MT, de Jongh HJ, ten Kate LP. The spectrum of splenogonadal fusion. Case report and review of 82 reported cases. Eur J Pediatr. 1985;144:316–23.
48. Hartwick RW, Ro JY, Srigley JR, Ordonez NG, Ayala AG. Adenomatous hyperplasia of the rete testis. A clinicopathologic study of nine cases. Am J Surg Pathol. 1991;15:350–7.
49. Nistal M, Castillo MC, Regadera J, Garcia-Cabezas MA. Adenomatous hyperplasia of the rete testis. A review and report of new cases. Histol Histopathol. 2003;18:741–52.
50. Ulbright TM, Gersell DJ. Rete testis hyperplasia with hyaline globule formation. A lesion simulating yolk sac tumor. Am J Surg Pathol. 1991;15:66–74.
51. Butterworth DM, Bisset DL. Cribriform intra-tubular epididymal change and adenomatous hyperplasia of the rete testis – a consequence of testicular atrophy? Histopathology. 1992;21:435–8.
52. Calder CJ, Aluwihare N, Graham CT. Cribriform intra-tubular epididymal change. Histopathology. 1993;22:406.
53. Sharp SC, Batt MA, Lennington WJ. Epididymal cribriform hyperplasia. A variant of normal epididymal histology. Arch Pathol Lab Med. 1994;118:1020–2.
54. Hirschowitz L, Rode J, Guillebaud J, Bounds W, Moss E. Vasitis nodosa and associated clinical findings. J Clin Pathol. 1988;41:419–23.
55. Lee LY, Tzeng J, Grosman M, Unger PD. Prostate gland-like epithelium in the epididymis: a case report and review of the literature. Arch Pathol Lab Med. 2004;128:60–2.
56. Nistal M, Paniagua R, Leon L, Regadera J. Ectopic seminiferous tubules in the tunica albuginea of normal and dysgenetic testes. Appl Pathol. 1985;3:123–8.

Paratesticular Soft Tissue Neoplasms

10

Alessandro Franchi, Raffaella Santi, and Gabriella Nesi

Introduction

Primary paratesticular soft tissue tumors are rare entities. Sarcomas have an estimated annual incidence of 0.3 cases per million [1] and represent 7–10 % of intrascrotal tumors [2]. However, among genitourinary sarcomas, the paratesticular region is the most commonly involved site [3]. They usually affect adult patients, with a median age at diagnosis of 65 years, even though rhabdomyosarcomas occur at a younger age (median 25 years) [1].

In recent years, the classification of soft tissue tumors has undergone major changes, mainly due to the introduction of new immunohistochemical markers and the identification of specific genetic alterations. Accordingly, the diagnostic category of malignant fibrous histiocytoma has been progressively abandoned, and paratesticular tumors previously diagnosed as such are now mainly considered in the spectrum of dedifferentiated liposarcoma [4]. Moreover, spindle cell rhabdomyosarcoma, which had been initially grouped under embryonal rhabdomyosarcoma, is now considered a separate entity based on the identification of different genetic characteristics [5–7].

Here we discuss the salient diagnostic features of the main mesenchymal lesions that may involve the paratesticular region.

Benign Entities

Lipoma

Lipoma accounts for approximately 90 % of benign paratesticular soft tissues tumors [8]. Grossly, lipomas are usually well circumscribed, unencapsulated, and lobulated. Size is variable but seldom exceeds 10 cm. Histologically, the majority of tumors consist of a uniform proliferation of mature univacuolated adipocytes with minimal or no variation in cell size. Variants of lipomas, including fibrolipoma and angiolipoma, may arise in the paratestis. Excision is an appropriate treatment for these tumors which have no tendency to recur.

Leiomyoma

Leiomyomas are the second most common benign mesenchymal neoplasm at this site, with a predilection for the epididymis [9]. They present as painless intrascrotal masses. On cut section, leiomyomas are firm, white-gray nodules with a whorled surface. Histologically, they consist of spindle-shaped cells arranged in fascicles. Similarly to uterine leiomyomas, bizarre and degenerative-

A. Franchi • R. Santi • G. Nesi (✉)
Division of Pathological Anatomy, University of Florence, Florence, Italy
e-mail: alessandro.franchi@unifi.it; raffaella.santi@yahoo.it; gabriella.nesi@unifi.it

M. Colecchia (ed.), *Pathology of Testicular and Penile Neoplasms*,
DOI 10.1007/978-3-319-27617-5_10

appearing "symplastic" changes have been described [10]. Smooth muscle actin, muscle-specific actin, desmin, and h-caldesmon are generally positive. CD34 and keratin may also be positive in some cases [11]. Surgical excision is curative.

Hemangioma

Paratesticular hemangiomas appear as a painless mass which occasionally may rapidly increase in size due to hemorrhage. Both cavernous and capillary type of hemangiomas may affect the spermatic cord or epididymis [12, 13]. Anastomosing hemangiomas consist of intersecting sinusoidal capillaries with occasional hobnail endothelial cells encompassed within a layer of pericytes [14].

Angiomyofibroblastoma

Angiomyofibroblastoma presents as a painless mass involving the scrotum or inguinal region in middle-aged and older men [15, 16]. It is usually superficial and well circumscribed, measuring 5–10 cm. Histologically it consists of rounded to slightly spindled cells dispersed in a collagenous stroma which may contain adipocytes. These tumors may typically exhibit a distinctive pattern of whorling cell growth around thick-walled vessels. Neoplastic cells show immunoreactivity for CD34, smooth muscle actin, desmin, and hormone receptors [17]. Angiomyofibroblastoma is adequately treated with local excision and recurrence is exceedingly rare.

Mammary-Type Myofibroblastoma

Mammary-type myofibroblastoma closely resembles spindle cell lipoma but differs on account of broader collagen bundles (Fig. 10.1) and desmin positivity [18]. It occurs in the inguinal region with a predilection for older men and presents either as a slowly growing painless mass or as an incidental finding at the time of surgery [19]. Local recurrence is very rare after complete resection.

Deep (Aggressive) Angiomyxoma

Deep ("aggressive") angiomyxoma occurs more frequently in females. In men it generally involves the spermatic cord or scrotum [20, 21]. Histology shows bland spindle or stellate cells in a myxoid matrix with dilated thin-walled blood vessels (Fig. 10.2). Some tumors may show features of both angiomyxoma and angiomyofibroblastoma. Immunohistochemistry does not play a role in the

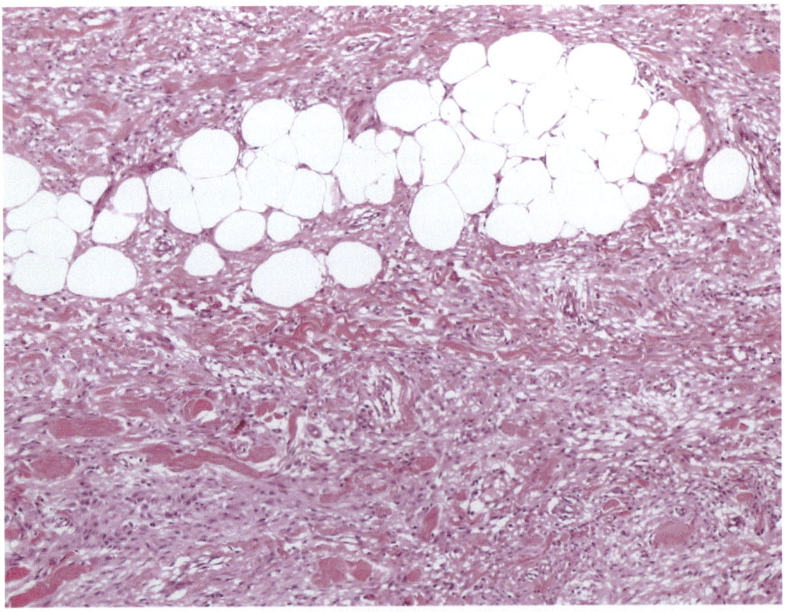

Fig. 10.1 Mammary-type myofibroblastoma is composed of bland spindle-shaped cells haphazardly arranged in fascicles in a collagenous background. Interspersed fat lobules are also noted

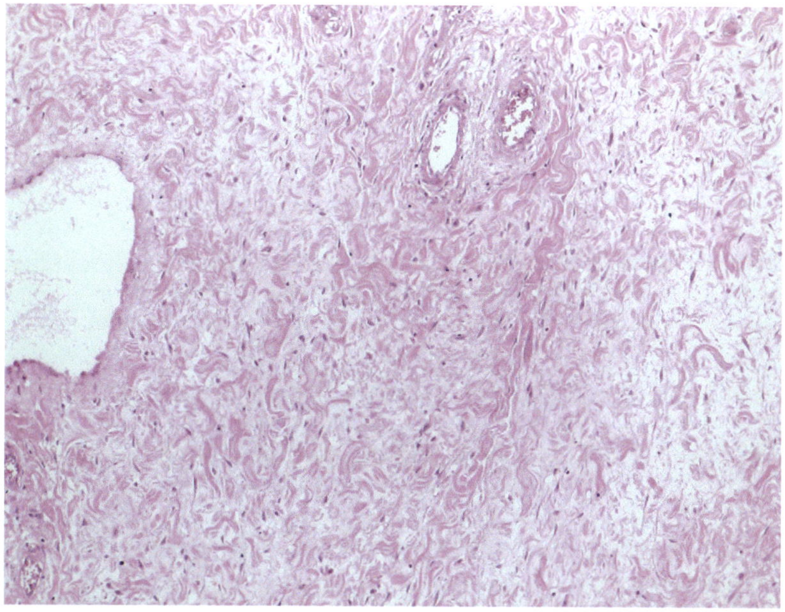

Fig. 10.2 Deep (aggressive) angiomyxoma consisting of spindle and stellate cells in an abundant myxoid matrix with dilated thin-walled blood vessels

differential diagnosis since the two lesions exhibit significantly overlapping immunophenotypes [22]. Angiomyxomas are locally aggressive and may recur, but do not metastasize. Wide resection with careful follow-up is recommended.

Schwannoma

Nerve sheath tumors in the paratesticular region are uncommon, and only a few cases have been reported. Regardless of their morphology, most of these tumors occur as a painless mass varying in size. The majority are benign schwannoma [23] and neurofibroma [24], while malignant peripheral nerve sheath tumor is exceedingly rare in this location [25].

Rhabdomyoma

Rhabdomyoma is extremely rare and typically affects young adults. In the paratesticular region, these tumors are distinctively composed of bundles of well-differentiated skeletal muscle cells embedded in a dense hyalinized collagenous stroma, often with adjacent prominent lymphoplasmacytic aggregates. These tumors lack nuclear atypia as well as mitotic figures. Desmin and muscle actin (HHF35) are diffusely positive. Nuclear positivity for myf-4 (myogenin) is highly specific [26].

Malignant Entities

Liposarcoma

Liposarcomas are the most frequently encountered sarcomas of the paratesticular region. Well-differentiated (WD) and dedifferentiated liposarcomas are by far the most common subtypes at this anatomical site, while the myxoid/round cell and pleomorphic subtypes are rare [27–30]. Liposarcoma typically affects adult patients (peak age in the sixth decade) and presents as a slowly growing paratesticular or inguinal mass that can be clinically mistaken for a hernia. Extension to the retroperitoneum through the inguinal canal may occur.

Grossly, WD liposarcoma appears as a large, well-circumscribed yellow mass, with variously sized areas of gray-white fibrous tissue. When present, the dedifferentiated component appears as a distinct white firm or tan/gray myxoid nodule (or multiple nodules). Histologically, it consists of mature adipocytes with marked variation in cell size, and at least focal nuclear atypia scattered hyperchromatic stromal cells are seen within irregular fibrous bands (Fig. 10.3). Lipoblasts may also occur, although they are not essential for the diagnosis. Other features include chronic inflammatory infiltrate that may occasionally obscure the adipocytic nature of the neoplasm and myxoid changes.

Dedifferentiated liposarcoma exhibits abrupt transition to a high-grade or, less frequently, low-grade sarcomatous component with features of undifferentiated pleomorphic sarcoma (formerly storiform and pleomorphic variant of malignant fibrous histiocytoma), myxofibrosarcoma, leiomyosarcoma, rhabdomyosarcoma or osteosarcoma (Fig. 10.4).

Immunohistochemically, the most useful diagnostic markers are MDM2 and CDK4, which allow distinguishing WD liposarcoma from benign lipomatous lesions and dedifferentiated liposarcoma from non-adipogenic sarcomas. WD and dedifferentiated liposarcomas are characterized by ring and/or giant marker chromosomes. Both rings and giant markers contain amplified

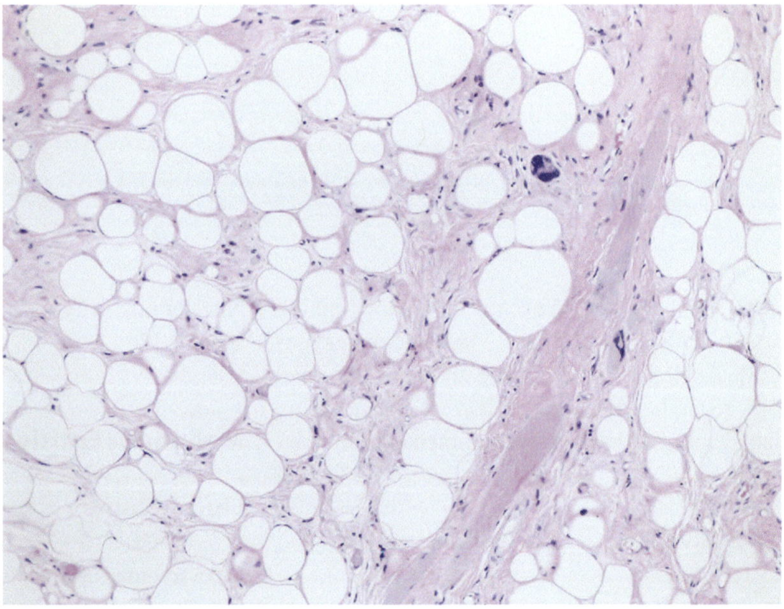

Fig. 10.3 Well-differentiated liposarcoma displaying lobules of relatively mature adipocytes with significant variation in cell size intersected by thick fibrous septa containing spindle cells with enlarged, hyperchromatic nuclei

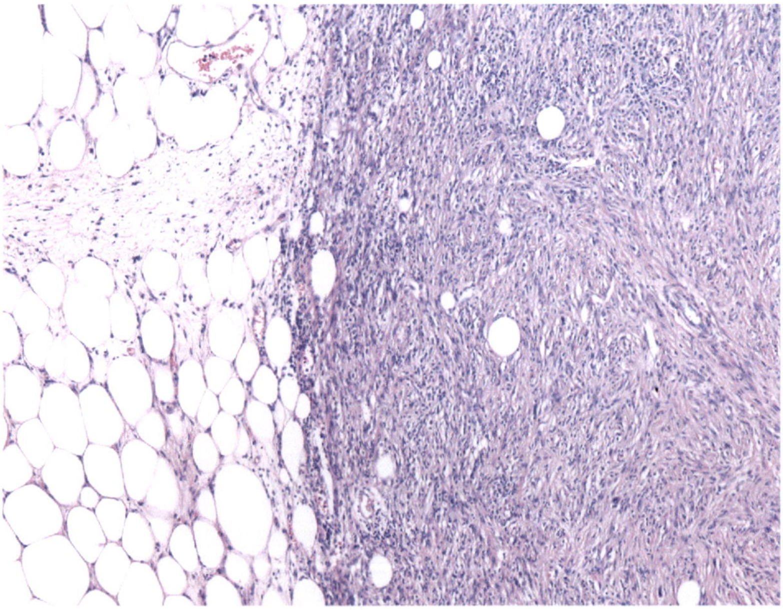

Fig. 10.4 Histology of dedifferentiated liposarcoma typically showing an abrupt shift from well-differentiated liposarcoma to dedifferentiated neoplastic tissue

sequences derived from the 12q13–15 chromosome region, which map several proto-oncogenes such as *MDM2*, *CDK4*, *HMGIC*, *CPM*, and *SAS*.

The clinical course of WD/dedifferentiated liposarcoma is characterized by frequent local recurrence, whereas distant spread is rare. Local recurrence is often repeated and may involve the inguinal canal, pelvis, and scrotum [29, 30].

The myxoid liposarcoma category currently includes more cellular, less differentiated tumors previously known as round cell liposarcoma and is characterized by the presence of the *FUS-DDIT3* or *EWSR1-DDIT3* rearrangement [31]. Myxoid liposarcoma appears as a well-circumscribed, multinodular, gelatinous lesion. The presence of round cell areas may confer a white fleshy appearance. Histologically, purely myxoid liposarcoma is a hypocellular proliferation of bland spindle cells in a myxoid background with a characteristic capillary network organized in a plexiform pattern. Lipoblasts are most often monovacuolated, tending to cluster around vessels or at the periphery of the lesion. High-grade lesions display undifferentiated round cell morphology ranging between 5 and 80 % in extent; pure round cell liposarcoma on the contrary is rare. High-grade areas reaching >5 % of the lesion predict unfavorable outcome.

Pleomorphic liposarcoma is a high-grade sarcoma with a variable number of lipoblasts. Lipoblasts frequently appear as large cells with a multivacuolated cytoplasm and irregular, hyperchromatic, scalloped nuclei with prominent nucleoli. The outcome is dismal, with a metastatic rate between 30 and 50 % and overall mortality between 40 and 50 %.

Leiomyosarcoma

Leiomyosarcoma is the second most frequent sarcoma of the paratesticular region, where it represents 20 % of all sarcomas [1]. Typically affecting adults, it presents as a firm, painless mass in the hemiscrotum. Most arise in the testicular tunics and in the spermatic cord [11]. Well-differentiated tumors consist of intersecting fascicles of spindle cells with brightly eosinophilic cytoplasm and cigar-shaped nucleus. Paranuclear vacuoles may be present. Poorly differentiated tumors consist of large pleomorphic cells with abundant eosinophilic cytoplasm and bizarre nuclei. Multinucleated cells can frequently be seen and mitotic activity is usually brisk (Fig. 10.5). Neoplastic cells are positive for smooth muscle actin, common muscle actin, desmin, and caldesmon, while S100, CD34, and myogenin are negative. Histologic grading is an

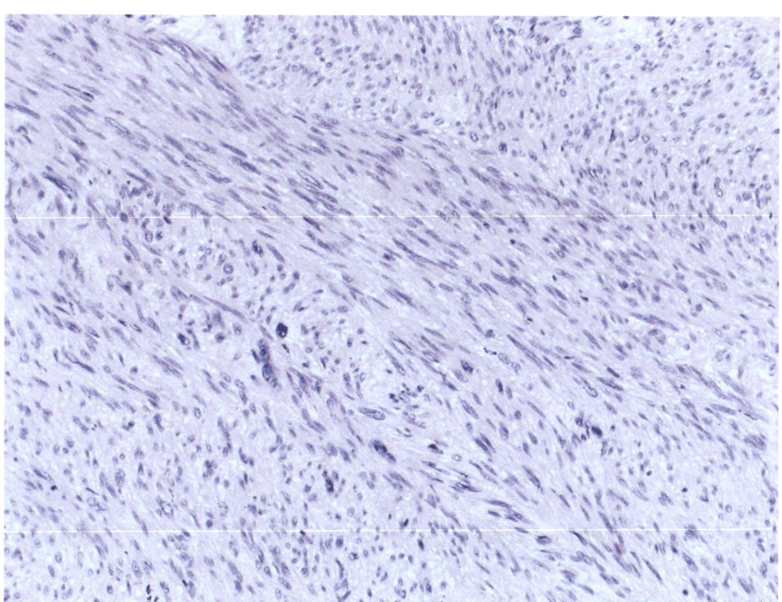

Fig. 10.5 A smooth muscle tumor with marked cytologic atypia and numerous mitoses diagnostic for leiomyosarcoma

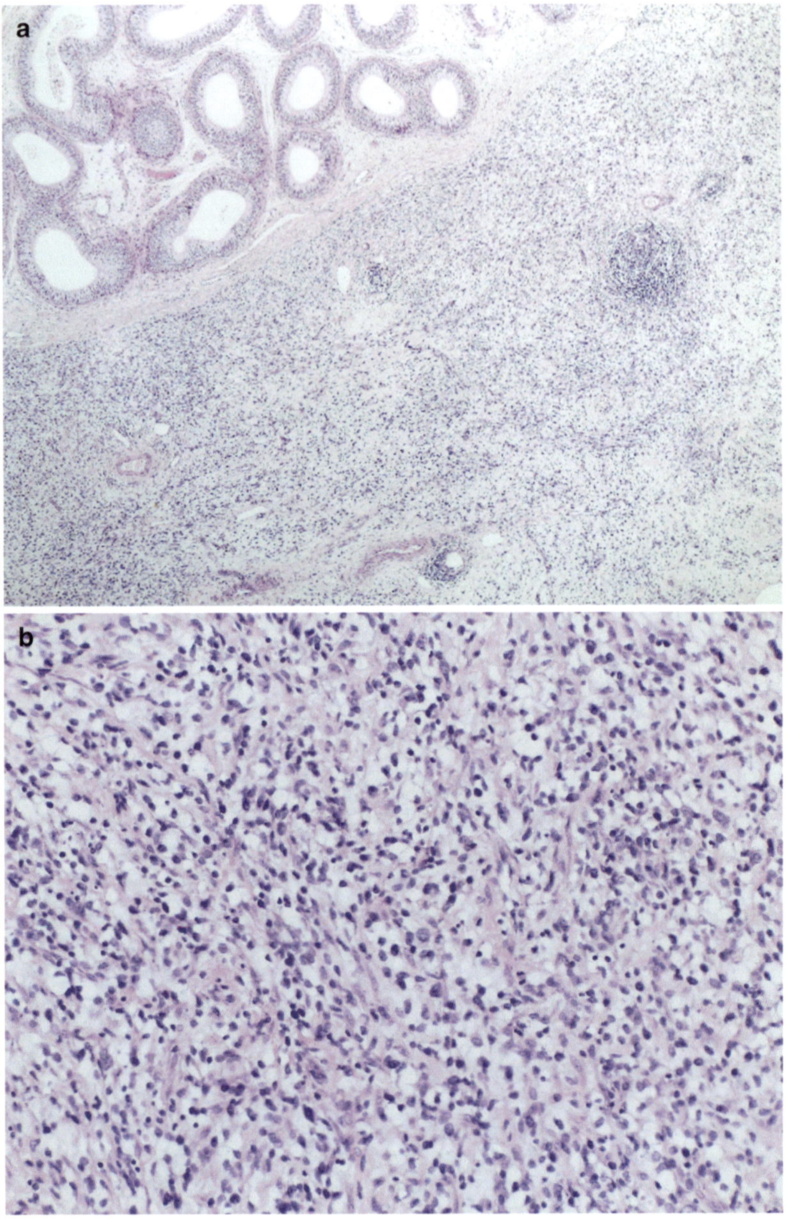

Fig. 10.6 Paratesticular embryonal rhabdomyosarcoma (**a**). A cell population consisting of small, round tumor cells with hyperchromatic nuclei may predominate (**b**)

important prognostic factor, as most low-grade leiomyosarcomas of the paratestis are indolent neoplasms while high-grade lesions behave aggressively [11].

Rhabdomyosarcoma

Rhabdomyosarcoma is the most common spermatic cord sarcoma in children, representing approximately 10 % of all sarcomas at this site [1]. Four subtypes are currently recognized: embryonal, alveolar, pleomorphic, and spindle cell/sclerosing [31]. The embryonal and the spindle cell/sclerosing subtypes are by far the most common in the paratestis.

Embryonal rhabdomyosarcoma is characterized by a mixture of undifferentiated small round cells (Fig. 10.6a, b) with a well-differentiated population of rhabdomyoblasts exhibiting an

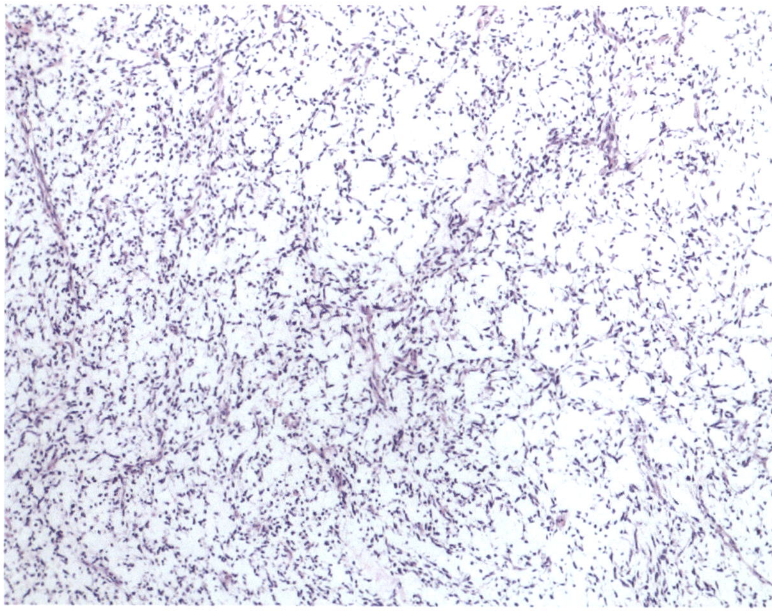

Fig. 10.7 Embryonal rhabdomyosarcoma showing neoplastic cells lying in a myxoid stroma

intensely eosinophilic cytoplasm, within a myxoid stroma (Fig. 10.7). Cross striations are sometimes present. The spindle cell/sclerosing subtype displays a fascicular proliferation of elongated cells with bright eosinophilic cytoplasm and cross striations, with focal to extensive stromal sclerosis (Fig. 10.8a). In the alveolar subtype, neoplastic cells grow in distinct nests separated by fibrous septa. They tend to be discohesive in the central part of the nest and aggregate at the periphery. Multinucleated giant cells may be seen. The pleomorphic subtype is only rarely detected in the paratesticular region and presents as a solid growth of highly pleomorphic cells with abundant eosinophilic cytoplasm.

The most useful immunohistochemical markers for skeletal muscle differentiation are desmin, myogenin, (myf-4), and MyoD1, which are both sensitive and specific (Fig. 10.8b). In addition, the majority of alveolar rhabdomyosarcomas present a PAX3-FOXO1 or PAX7-FOXO1 gene fusion, which can be searched for diagnostic purposes.

The outcome for pediatric patients affected with localized paratesticular rhabdomyosarcoma, including the alveolar subtype, is excellent [32].

Desmoplastic Small Round Cell Tumor

Desmoplastic small round cell tumor (DSRCT) is an aggressive tumor that typically occurs in the abdomen, but it may also involve the paratestis of children and young adults [33, 34]. It is composed of multiple nodules, each consisting of nests of uniform small cells with scant cytoplasm, separated by dense bands of collagen (Fig. 10.9). Immunohistochemically, this tumor is polyphenotypic, staining for vimentin, keratins, EMA, desmin, and NSE. DSRCT harbors a characteristic chromosomal abnormality, i.e., t(11;22)(p13;q12), which results in *EWSR1-WT1* fusion. Nuclear WT1 positivity can be observed using an antibody directed against the C-terminus. Similar to their intra-abdominal counterparts, paratesticular DSCRTs behave in a clinically aggressive fashion, spreading to the lungs and retroperitoneal lymph nodes.

Melanotic Neuroectodermal Tumor of Infancy

Melanotic neuroectodermal tumor of infancy (MNTI) is an uncommon tumor that typically affects infants under 1 year of age. It usually

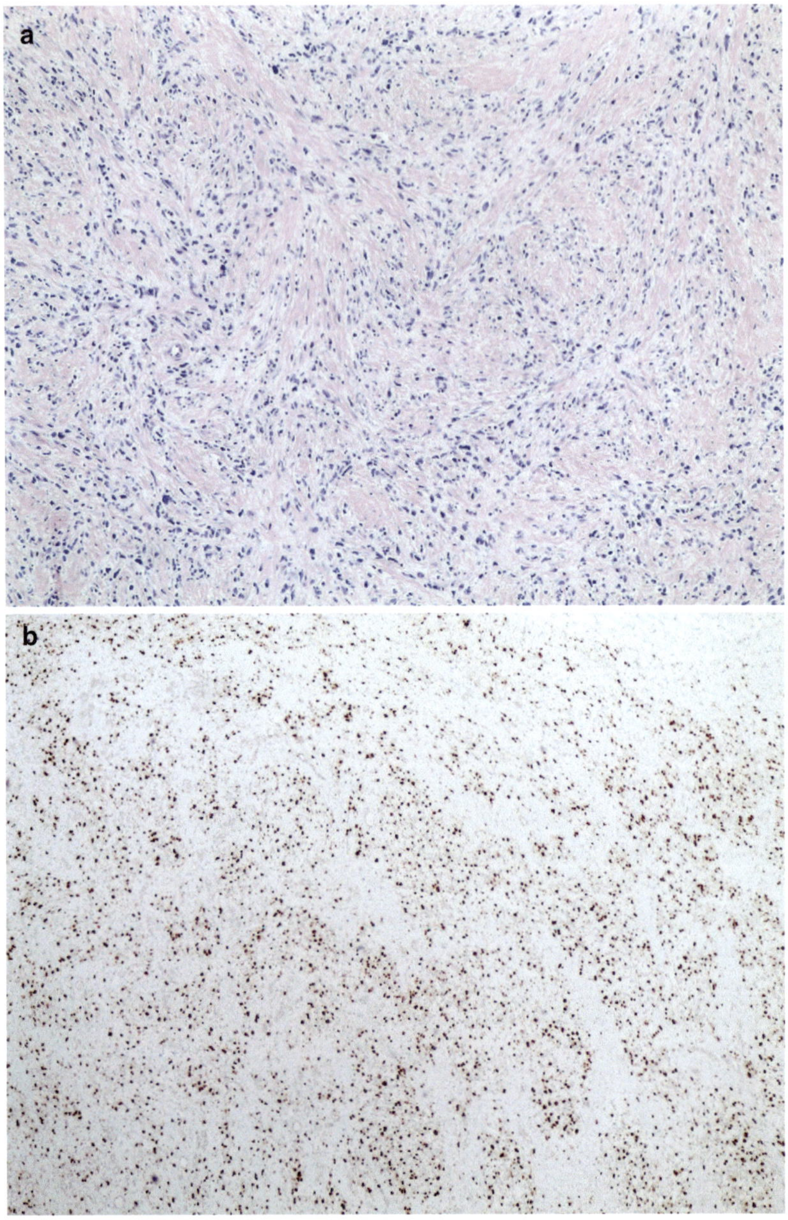

Fig. 10.8 A dense hyalinized stroma characterizes the sclerosing variant of rhabdomyosarcoma (**a**). Positive staining for myogenin (myf-4) assists in the diagnosis (**b**)

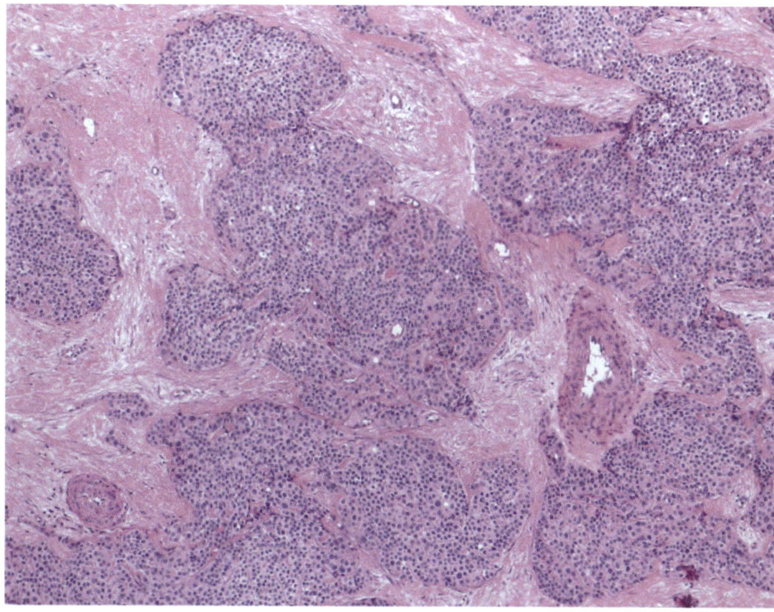

Fig. 10.9 Desmoplastic round cell tumor consisting of small round/oval cells arranged in solid nests embedded in a dense desmoplastic stroma

arises in the maxilla, but may occasionally involve the epididymis and paratesticular region (Fig. 10.10a) [35]. Histologically, it consists of two admixed populations: immature small, ovoid neuroblast-like cells and larger clusters of pigmented epithelioid cells (Fig. 10.10b). The small-cell component shows neural differentiation and stains for NSE, neurofilament, glial fibrillar acidic protein, and chromogranin. The large cells are immunoreactive for HMB45 and cytokeratin. Differential diagnosis for round cell malignancies, particularly embryonal rhabdomyosarcoma, may be challenging, especially in small biopsies that do not include both components. MNTI is considered an indolent tumor, but it may occasionally recur locally and spread to lymph nodes and distant sites [36, 37].

Fig. 10.10
Paratesticular melanotic neuroectodermal tumor of infancy (**a**). At higher magnification, small, neuroblast-like cells and melanin-containing epithelioid cells can be distinguished. Mitotic activity is minimal, and cytologic atypia is lacking (**b**)

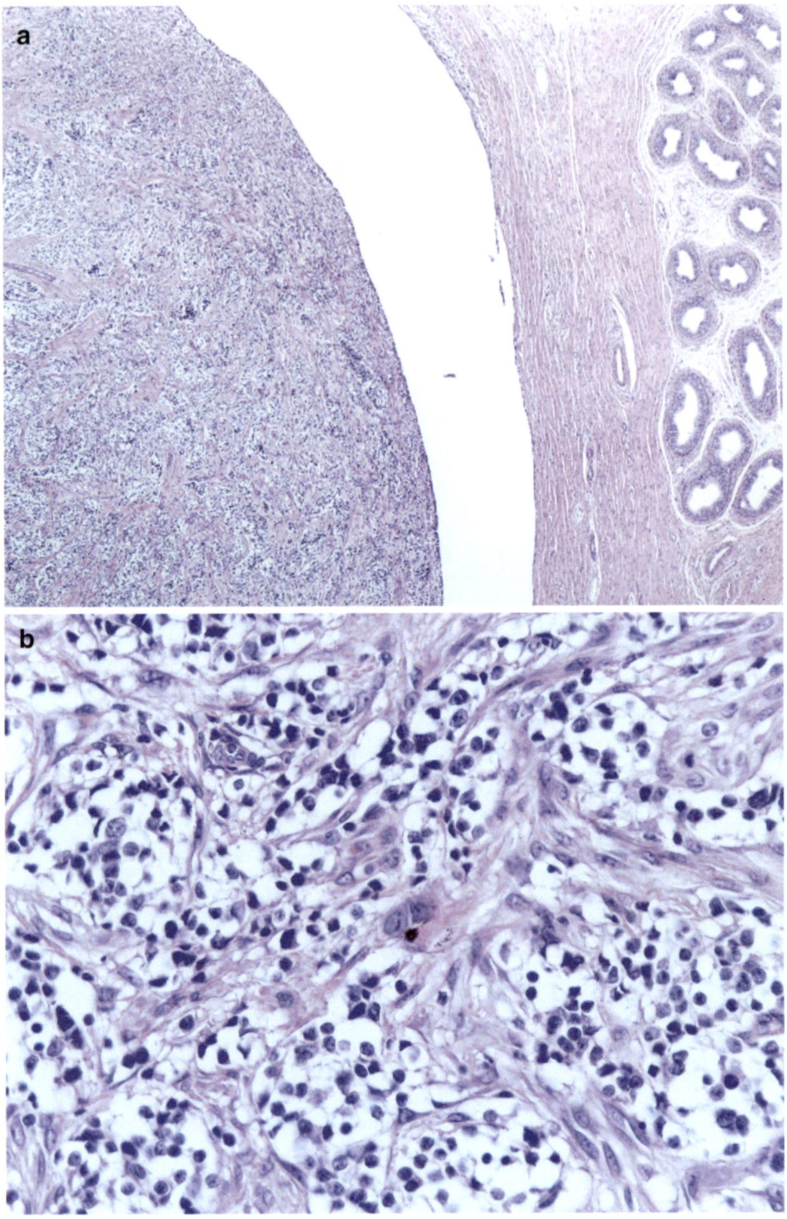

References

1. Rodríguez D, Barrisford GW, Sanchez A, Preston MA, Kreydin EI, Olumi AF. Primary spermatic cord tumors: disease characteristics, prognostic factors, and treatment outcomes. Urol Oncol. 2014;32:52.e19–25.
2. Sogani PC, Whitmore WF, Grabstald Jr H. Spermatic cord sarcoma in adults. J Urol. 1978;120:301–5.
3. Mondaini N, Palli D, Saieva C, Nesi G, Franchi A, Ponchietti R, Tripodi S, Miracco C, Meliani E, Carini M, Livi L, Zanna I, Trovarelli S, Marino V, Vignolini G, Pomara G, Orlando V, Giubilei G, Selli C, Rizzo M. Clinical characteristics and overall survival in genitourinary sarcomas treated with curative intent: a multicenter study. Eur Urol. 2005;47:468–73.
4. Coindre JM, Mariani O, Chibon F, Mairal A, De Saint Aubain Somerhausen N, Favre-Guillevin E, Bui NB, Stoeckle E, Hostein I, Aurias A. Most malignant fibrous histiocytomas developed in the retroperitoneum are dedifferentiated liposarcomas: a review of 25 cases initially diagnosed as malignant fibrous histiocytoma. Mod Pathol. 2003;16:256–62.
5. Alaggio R, Zhang L, Sung YS, Huang SC, Chen CL, Bisogno G, Zin A, Agaram NP, LaQuaglia MP, Wexler LH, Antonescu CR. A molecular study of pediatric spindle and sclerosing rhabdomyosarcoma: identification of novel and recurrent VGLL2-related fusions in infantile cases. Am J Surg Pathol. 2016;40:224–35.
6. Agaram NP, Chen CL, Zhang L, LaQuaglia MP, Wexler L, Antonescu CR. Recurrent MYOD1 mutations in pediatric and adult sclerosing and spindle cell rhabdomyosarcomas: evidence for a common pathogenesis. Genes Chromosomes Cancer. 2014;53:779–87.
7. Mosquera JM, Sboner A, Zhang L, Kitabayashi N, Chen CL, Sung YS, Wexler LH, LaQuaglia MP, Edelman M, Sreekantaiah C, Rubin MA, Antonescu CR. Recurrent NCOA2 gene rearrangements in congenital/infantile spindle cell rhabdomyosarcoma. Genes Chromosomes Cancer. 2013;52:538–50.
8. Vagnoni V, Brunocilla E, Schiavina R, Borghesi M, Passaretti G, Gentile G, Fiorentino M, Martorana G. Inguinal canal tumors of adulthood. Anticancer Res. 2013;33:2361–8.
9. Roman Birmingham PI, Navarro Sebastian FJ, Garcia Gonzalez J, Romero Barriuso G, Guijarro Espadas A. Paratesticular tumors. Description of our case series through a period of 25 years. Arch Esp Urol. 2012;65:609–15.
10. Borri A, Nesi G, Bencini L, Pernice LM. Bizarre leiomyoma of the epididymis. A case report. Minerva Urol Nefrol. 2000;52:29–31.
11. Fisher C, Goldblum JR, Epstein JI, Montgomery E. Leiomyosarcoma of the paratesticular region: a clinicopathologic study. Am J Surg Pathol. 2001;25:1143–9.
12. Jeon YS, Cho SG, Kim WH, Choi SJ. Cavernous haemangioma of the spermatic cord in a child. Pediatr Radiol. 2006;36:1323–5.
13. Liokumovich P, Herbert M, Sandbank J, Schvimer M, Dolberg L. Cavernous hemangioma of spermatic cord: report of a case with immunohistochemical study. Arch Pathol Lab Med. 2002;126:357–8.
14. Montgomery E, Epstein JI. Anastomosing hemangioma of the genitourinary tract: a lesion mimicking angiosarcoma. Am J Surg Pathol. 2009;33:1364–9.
15. Laskin WB, Fetsch JF, Mostofi FK. Angiomyofibroblastomalike tumor of the male genital tract: analysis of 11 cases with comparison to female angiomyofibroblastoma and spindle cell lipoma. Am J Surg Pathol. 1998;22:6–16.
16. Iwasa Y, Fletcher CD. Cellular angiofibroma: clinicopathologic and immunohistochemical analysis of 51 cases. Am J Surg Pathol. 2004;28:1426–35.
17. Folpe AL, Weiss SW. Paratesticular soft tissue neoplasms. Semin Diagn Pathol. 2000;17:307–18.
18. Mukonoweshuro P, McCormick F, Rachapalli V, Natale S, Smith ME. Paratesticular mammary-type myofibroblastoma. Histopathology. 2007;50:396–7.
19. McMenamin ME, Fletcher CD. Mammary-type myofibroblastoma of soft tissue: a tumor closely related to spindle cell lipoma. Am J Surg Pathol. 2001;25:1022–9.
20. Tsang WY, Chan JK, Lee KC, Fisher C, Fletcher CD. Aggressive angiomyxoma. A report of four cases occurring in men. Am J Surg Pathol. 1992;16:1059–65.
21. van Roggen JF, van Unnik JA, Briaire-de Bruijn IH, Hogendoorn PC. Aggressive angiomyxoma: a clinicopathological and immunohistochemical study of 11 cases with long-term follow-up. Virchows Arch. 2005;446:157–63.
22. Granter SR, Nucci MR, Fletcher CD. Aggressive angiomyxoma: reappraisal of its relationship to angiomyofibroblastoma in a series of 16 cases. Histopathology. 1997;30:3–10.
23. Montgomery JS, Hollenbeck BK, Fisher PC, Murphy HS, Underwood 3rd W. Benign paratesticular schwannoma. Can J Urol. 2004;11:2393–5.
24. Milathianakis KN, Karamanolakis DK, Mpogdanos IM, Trihia-Spyrou EI. Solitary neurofibroma of the spermatic cord. Urol Int. 2004;72:271–4.
25. Banks E, Yum M, Brodhecker C, Goheen M. A malignant peripheral nerve sheath tumor in association with a paratesticular ganglioneuroma. Cancer. 1989;64:1738–42.
26. Jo VY, Reith JD, Coindre JM, Fletcher CD. Paratesticular rhabdomyoma: a morphologically distinct sclerosing variant. Am J Surg Pathol. 2013;37:1737–42.
27. Schwartz SL, Swierzewski 3rd SJ, Sondak VK, Grossman HB. Liposarcoma of the spermatic cord: report of 6 cases and review of the literature. J Urol. 1995;153:154–7.
28. Montgomery E, Fisher C. Paratesticular liposarcoma: a clinicopathologic study. Am J Surg Pathol. 2003;27:40–7.
29. Khandekar MJ, Raut CP, Hornick JL, et al. Paratesticular liposarcoma: unusual patterns of recur-

rence and importance of margins. Ann Surg Oncol. 2013;20:2148–55.

30. Kryvenko ON, Rosenberg AE, Jorda M, Epstein JI. Dedifferentiated liposarcoma of the spermatic cord: a series of 42 cases. Am J Surg Pathol. 2015;39:1219–25.
31. Fletcher CD, Bridge JA, Hogendoorn PCW, Mertens F, editors. WHO classification of tumours of soft tissue and bone. Lyon: IARC Press; 2013.
32. Ferrari A, Bisogno G, Casanova M, Meazza C, Piva L, Cecchetto G, Zanetti I, Pilz T, Mattke A, Treuner J, Carli M. Paratesticular rhabdomyosarcoma: report from the Italian and German Cooperative Group. J Clin Oncol. 2002;20:449–55.
33. Cummings OW, Ulbright TM, Young RH, Dei Tos AP, Fletcher CD, Hull MT. Desmoplastic small round cell tumors of the paratesticular region. A report of six cases. Am J Surg Pathol. 1997;21:219–25.
34. Thuret R, Renaudin K, Leclere J, Battisti S, Bouchot O, Theodore C. Uncommon malignancies: case 3. Paratesticular desmoplastic small round-cell tumor. J Clin Oncol. 2005;23:6253–5.
35. Calabrese F, Danieli D, Valente M. Melanotic neuroectodermal tumor of the epididymis in infancy: case report and review of the literature. Urology. 1995;46:415–8.
36. De Chiara A, Van Tornout JM, Hachitanda Y, Ortega JA, Shimada H. Melanotic neuroectodermal tumor of infancy. A case report of paratesticular primary with lymph node involvement. Am J Pediatr Hematol Oncol. 1992;14:356–60.
37. Ulbright TM, Young RH. Testicular and paratesticular tumors and tumor-like lesions in the first 2 decades. Semin Diagn Pathol. 2014;31:323–81.

Frozen Section in Testicular Pathology

11

Maurizio Colecchia and Nicola Nicolai

Introduction

Intraoperative examination of testicular nodules by frozen section was rarely used in the past because of the inherent diagnostic uncertainty [1, 2]. In recent years, it has been more widely used for the diagnosis of small nodules detected by ultrasonography. A diagnostic issue the pathologist is less frequently asked to resolve by frozen section is the assessment of resection margins in partial tumor resection. Further reasons for frozen section examination are generally related to partial orchiectomies performed in monorchid individuals: urologists typically ask for a conservative approach when there are synchronous bilateral germ cell tumors or a unilateral germ cell tumor with a history of contralateral orchiectomy for germ cell tumor.

Tumor masses in prepubertal patients and frozen section or touch preparation of testicular biopsies for infertility are less common reasons for requesting the exam. In this chapter, we describe the usefulness and limits of frozen sections in the oncological setting and the importance of effective communication with urologists in cases where we are asked to guide their surgical hands.

M. Colecchia (✉)
Uropathology Unit, Department of Pathology, Fondazione IRCCS Istituto Nazionale dei Tumori di Milano, Milan, Italy
e-mail: maurizio.colecchia@istitutotumori.mi.it

N. Nicolai
Testis Surgery Unit, Fondazione IRCCS Istituto Nazionale dei Tumori di Milano, Milan, Italy
e-mail: nicola.nicolai@istitutotumori.mi.it

Clinical Background for Gross Consultation on Radical Orchiectomy Specimen

The diagnosis of a testicular germ cell tumor is often clear prior to orchiectomy. A testicular swelling with elevation of the serum tumor markers alpha-fetoprotein (AFP) and/or beta-subunit of human chorionic gonadotropin (β-hCG) is a very frequent scenario. In such cases, radical orchiectomy can be performed immediately, without any intraoperative macroscopic or frozen section examination. When a testicular swelling is found but serum tumor markers are normal and there is no evidence of metastases, surgical exploration through an inguinal incision is indicated, followed by exteriorization of the testis within its tunics. Orchiectomy with division of the spermatic cord at the internal inguinal ring must be performed if a gross neoplastic mass is found in the testicular parenchyma [1]. Basically, there is no specific indication for macroscopic consultation once the orchiectomy specimen has been removed.

M. Colecchia (ed.), *Pathology of Testicular and Penile Neoplasms*,
DOI 10.1007/978-3-319-27617-5_11

Consultation for a Specific Diagnosis Prior to Surgery for Possible Testis-Sparing Operation

An increasing proportion of patients present with small intratesticular masses detected during transscrotal ultrasonography. The most common indication for this examination includes the workup of men in infertile/subfertile couples or patients with some testicular discomfort. Most of these men have no marker elevation and almost all have no signs of metastatic deposits. Until a couple of decades ago, surgical exploration was mandatory in case of an intratesticular mass. Nowadays, this recommendation conflicts with the evidence that very small testicular lesions may not contain tumor. There is a direct relationship between increasing lesion size and the likelihood of a malignant tumor. In a series of 80 patients presenting testicular masses up to 50 mm, normal serum tumor markers and no evidence of metastases, only 3 (23 %) of those with a lesion up to 10 mm had a malignant tumor versus 100 % of 26 with a lesion exceeding 30 mm [3]. In a more recent series of 103 solid testicular nodules, as many as 67 (94.4 %) of 71 cases with a nodule up to 5 mm did not contain malignant tumor, versus only four (19 %) of 19 cases with a nodule between 5 and 10 mm, and none of the 11 cases with a solid testicular mass >10 mm, while in two cases the nodules were missed [4]. Although these series as well as others are not perfectly matched in terms of case selection, identification of small lesions not exceeding 5 mm in diameter should be regarded as a low-relevance clinical finding, because the vast majority of such lesions do not contain malignant cells. Nonetheless, once physicians have decided on surgical exploration of a testis which contains a nodule in a patient without any other signs of malignancy, a biopsy should be taken (along with enucleation of the intraparenchymal tumor) for frozen section analysis if the diagnosis remains unclear after exposition of the testis. Enucleation alone may even be sufficient treatment for a small single lesion in the case of testicular sex cord-stromal tumors. In the last decade, several studies reported on the feasibility and safety of testis-sparing surgery in testicular sex cord-stromal tumors [5–7]. From a theoretical point of view, different aspects seem to be proper premises to justify testis-sparing surgery in the case of testicular sex cord-stromal tumors. These tumors differ from germ cell tumors in that they do not display multifocal disease, are not associated with precancerous lesions that could herald invasive cancer (like intratubular neoplasia in germ cell tumors), and show a low rate of local recurrence. Although no prospective comparative data are available to make a comparison between radical orchiectomy and testis-sparing surgery in case of testicular sex cord-stromal tumors, the available data following testis-sparing surgery evince that local recurrences are very rare [7], whereas metastatic spread was not reported in any of the most recent studies including a total of 84 cases [5, 8, 9].

Specimen Handling

To date there has been no general consensus about the way testis specimens for frozen section should be handled. After surgical excision, it is important that the sample be transferred to the frozen section room as entire as possible. The pathologist needs a fresh specimen, without incisions or fragmentations that should be measured and examined very accurately, paying attention to color and shape. Necrotic or hemorrhagic areas that may harbor germ cell components must be sampled as well, and the urologist should include such foci in the sample sent for intraoperative consultation [10]. A specimen consisting of small nodules should be examined in toto: after inking, it is serially sectioned to identify the lesion and assess its distance to the surgical margins.

Specimen Interpretation

Few studies have investigated the accuracy of frozen section examination of testicular lesions. The distinction between benign and malignant lesions was highly accurate in one study (86.7 %), but an inconclusive diagnosis for nonpalpable incidental tumors was reported in 13.3 % of cases [11]. In another study, the percentage of wrong diagnoses in Leydig cell tumor nodules was 10 % [12].

Stromal Tumors

Stromal tumors sometimes present with equivocal features, and frozen section analysis can be used for the differential diagnosis between Leydig and Sertoli cell tumors on the one hand and tumors of germ cell origin on the other. The more common stromal tumor, Leydig cell tumor, is characterized by solid growth of uniform, polyhedral cells showing no atypia, with granular eosinophilic cytoplasm and no lymphocytic background (Fig. 11.1).

Sertoli cell tumor can be more difficult to distinguish because of the clear cytoplasm and variable growth pattern (Fig. 11.2). In rare cases diagnosis by frozen section can be difficult due to microscopic characteristics of atypia. Given the pressure for a quick diagnosis without the help of histochemical and immunohistochemical findings, the unexperienced pathologist may suggest a diagnosis of a stromal tumor, deferring the final diagnosis until examination of the definitive preparation. This is an important issue, especially considering that testis-sparing surgery for Leydig cell tumors is justified by long-term follow-up data showing no recurrence in the majority of cases [12].

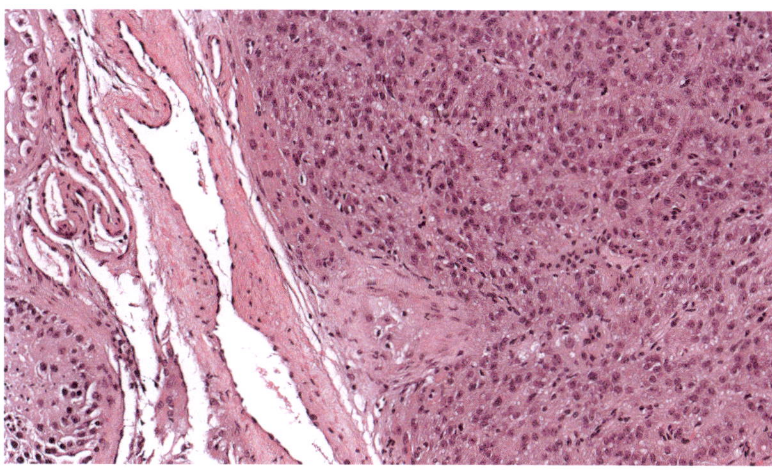

Fig. 11.1 Leydig cell tumor. Leydig cell tumors have uniform cells without atypia, showing small nucleoli and granular eosinophilic cytoplasm. The absence of lymphocytes is a characteristic feature differentiating Leydig cell tumor from seminoma (Published with kind permission of ©Maurizio Colecchia 2015. All Rights Reserved)

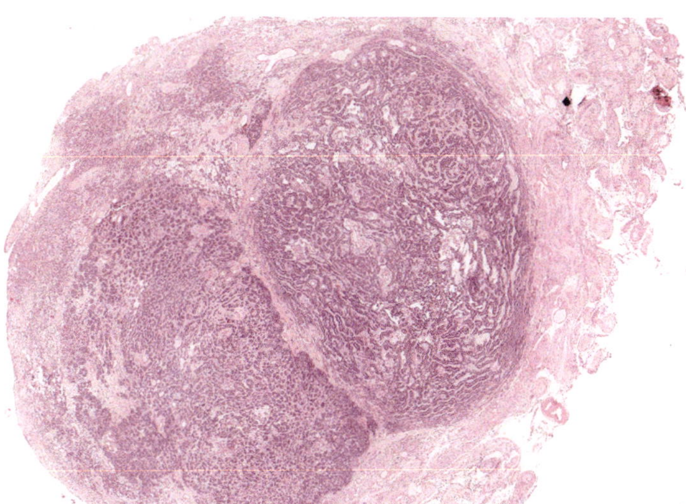

Fig. 11.2 Sertoli cell tumor. Low-power magnification of Sertoli cell tumor on frozen section shows tubules and nests of this stromal benign-appearing neoplasm. Recognition of this entity allows conservative surgery

Malignant cases may occur, but it may not be possible to identify them by morphology alone in frozen tissue [10]. Cases of malignant Sertoli cell tumors with an infiltrative growth pattern and severe atypia with mitotic figures necessitate a differential diagnosis with seminoma, which can be problematic.

Diagnostic Pitfalls in Seminoma Recognition

A diagnostic problem may present itself when there is granulomatous or lymphocytic infiltration with scattered plasma cells and benign spindle cells in chronic or granulomatous orchitis (Fig. 11.3). This occurrence shows morphologic overlap with seminoma with granulomatous infiltration, where the lymphocytic infiltrate is so abundant that it obliterates the germ cell component and the neoplastic proliferation could be missed (Fig. 11.4). The main cytological features of seminoma cells are abundant but ill-defined cytoplasm, large nuclei, and prominent nucleoli; in limited areas, crush artifacts occur consisting of clumping of the nuclei and hematoxylin stripes. Atypical intratubular germ cells are present in the surrounding testicular parenchyma (Fig. 11.5).

Lymphocytic infiltrates are prevalent in viral-type orchitis [13] and have recently been reported

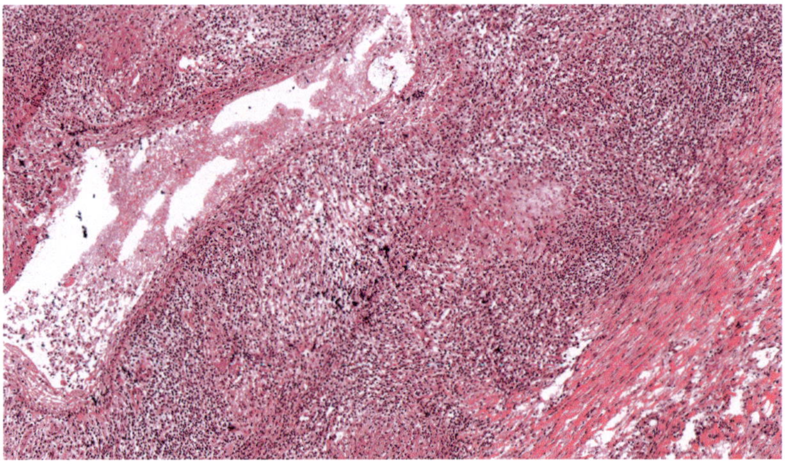

Fig. 11.3 Chronic orchitis. Small lymphoid cells, plasma cells, and fibrosis in the hilum of the testis

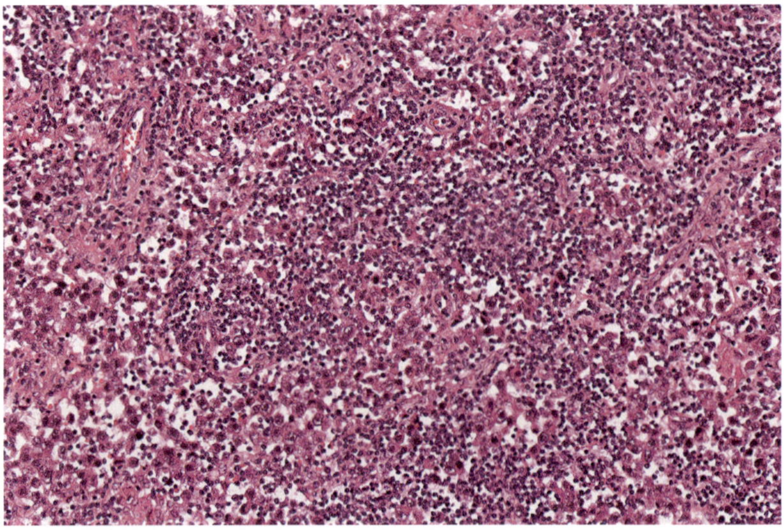

Fig. 11.4 Seminoma with granulomatous reaction. The inflammatory infiltrate is so abundant that it masks the neoplastic cells

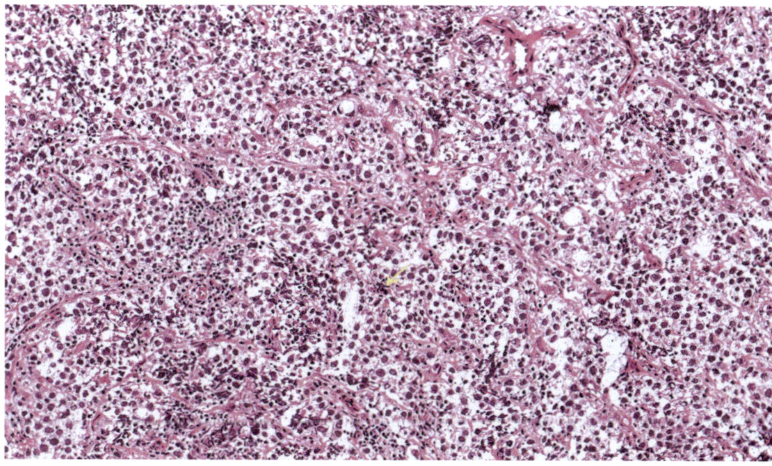

Fig. 11.5 Seminoma. Large nuclei with prominent nucleoli are characteristic features of seminomatous cells with intermixed small lymphocytes; crush artifacts and clumping of the nuclei are present in this frozen section (*arrow*)

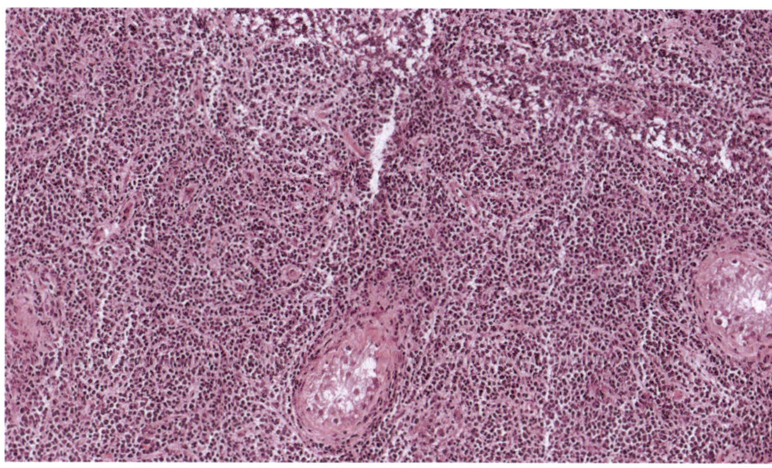

Fig. 11.6 Lymphoma. Radical orchiectomy in a 60-year-old man. The interstitium is expanded by monotonous lymphoid cells. The seminiferous tubule is surrounded by lymphoid cells. The differential diagnosis in this case includes chronic orchitis and seminoma

as diagnostically problematic in an intraoperative consultation performed in four of ten cases of viral-type orchitis [14]. Based on frozen section analysis, acute orchitis with possible intratubular tumor suspicious for lymphoma in one case and seminoma in another was diagnosed. The interpretation of the ten cases was difficult also on permanent sections, and they were sent for a second opinion, which resulted in a final diagnosis of viral-type orchitis [14].

Supporting this diagnosis is the presence of bands of inflamed seminiferous tubules flanked by uninvolved tubules where the inflammatory infiltrate contains primarily lymphocytes and histiocytes. Numerous histiocytes occupy the seminiferous tubules and are easily mistaken for a neoplasm, while small lymphocytes predominate in the interstitium. The tubules away from the inflammation are atrophic, with hypospermatogenesis or containing only Sertoli cells [13, 14], and the distension of the tubules by inflammatory cells is the more striking feature. The most challenging problem in frozen section analysis is the suspicion of a seminoma with a purely intertubular growth pattern that lacks a mass lesion on gross examination similar to viral-type orchitis [15]. For this differential diagnosis, it is necessary to exclude the presence of seminoma cells within the lymphocytic interstitial infiltrate.

Other differential diagnoses with uncommon hematopoietic neoplasms, mainly lymphomas (Fig. 11.6), have been discussed in Chap. 6. Less common inflammatory lesions are bacterial orchitis secondary to *Neisseria gonorrhea* or

Chlamydia trachomatis infection in sexually active individuals, which are generally secondary to bacterial spread from the epididymis. A very uncommon occurrence is Rosai-Dorfman disease of the testis [16].

Teratomatous Components

Typical clinical ambiguity regarding the nature of a testicular mass requiring frozen section examination occurs in the case of an epidermoid cyst [17]. This is a single cystic lesion composed of a mature squamous epithelial lining containing abundant amounts of keratin without skin adnexal structures (Fig. 11.7). The latter finding is suggestive of an epidermoid cyst because dermoid cysts of the testis contain hair follicles with sebaceous glands. However, the distinction on frozen examination has no important clinical consequences given the benign course of both lesions [18].

Unlike postpubertal teratomas, which are more complex, typically solid tumors with multiple cysts, epidermoid cysts lack intratubular germ cell neoplasia in the adjacent tissue [19]. The diagnosis of teratoma, regardless of its maturity, is important in light of the reported metastatic potential in the majority of cases occurring in postpubertal testes (Fig. 11.8).

Other Germ Cell Tumors

Definitive histotyping of germ cell tumors on frozen section is unnecessary because their treatment is generally the same, i.e., radical orchiectomy. This is underlined by Juan Rosai in the introduction to his textbook on surgical pathology, where he mentions that when frozen section analysis does not influence the surgical procedure, it is not indicated. Using this criterion, Dr Rosai estimated that almost half of the frozen sections done at a particular institution could be avoided [20].

Fibrous Scar-Like Tissue

Collagenous scar-like tissue with only few seminiferous tubules containing Sertoli cells but no viable tumor is sometimes the presentation of a testicular lesion thought to be benign and sent for intraoperative examination (Fig. 11.9). The possibility of a "burned-out" germ cell tumor (see Chap. 6) or the occurrence in a sclerotic/atrophic testis must be ruled out on permanent sections, where the presence of intratubular germ cell neoplasia near a regressed germ cell tumor should be investigated and the clinical history of the patient be taken into account.

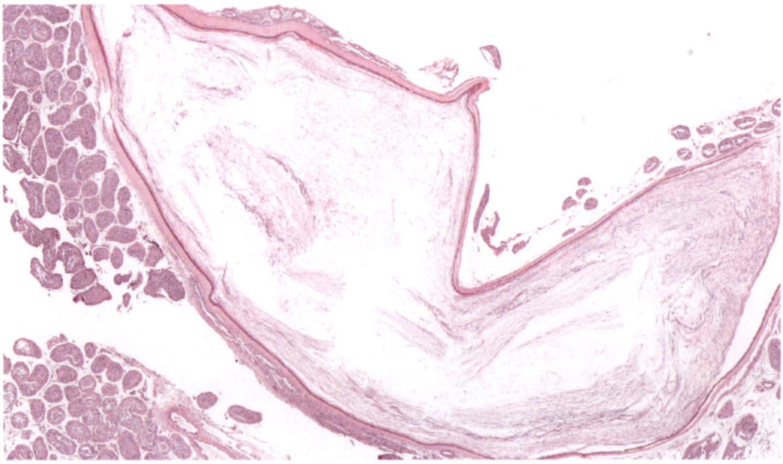

Fig. 11.7 Epidermoid cyst. A single cyst composed of mature squamous lining containing keratinous material. The absence of intratubular germ cell neoplasia in the surrounding testis is a hallmark of this benign lesion

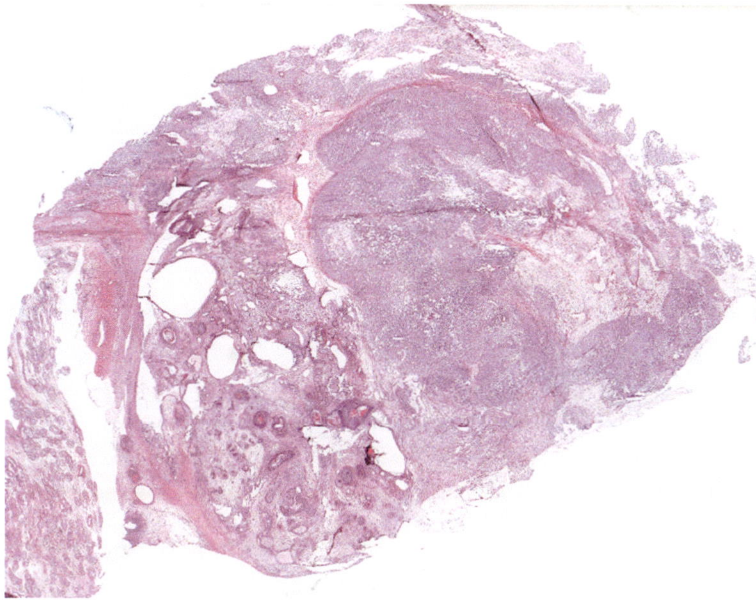

Fig. 11.8 Teratoma. Whichever mature or immature components make up this teratoma, this intraoperative finding prompts a radical orchiectomy given the metastatic potential of teratoma occurring in postpubertal testes

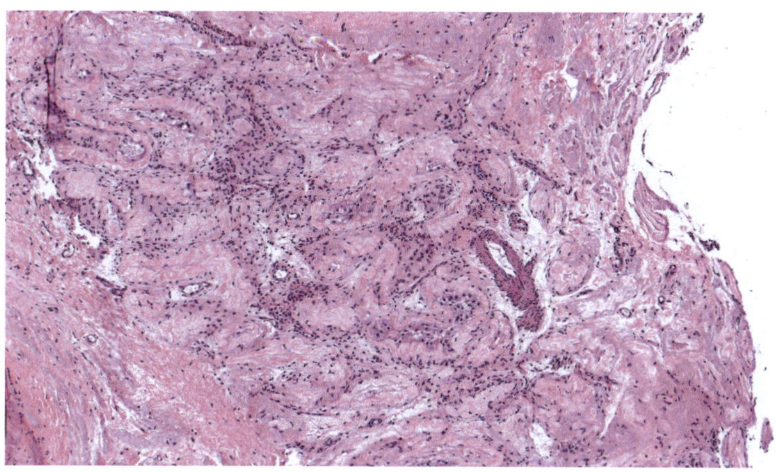

Fig. 11.9 Fibrous scar-like tissue. Collagenous scar-like tissue with few atrophic tubules with Sertoli cells only

Adenomatoid Tumor

The typically innocuous microscopical appearance and the presentation as a solitary, small, epididymal nodule can help in the diagnosis of this benign tumor. The gross appearance of malignant mesothelioma as a large tumor pervasively infiltrating the testicular parenchyma is in contrast to the appearance of an adenomatoid tumor. The neoplasm consists of gland-like structures, tubules, and vacuoles in a fibrous stroma (Fig. 11.10a). The vacuolization can be reminiscent of metastatic adenocarcinoma (i.e., signet-ring cell adenocarcinoma) but may also be an unusual feature in Sertoli cell tumors (Fig. 11.10b) and in cases of yolk sac tumor with a microvacuolated pattern. The final diagnosis will be based on the location of the tumor and immunohistochemical staining of permanent sections [21]. When an adenomatoid tumor is not radically resected, there is no need for additional excision because of its benign nature.

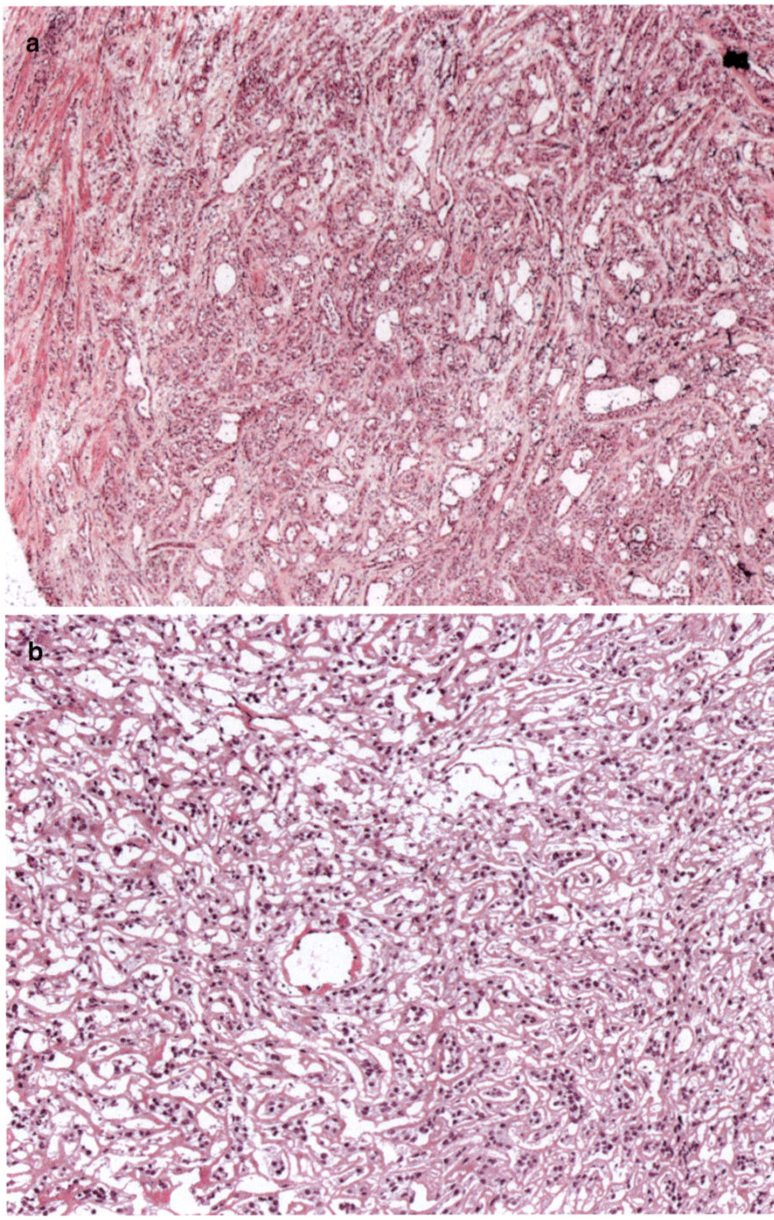

Fig. 11.10 (**a**) Adenomatoid tumor and (**b**) Sertoli cell tumor. Comparing the microscopic features of adenomatoid tumor (**a**) with those of Sertoli cells with prominent vacuoles (**b**) makes it easy to recognize the two lesions, which can be hard to distinguish on frozen sections

Frozen Section of Lymph Nodes in Retroperitoneal Nodal Dissection

In patients with clinical retroperitoneal metastasis, nodal dissection may be performed [22, 23]. The pathologist must be aware of any neoadjuvant chemotherapy administered to the patient before the request of frozen examination of the lymphadenectomy specimen. Examination of the gross specimen before frozen section can be conclusive in many cases (Fig. 11.11). When multiple nodes are submitted, the largest is often the most suspicious to examine for a fast diagnosis of malignancy.

Histopathological examination allows the diagnosis of metastatic germ cell malignancy and the establishment of a presumptive histological type (Fig. 11.12). If the grossly abnormal areas

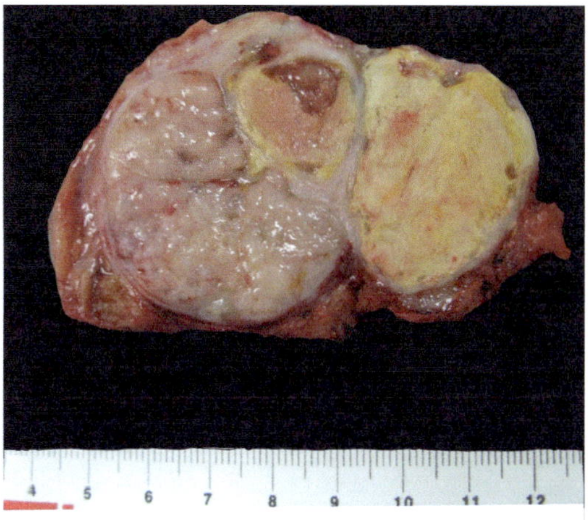

Fig. 11.11 Gross specimen of retroperitoneal lymph node. Macroscopic examination of the gross specimen allows easy detection of metastasis

are fibrotic without viable tumor cells, the pathologist provides a preliminary report, deferring the final diagnosis until permanent sections will be available.

The presence of unilateral lymph node metastases does not justify bilateral retroperitoneal node dissection. Immunohistochemical quick staining has been reported to be a useful adjunctive tool during frozen section examination in retroperitoneal lymphadenectomy [24].

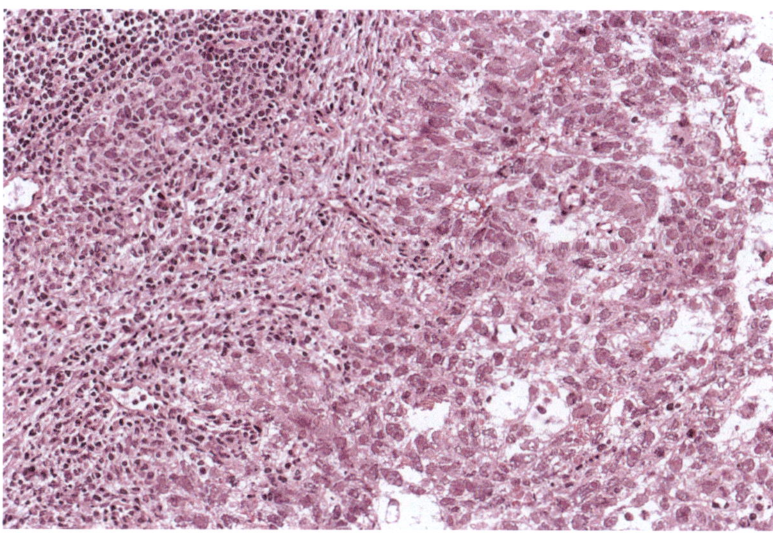

Fig. 11.12 Lymph node metastasis of germ cell tumor. Embryonal carcinomatous cells in a lymph node metastasis. Surgeons rarely ask for intraoperative examination during retroperitoneal nodal dissection for a metastatic germ cell malignancy previously detected by tomography

References

1. Albers P, Albrecht W, Algaba F, Bokemeyer C, Cohn-Cedermark G, Fizazi K, Horwich A, Laguna MP, European Association of Urology. EAU guidelines on testicular cancer: 2011 update. Eur Urol. 2011;60:304–19.
2. Shilo Y, Zisman A, Lindner A, Raz O, Strauss S, Siegel YI, Segal M, Sandbank J, Leibovici DT. The predominance of benign histology in small testicular masses. Urol Oncol. 2012;30:719–22.
3. Connolly SS, D'Arcy FT, Bredin HC, Callaghan J, Corcoran MO. Value of frozen section analysis with suspected testicular malignancy. Urology. 2006;67:162–5.
4. Goddi A, Sacchi A, Magistretti G, Almolla J, Salvadore M. Real-time tissue elastography for testicular lesion assessment. Eur Radiol. 2012;22:721–30.
5. Bozzini G, Picozzi S, Gadda F, Colombo R, Decobelli O, Palou J, Colpi G, Carmignani L. Long-term follow-up using testicle-sparing surgery for Leydig cell tumor. Clin Genitourin Cancer. 2013;11:321–4.
6. Carmignani L, Colombo R, Gadda F, Galasso G, Lania A, Palou J, Algaba F, Villavicencio H, Colpi GM, Decobelli O, Salvioni R, Pizzocaro G, Rigatti P, Rocco F. Conservative surgical therapy for Leydig cell tumor. J Urol. 2007;178:507–11.
7. Loeser A, Vergho DC, Katzenberger T, Brix D, Kocot A, Spahn M, Gerharz EW, Riedmiller H. Testis-sparing surgery versus radical orchiectomy in patients with Leydig cell tumors. Urology. 2009;74:370–2.
8. Giannarini G, Mogorovich A, Menchini Fabris F, Morelli G, De Maria M, Manassero F, Loggini B, Pingitore R, Cavazzana A, Selli C. Long-term followup after elective testis sparing surgery for Leydig cell tumors: a single center experience. J Urol. 2007;178:872–6.
9. Suardi N, Strada E, Colombo R, Freschi M, Salonia A, Lania C, Cestari A, Carmignani L, Guazzoni G, Rigatti P, Montorsi F. Leydig cell tumour of the testis: presentation, therapy, long-term follow-up and the role of organ-sparing surgery in a single-institution experience. BJU Int. 2009;103:197–200.
10. Algaba F, Ro JY, Shen SS, Truong LD. Testis. In: Frozen section library: genitourinary tract. New York: Springer; 2009. p. 137–59.
11. Leroy X, Rigot JM, Aubert S, Ballereau C, Gosselin B. Value of frozen section examination for the management of nonpalpable incidental testicular tumors. Eur Urol. 2003;44:458–60.
12. Carmignani L, Salvioni R, Gadda F, Colecchia M, Gazzano G, Torelli T, Rocco F, Colpi GM, Pizzocaro G. Long-term follow up and clinical characteristics of testicular Leydig cell tumor: experience with 24 cases. J Urol. 2006;176:2040–3.
13. Braaten KM, Young RH, Ferry JA. Viral-type orchitis: a potential mimic of testicular neoplasia. Am J Surg Pathol. 2009;33:1477–84.
14. Agarwal V, Li JK, Bard R. Lymphocytic orchitis: a case report. Hum Pathol. 1990;21:1080–2.
15. Henley JD, Young RH, Wade CL, Ulbright TM. Seminomas with exclusive intertubular growth: a report of 12 clinically and grossly inconspicuous tumors. Am J Surg Pathol. 2004;28:1163–8.
16. Fernandopulle SM, Hwang JS, Kuick CH, Lui J, Tan PH, Siow WY, Wong M. Rosai-Dorfman disease of the testis: an unusual entity that mimics testicular malignancy. J Clin Pathol. 2006;59:325–7.
17. Heidenreich A, Zumbé J, Vorreuther R, Klotz T, Vietsch H, Engelmann UH. Testicular epidermoid cyst: orchiectomy or enucleation resection? Urologe A. 1996;35:1–5.
18. Ulbright TM, Srigley JR. Dermoid cyst of the testis: a study of five postpubertal cases, including a pilomatrixoma-like variant, with evidence supporting its separate classification from mature testicular teratoma. Am J Surg Pathol. 2001;25:788–93.
19. Wiesenthal JD, Ettler H, Razvi H. Testicular epidermoid cyst: a case report and review of the clinicopathologic features. Can J Urol. 2004;11:2133–5.
20. Rosai J. Introduction chapter 1. In: Rosai and Ackerman's surgical pathology. 10th ed. New York: Mosby; 2011. p. 12.
21. Delahunt B, Eble JN, King D, Bethwaite PB, Nacey JN, Thornton A. Immunohistochemical evidence for mesothelial origin of paratesticular adenomatoid tumour. Histopathology. 2000;36:109–15.
22. Algaba F, Arce Y, López-Beltrán A, Montironi R, Mikuz G, Bono AV, European Society of Uropathology; Uropathology Working Group. Intraoperative frozen section diagnosis in urological oncology. Eur Urol. 2005;47:129–36.
23. Subik MK, Gordetsky J, Yao JL, di Sant'Agnese PA, Miyamoto H. Frozen section assessment in testicular and paratesticular lesions suspicious for malignancy: its role in preventing unnecessary orchiectomy. Hum Pathol. 2012;43:1514–9.
24. Stosiek P, Wodke A, Kasper M. Immunohistological detection of lymph node metastases in the testicular center as quick section diagnosis during retroperitoneal lymphadenectomy. Pathol Res Pract. 1993;189:1010–4.

Part III

Pathology of Precancerous Lesions and Tumors of the Penis

Precancerous Lesions of the Penis 12

Maurizio Colecchia and Biagio Paolini

A heterogeneous group of precancerous lesions affect the penis, consisting of cellular alterations of the squamous epithelium: proliferation, loss of polarity, and nuclear atypia of varying degrees [1].

The guidelines on penile cancer of the European Association of Urology (EAU) classify premalignant lesions of the penis into different categories according to the probability of developing into squamous cell carcinoma (SCC): (a) lesions sporadically associated with SCC of the penis (cutaneous horn and bowenoid papulosis), (b) lesions at intermediate risk of progression to SCC (balanitis xerotica obliterans/lichen sclerosus et atrophicus), and (c) lesions at high risk of developing into SCC (penile intraepithelial neoplasia (PeIN), Bowen disease, and erythroplasia of Queyrat) [2]. A 2014 update of the guidelines has included giant condylomata and Paget's disease among the lesions with up to one-third transformation into invasive SCC [3]. Very few pathologic studies of penile precancerous lesions have been reported, mostly related to carcinoma in situ (CIS) and HPV, and there is limited information about low-grade atypical lesions [4].

The tools for an early diagnosis based on accurate physical examination should include inspection of the penis with visual magnification (peniscopy). Peniscopy is an examination through a microscope, very similar to colposcopy, although it does not have the same standards of performance. It allows magnification of the penile surface of up to ten times. Evaluation of the glans mucosa and the preputial skin should be done with 5 % acetic acid application. A peniscopic classification considers the shape, color, borders, and elevation of the lesion [5]. A biopsy is required in case of any suspicious lesions or in those that do not heal following topical therapy. Delayed diagnosis of penile cancer is still a problem and may occur due to the reluctance of patients to undergo medical evaluation but also as a consequence of a delayed biopsy. Accurate inspection allows the detection of macroscopic lesions such as condyloma acuminatum, which is the most common epithelial proliferation in the anogenital area and the most common benign penile tumor.

Condyloma Acuminatum

Condyloma acuminatum is a highly contagious disease caused by the human papillomavirus (HPV), specifically by the more frequently

M. Colecchia (✉)
Uropathology Unit, Department of Pathology, Fondazione IRCCS Istituto Nazionale dei Tumori di Milano, Milan, Italy
e-mail: maurizio.colecchia@istitutotumori.mi.it

B. Paolini
Department of Pathology, Fondazione IRCCS Istituto Nazionale dei Tumori di Milano, Milan, Italy
e-mail: biagio.paolini@istitutotumori.mi.it

M. Colecchia (ed.), *Pathology of Testicular and Penile Neoplasms*,
DOI 10.1007/978-3-319-27617-5_12

detected HPV-6 and HPV-11 serotypes, although high-risk HPV types (16, 18, 31, 33 and 35) have been demonstrated in condyloma-like lesions [6]. At gross examination condyloma acuminatum is a white, exophytic, cauliflower-like lesion (Fig. 12.1). The clinical presentation with small, flat, inconspicuous lesions (Fig. 12.2) has microscopic features in common with hyperparakeratosis, acanthosis, and superficial koilocytosis, typically showing papillomatous proliferation of condylomatous papillae (Fig. 12.3). The virus can be demonstrated by immunohistochemistry and in situ hybridization techniques; cytologically, cytoplasmic vacuolization, binucleation, and hyperchromasia with typical "wrinkled," irregular nuclei are the hallmarks of infected cells (Fig. 12.4). The papillae are broad-based and rounded. Unlike warty SCC, condyloma acuminatum does not infiltrate into the corpus

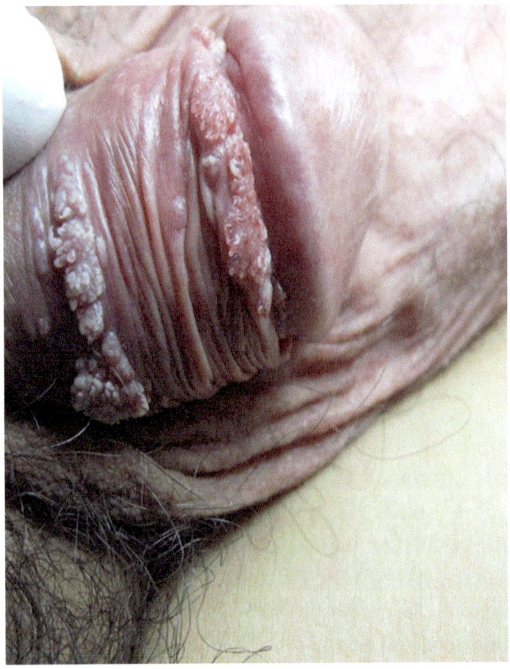

Fig. 12.1 Condyloma acuminatum. Filiform and papular lesions in the foreskin of the penis

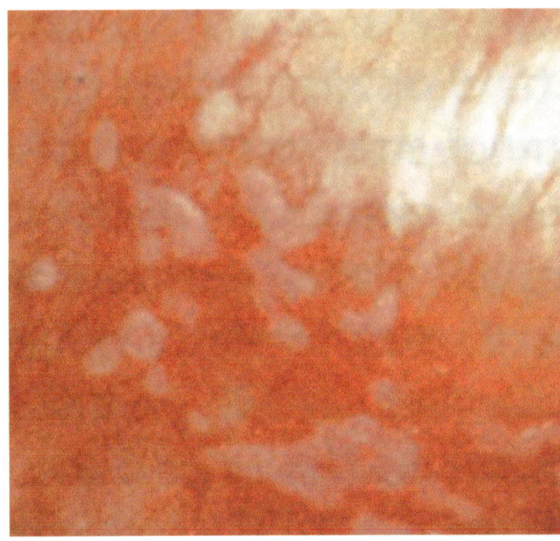

Fig. 12.2 Flat condylomata. Macroscopic appearance of flat lesions at high magnification

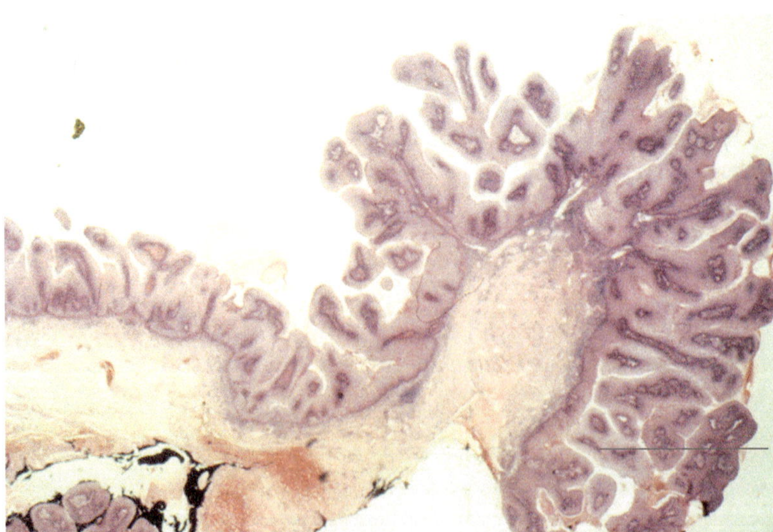

Fig. 12.3 Condyloma. Treelike pattern with a prominent fibrovascular core in a papillomatous pattern of growth

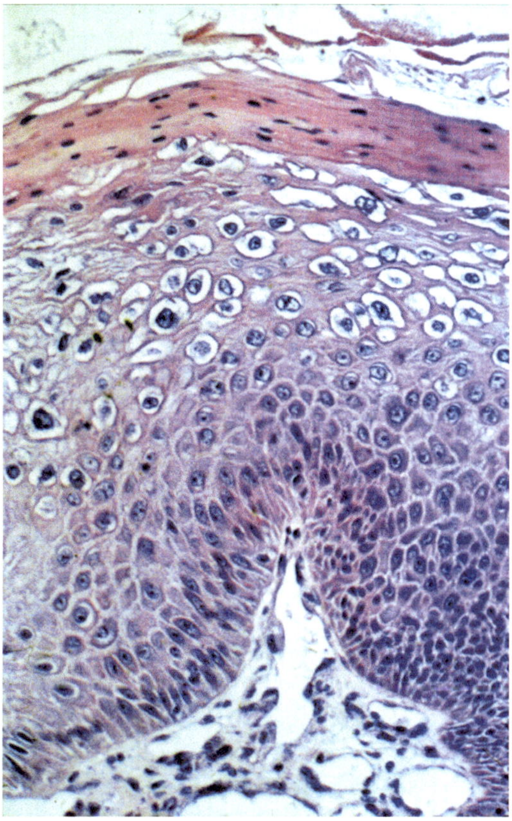

Fig. 12.4 Condyloma. Wrinkled enlarged nuclei surrounded by perinuclear halo (koilocytes) in the full-thickness epithelium

spongiosum and corpora cavernosa. Clinically there is overlapping with molluscum contagiosum, but the two entities are easy to differentiate by microscopy. Even if condylomata are associated with an increased risk of cancer, only a small minority develop into SCC [7].

Cutaneous Horn of the Penis

This is the clinical term for a benign tumor consisting usually of a solitary, hyperkeratotic, papillomatous lesion [8]; multiple lesions also occur but less frequently [9]. It shows the microscopic features of florid epithelial hyperplasia, with hyperparakeratosis lacking atypical cells. One-third of penile horn lesions are associated with malignant tumors of different morphologies including verrucous carcinoma [10] and SCC [11].

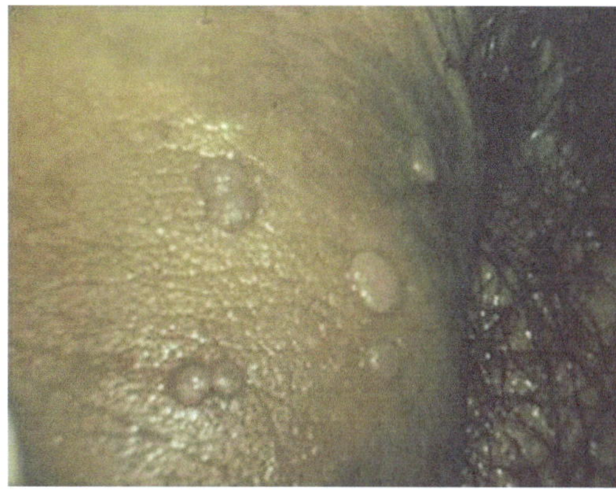

Fig. 12.5 Bowenoid papulosis. Smooth-topped brown aspect of a bowenoid papulosis lesion

Bowenoid Papulosis

This term has been proposed for a set of morphologic features similar to those of Bowen disease with a different clinical presentation. Bowenoid papulosis is characterized by small (2–10 mm), multicentric, smooth, velvety, maculopapular, reddish-brown or grayish-white lesions, sometimes verrucoid, on the shaft, foreskin, or scrotum of young males [12] (Fig. 12.5). The lesions typically undergo spontaneous resolution without sequelae. It is an HPV-related condition, with an 80 % detection rate of HPV-16 in the series reported by Ikenberg [13]. Bowenoid papulosis may occur together with condyloma, and the two have been confirmed to be related [14]. The microscopy is so similar to that of the precursor of penile SCC that some authors prefer to group it under the term of bowenoid dysplasia/PeIN. A lesser degree of cytologic atypia and a lower mitotic count than in high-grade PeIN are commonly observed. The atypical cells tend to have a more patchy disposition compared with CIS, and there may be a variably increased pigmentation of the basal layer [15] (Fig. 12.6).

Lichen Sclerosus Et Atrophicus

Lichen sclerosus (LS) is a chronic inflammatory skin condition of unknown cause, first described by Stühmer as balanitis xerotica obliterans

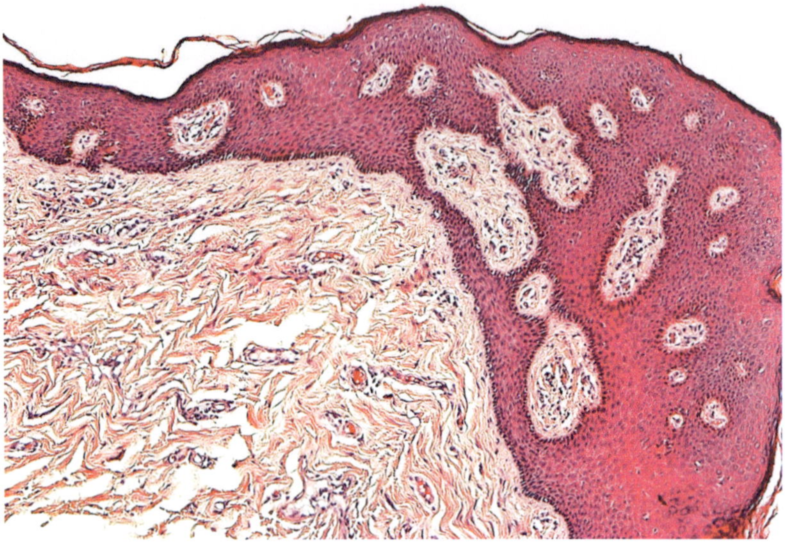

Fig. 12.6 Bowenoid papulosis. Scattered atypical keratinocytes with patchy disposition and variably increased pigmentation of the basal layer

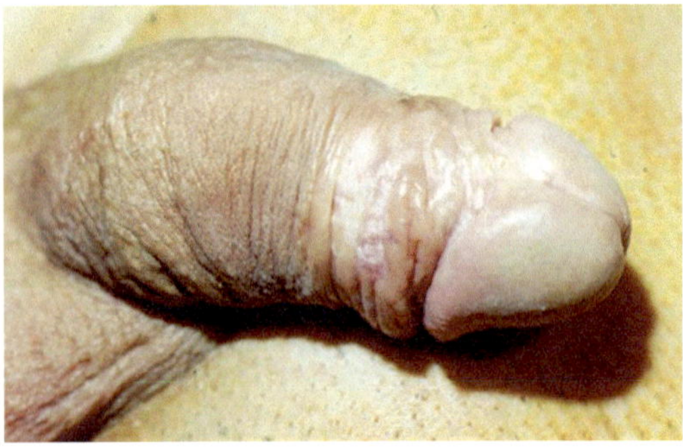

Fig. 12.7 Lichen sclerosus. Typical white sclerotic area at the tip of the foreskin (Courtesy Dr. G. Bandieramonte. Published with kind permission of ©Maurizio Colecchia 2015. All Rights Reserved)

affecting the glans and prepuce [16]. On clinical examination there are areas of pallor, atrophy, and sclerotic ivory-white plaques involving the glans and prepuce, often with a nonretractile prepuce (Fig. 12.7). Patients commonly present with pruritus, soreness, difficulty retracting the foreskin, burning with urination, poor urinary stream, and painful erections. LS is microscopically characterized by atrophic epithelium frequently intermixed with hyperplastic areas, vacuolar degeneration of the basal cell layer (blisters), and thickened lamina propria with edema and band-like keratinization (sclerosis) or hyalinization (Fig. 12.8). The presence of a lymphocytic inflammatory infiltrate and melanophages is variable [17]. Early lesions show a superficial lymphoid infiltrate underneath the epithelium without sclerosis, but late lesions are sclerotic without or with minimal inflammation. In a recent study, a French group observed the alterations adjacent to invasive SCC and reported LS associated with carcinoma of either usual (19 cases) or verrucous type (eight cases) [18], so that LS-linked penile SCC represented 51 % (27/53) of penile cancers belonging to non-HPV-related histotypes. Cases of LS associated with atypical foci in epithelium raising concern of epithelial dysplasia have been reported: squamous cell atypia in the epithelium immediately above the sclerotic stroma was observed by Velazquez and Cubilla in 52/68 cases of LS [17]. These authors observed the preferential association of LS with hyperplastic and low-grade squamous intraepithelial lesions as well as with special keratinizing subtypes of SCC, tumors usually not associated with HPV, suggesting a specific carcinogenic role for LS. In the literature this association has been variably reported in 5.8–50 % of cases [19–26], and this figure was much higher (69 %) when considering carcinomas affecting exclusively the foreskin [24]. The variability could be explained by the difficulty in recognizing LS histology [27].

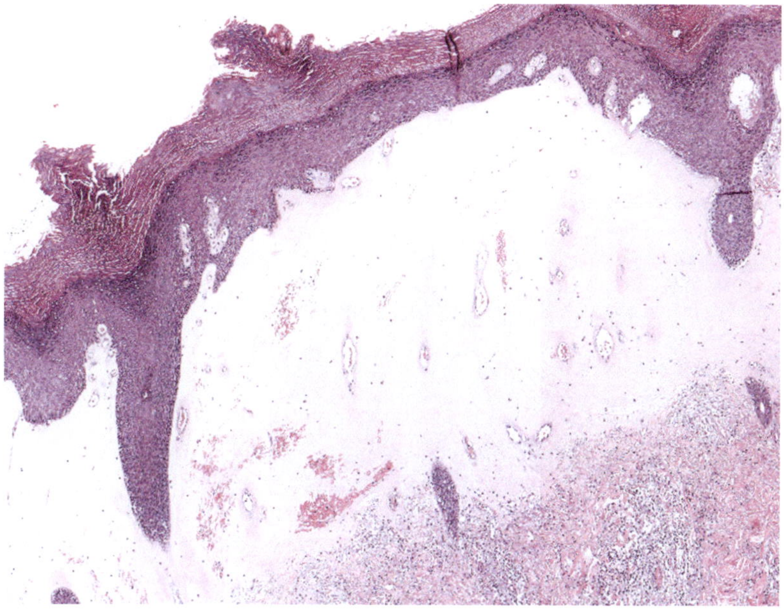

Fig. 12.8 Lichen sclerosus. Thickened lamina propria with extensive hyalinization and marked edema; the lesion is characterized by an atrophic epithelium presenting vacuolar alteration of the basal layer

Squamous Hyperplasia

Squamous hyperplasia (SH) is an epithelial abnormality characterized by acanthotic thickening of the epithelium of the glans, coronal sulcus, or foreskin without atypia. It is the most commonly found epithelial lesion associated with usual, papillary, and verrucous-type SCC [25]. It seems to be a reactive condition rather than a specific entity. In a study by Velazquez and Cubilla [4], SH was found in 83 % of usual-type SCC cases, followed in frequency by low-grade squamous intraepithelial lesions (57 % of cases) and high-grade squamous intraepithelial lesions (44 %). This feature and the commonly found continuity with invasive tumor suggest that SH may be a precursor of penile carcinoma (Fig. 12.9). Macroscopically, the lesion may be a linear, pearly white thickening on the cut surface, and clinically it may be difficult to distinguish from PeIN [26]. The acanthotic thickening characterizing SH may be more than 15 layers thick and have irregular borders. Orthokeratosis, minimal to absent parakeratosis, and normal epithelial maturation are common microscopic features. There is absence of cytologic atypia, koilocytosis, and intraepithelial keratin pearls.

The differential diagnosis of SH from differentiated PeIN or extremely low-grade invasive neoplasms (e.g., pseudohyperplastic and verrucous carcinomas) may be particularly difficult, with the lack of basal atypia and inflammatory changes supporting the diagnosis of SH.

Histologic Subtypes of SH

Flat SH is the most common type: hyperkeratosis with orthokeratosis and a linear interface between the basal layer and the stroma are frequently present (Fig. 12.10). The mixed form is the second most common type, with mixed areas of flat and papillary SH. Pseudoepitheliomatous SH is an uncommon pattern. There is downward elongated proliferation of rete ridges that appear detached from the epithelium. Regular epithelial nests with peripheral palisading and stromal reaction are not prominent. The most distinctive feature of pseudoepitheliomatous SH with respect to pseudoepitheliomatous SCC is the presence of nests and columns reaching a superficial level of depth with a limiting front of epithelial stromal interface paralleling the epithelial surface. Some cases of flat SH are associated with papillary SH.

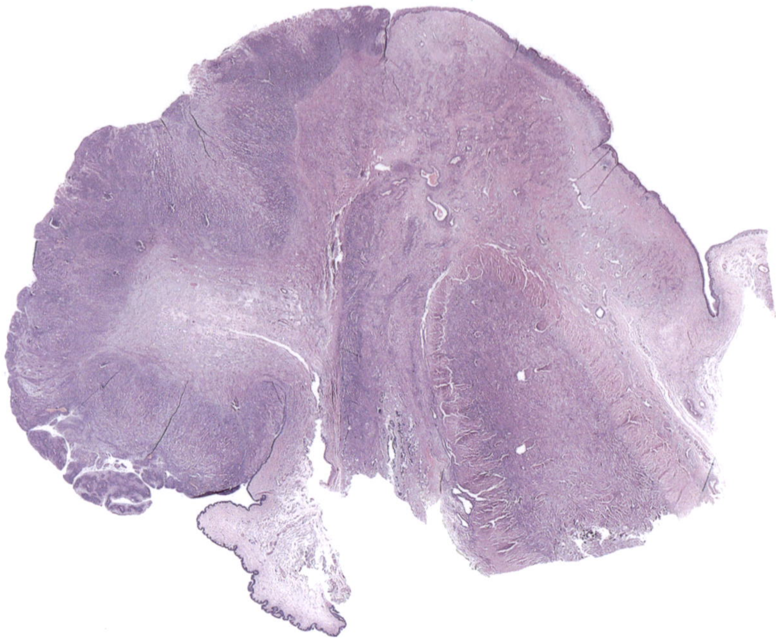

Fig. 12.9 Squamous hyperplasia and cancer. At this low-power magnification, squamous cell carcinoma deeply invades the glans associated with squamous hyperplasia of the adjacent mucosa (Published with kind permission of ©Maurizio Colecchia 2015. All Rights Reserved)

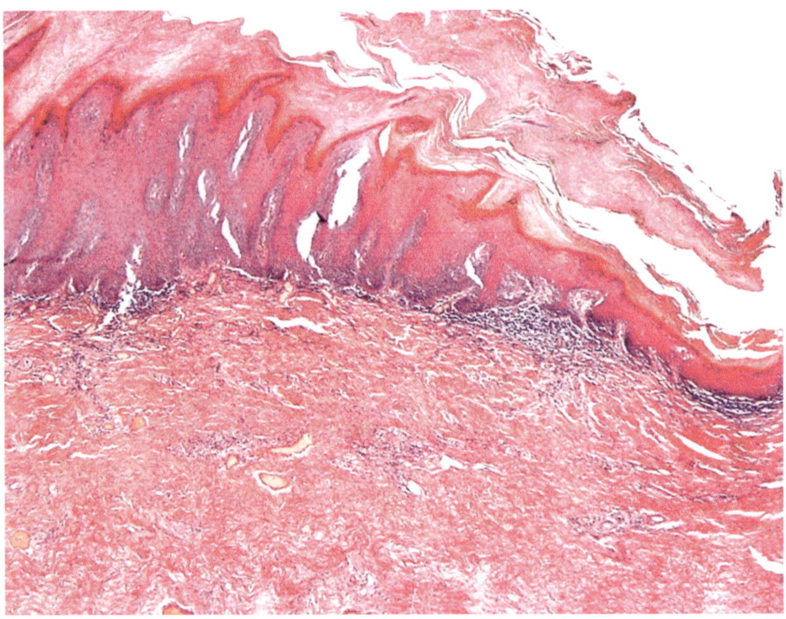

Fig. 12.10 Squamous hyperplasia. There is acanthosis with hyperorthokeratosis without atypia of the epithelium

Penile Intraepithelial Lesions

Penile intraepithelial neoplasia (PeIN) is an alteration of the penile squamous epithelium characterized by dysplastic changes with an intact basement membrane. PeIN may present as single or multiple clinically localized lesions and may be detected by peniscopy as a neoplastic squamous intraepithelial proliferation with variable keratinization and epithelial atypia [5]. Various terms are in use for PeIN, the most common of which are CIS, low- and high-grade intraepithelial dysplasia, low- and high-grade intraepithelial neoplasia, Bowen disease, and erythroplasia of Queyrat.

Bowen disease is characterized by well-circumscribed scaly lesions of the skin of the shaft of the penis and erythroplasia of Queyrat by irregular velvety red lesions of the glans. Both are HPV-related lesions with microscopic features of PeIN.

PeIN can be classified in HPV-related and non-HPV-related (differentiated PeIN) intraepithelial neoplasia as reported in the new WHO 2016 classification [27] (Table 12.1).

The usual and low-grade subtypes of SCC are associated with differentiated PeIN. For classification purposes and morphologic standardization of PeIN, use of the p16/p53/Ki67 immunohistochemical panel has been suggested by Chaux et al. [25].

Table 12.1 Proposal of pathological classification of penile intraepithelial neoplasia

1.	Non-HPV-related PeIN
	Differentiated (simplex) PeIN
2.	HPV-related PeIN
	Basaloid PeIN
	Warty PeIN
	Warty–basaloid PeIN
3.	Other rare patterns (pleomorphic, spindle, clear cell pagetoid)

Modified from Velazquez [27]

Differentiated PeIN

In its typical form, differentiated PeIN has acanthotic epithelium with elongated rete ridges, abnormal keratinocyte maturation, and parakeratosis (Fig. 12.11). Koilocytes are typically absent. Occasionally in the basal layers, atypical basal cells and sometimes keratin pearls are present. There are prominent intercellular bridges with spongiosis and sometimes acantholysis. Epithelial thickening with minimal atypia is sometimes present closer to the invasive carcinoma, and papillary, pseudohyperplastic, and verrucous features may be noted. Parakeratosis is common. There is an association of differentiated PeIN with atypical LS, and the differentiated PeIN commonly affects the foreskin and less commonly the glans or the coronal sulcus with a background of long-standing lichen sclerosus [25–30]. In the WHO 2016 classification, the authors about the grading claim that it is optional to grade differentiated PeIN in low- and high-grade categories [27].

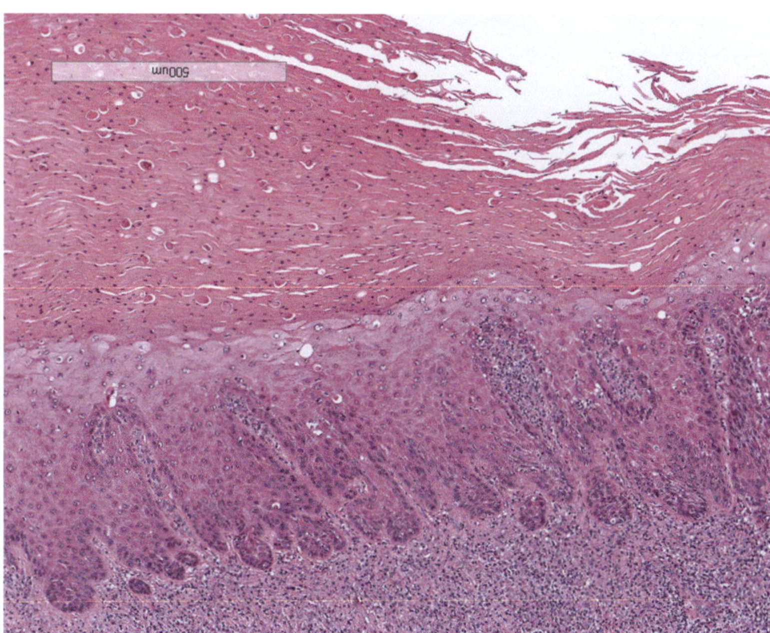

Fig. 12.11 Differentiated penile intraepithelial neoplasia. The epithelium shows thick parakeratosis, elongation of rete ridges, enlarged keratinocytes, and keratin pearl formation. Note the atypical hyperchromatic nuclei of the basal cell layers (Published with kind permission of ©Maurizio Colecchia 2015. All Rights Reserved)

HPV-Related PeIN: Basaloid and Warty PeIN

Basaloid PeIN is a high-grade PeIN lesion (PeIN III) where the epithelium is replaced by a monotonous population of small or intermediate-sized immature cells with numerous mitoses and isolated koilocytes (Fig. 12.12). Apoptotic bodies are prominent and there is a thin parakeratotic layer. Spindle, polyhedral, or pleomorphic cells can be observed. HPV 16 is frequently detected in basaloid PeIN. An intraepithelial lesion close to the meatus is sometimes suggestive of urothelial origin. The papillary shape and the presence of a fibrovascular core is an overlapping feature of urothelial carcinoma and papillary basaloid PeIN (Fig. 12.13a). Presence of p16 immunoreactiv-

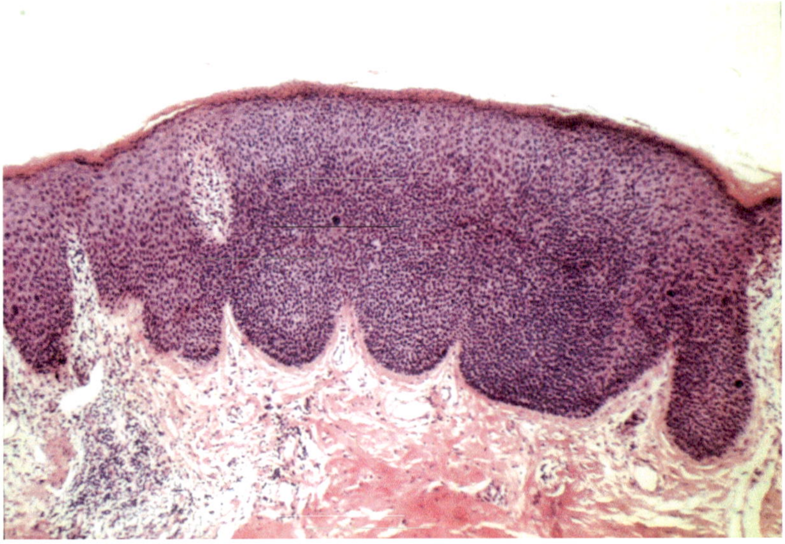

Fig. 12.12 Basaloid penile intraepithelial neoplasia. The entire thickness of the epithelium shows small round blue cells with a high nuclear/cytoplasmic ratio suggestive of a high-grade lesion (Published with kind permission of ©Maurizio Colecchia 2015. All Rights Reserved)

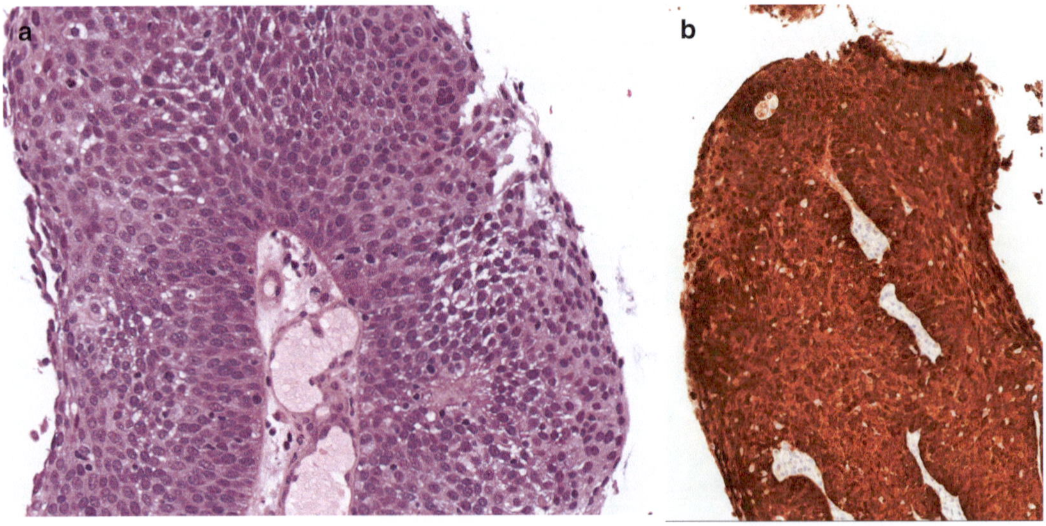

Fig. 12.13 Penile intraepithelial neoplasia, papillary basaloid type. (**a**) The transitional-like resemblance of the papillary growth of this basaloid intraepithelial neoplasia calls for a differential diagnosis between urothelial papillary carcinoma and penile neoplasia (Published with kind permission of ©Maurizio Colecchia 2015. All Rights Reserved). (**b**) Marked positivity for p16 associated with negative immunostain for p63 prompts the diagnosis of basaloid (papillary) penile intraepithelial neoplasia

ity and absence of p63 nuclear expression are mandatory to confirm basaloid SCC. In Fig. 12.13b, the papillary growth displays strong diffuse positivity for p16 in malignant cells with transitional-like features.

In warty PeIN, the epithelium has an undulating or flat surface with atypical parakeratosis, cellular pleomorphism, and koilocytic changes (Fig. 12.14). Unlike in basaloid PeIN, there is squamous maturation in warty PeIN. HPV is generally positive with different genotypes detected. It may be isolated or associated with an invasive component [31–34]. Lesions frequently have combined features of the basaloid and warty types (warty–basaloid penile intraepithelial neoplasia): the superficial epithelium shows features of warty PeIN, while the deeper layers are replaced by small basaloid cells. Other less frequently observed patterns of PeIN are pleomorphic, spindle, clear cell, and pagetoid [27] (Table 12.1).

Correlation of different histologic types of invasive carcinomas with subtypes of PeIN has revealed a morphologic correspondence between the invasive tumor and the associated intraepithelial lesion.

In a study of 288 carcinomas, the entire surface of the penile specimen was microscopically examined to describe the morphologic features of all epithelial alterations and to investigate their relation with early carcinoma and subtypes of invasive carcinoma [26]. SH, the most common lesion, was found in 83 % of cases. In many cases, the authors reported a morphologic transition from SH to low-grade PeIN, while the association of SH and PeIN II–III was infrequent and discontinuous. PeIN I was associated with invasive SCC in 57 % of cases and PeIN II–III in 44 %. In 62 % of cases, there was more than one associated lesion per specimen. The high frequency of SH and PeIN I and the preferential association with usual, verrucous, and papillary carcinomas suggest that despite its benign appearance, SH may be a precursor of the aforementioned carcinomas. The association of basaloid, warty, or mixed forms of PeIN II–III with their invasive counterparts indicates these are their likely precursors [4, 25–27, 29].

Giant Condyloma

Giant condyloma, also known as Buschke-Löwenstein tumor, is an uncommon HPV-related lesion with a cobblestone, verruciform appearance, mostly affecting the foreskin and coronal sulcus (Fig. 12.15). The endophytic growth pattern causes deep invaginations in the underlying tissues and the formation of cutaneous fistulae.

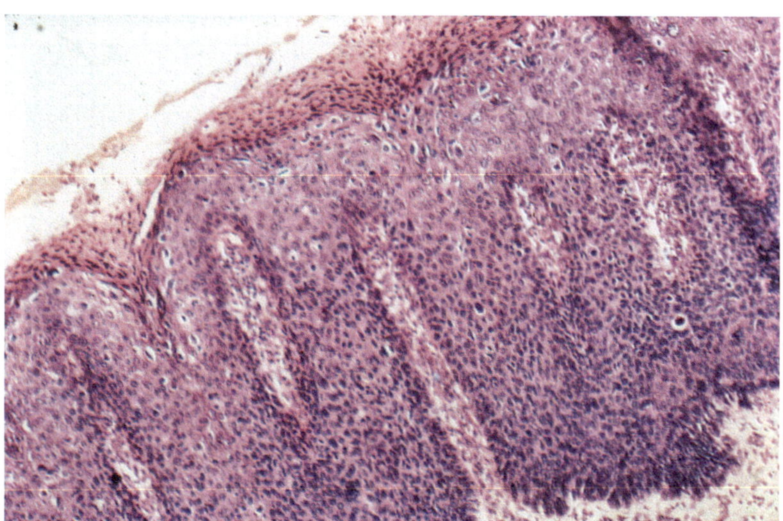

Fig. 12.14 Warty penile intraepithelial neoplasia. Striking pleomorphic cellular atypia with full-thickness koilocytosis. The epithelium shows a spiking surface and atypical parakeratosis

Giant condyloma is microscopically similar to condyloma acuminatum, and this explains the inappropriate and misleading use of this term in the literature [35]. There is profuse papillomatous growth, and different degrees of atypia in the same lesion – from typical condyloma to CIS or invasive carcinoma – are not uncommon. The main differential diagnosis is with warty carcinoma [36].

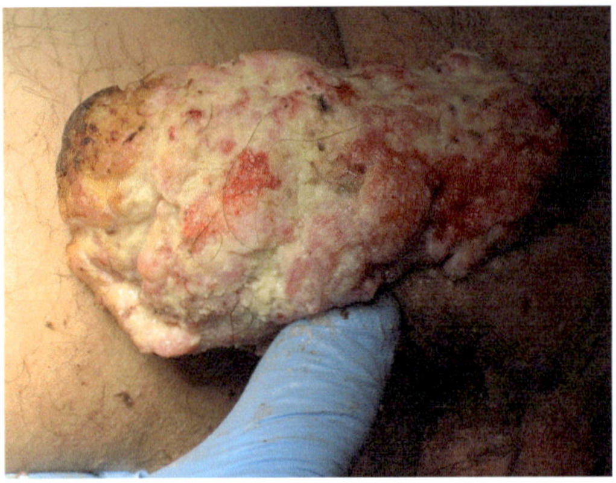

Fig. 12.15 Giant condylomata. Gross appearance of giant condylomata (>5 cm in diameter): monocentric verruciform tumors with a "cobblestone" surface

Paget's Disease

Primary Paget's disease is an adenocarcinoma originating from intraepithelial ducts involving the skin of the shaft, often associated with scrotal, inguinal, and perianal lesions. Paget's disease is uncommonly limited to the penis and usually occurs as a multidistrict disease [37]. It should be distinguished from SCC in situ with pagetoid features (Fig. 12.16) and pagetoid spread of urothelial carcinoma [38, 39]. Immunohistochemically, Paget's disease expresses CEA, EMA, low-molecular-weight cytokeratin, and GFCDP-15 [40].

The squamous differentiation in pagetoid squamous CIS is recognized by immunohistochemical expression of p63, as reported in 30 cases of pagetoid squamous CIS by Chang et al. [41]. The same authors found no p63 positivity in 40 cases of primary extramammary Paget's disease, providing strong evidence on the diagnostic use of p63 for this differential diagnosis. Paget's disease secondary to transitional cell carcinoma occurs in elderly patients with a known history of urothelial carcinoma [42], when positivity for CK7 and CK20 and negativity for CEA provide the evidence to differentiate this lesion from Paget's disease.

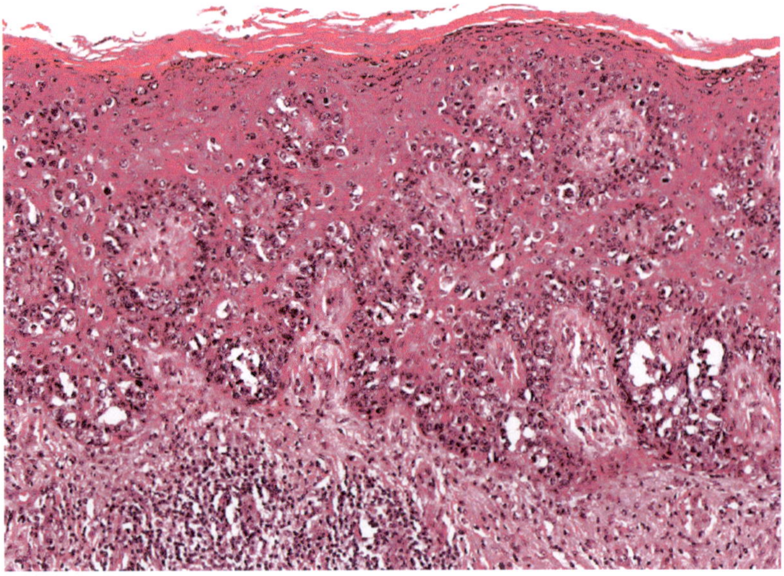

Fig. 12.16 Pagetoid spread of squamous cell carcinoma. Intraepithelial proliferation of large atypical cells with pale cytoplasm (Published with kind permission of ©Maurizio Colecchia 2015. All Rights Reserved)

Treatment

The ideal treatment of preinvasive lesions should be able to eradicate the disease, prevent recurrences and progression, and preserve anatomy and function. Both medical and surgical treatments have been used to this end. Many topical agents applied in the last decades have yielded heterogeneous results. In recent years imiquimod, a biological response modifier commonly used to treat genital warts, has been employed in different preinvasive anogenital lesions. A recent review [43] addressed this issue: 27 patients with different penile intraepithelial lesions were identified of whom 21 (78 %) achieved a complete response and 5 (19 %) achieved partial responses. Most patients were described in case reports, and lesions were widely heterogeneous, including Bowen disease and erythroplasia of Queyrat and bowenoid papulosis. Moreover, follow-up was immature in many of the cases and the therapy schedules extremely diverse. Considerable caution is therefore warranted in considering this drug as a standard choice for preinvasive penile lesions.

Physical removal of diseased tissue includes surgery, photodynamic therapy, and laser excision [2, 3]. Surgery may either be micrographic surgery or dissection of the glans followed by resurfacing. Mohs micrographic surgery (MMS) consists of immediate frozen sectioning of the specimen and identification and mapping of positive margins followed by repeated excision until tumor clearance. This technique permits total removal of disease, while sparing the unaffected portions of the penis. Sharp dissection of the glans with a cold knife followed by resurfacing with a skin graft from the thigh is a more recent alternative, associated with very good cosmetic results. Judging by recent publications on small cohorts, both techniques seem effective and safe. MMS necessitated repeated treatments, but no progression was documented. Importantly, both techniques provide the pathologist with a specimen for reading.

Photodynamic therapies use photosensitizers that are applied to the surface of the penis. The photosensitizers are metabolized differently by normal and affected cells, where the substance remains longer. By application of a specific light, the technique can facilitate lesion identification, thereby permitting accurate removal of disease or direct destruction of affected tissue. A recent publication on photodynamic diagnosis included 11 patients in whom the identified areas were treated with Nd:YAG laser; all patients were rendered disease-free and no recurrence was recorded [44]. Application of a photosensitizer followed by illumination in another study on ten patients showed that multiple treatments were necessary (two to eight), and three patients were not rendered definitively disease-free [45]. An important drawback of these techniques is that there is no definitive specimen for pathologic reading. Two recent reports addressed the use of Nd:YAG laser in 2 small series of 17 [46] and 6 [47] patients with PeIN. The immediate efficacy was very good, although recurrences occurred in 2 of 17 and 4 of 6 patients, respectively. Moreover, one patient in each series progressed to invasive cancer and one in each series developed nodal metastases. With Nd:YAG laser tissue destruction, definitive specimens are not available. Bandieramonte et al. [5] published in 2008 the largest experience with laser therapy in intraepithelial neoplasia. As many as 106 patients were treated with CO_2 laser: 103 remained free of disease at a median follow-up of 66 months (IQR 35–132 months). Recurrences were recorded in 11.3 % of cases, multiple recurrences in 4.7 %. Two patients progressed and needed partial amputation, while none had nodal metastasis. This technique allowed the authors to obtain a definitive pathology result with good concordance between the first and final diagnoses (77 %), while in the remaining cases complete excision showed unexpected invasion of the lamina propria [5]. The limitation in the interpretation of biopsies in patients with penile SCC has been stressed in several reports [48–50], emphasizing the importance of evaluating the involvement of excision margins to avoid recurrences [48, 50].

References

1. Cubilla AL, Meijer CJ, Young RH. Morphological features of epithelial abnormalities and precancerous lesions of the penis. Scand J Urol Nephrol Suppl. 2000;205:215–9.
2. Pizzocaro G, Algaba F, Horenblas S, Solsona E, Tana S, Van Der Poel H, Watkin NA, European Association

of Urology (EAU) Guidelines Group on Penile Cancer. EAU penile cancer guidelines 2009. Eur Urol. 2010;57:1002–12.
3. Hakenberg OW, Compérat EM, Minhas S, Necchi A, Protzel C, Watkin N. EAU guidelines on penile cancer: 2014 update. Eur Urol. 2014;67:142–50.
4. Velazquez EF, Cubilla AL. Penile squamous cell carcinoma: anatomic, pathologic and viral studies in Paraguay (1993–2007). Anal Quant Cytol Histol. 2007;29:185–98.
5. Bandieramonte G, Colecchia M, Mariani L, Lo Vullo S, Pizzocaro G, Piva L, Nicolai N, Salvioni R, Lezzi V, Stefanon B, De Palo G. Peniscopically controller CO2 laser excision for conservative treatment of in situ and T1 penile carcinoma: report on 224 patients. Eur Urol. 2008;54:875–82.
6. Löwhagen GB, Bolmstedt A, Ryd W, Voog E. The prevalence of "high-risk" HPV types in penile condyloma-like lesions: correlation between HPV type and morphology. Genitourin Med. 1993;69:87–90.
7. Nordenvall C, Chang ET, Adami HO, Ye W. Cancer risk among patients with condylomata acuminata. Int J Cancer. 2006;119:888–93.
8. Mastrolorenzo A, Tiradritti L, Locunto U, Carini M, Massi D, Zuccati G. Incidental finding: a penile cutaneous horn. Acta Derm Venereol. 2005;85:283–4.
9. Hernandez-Graulau JM, Fiore A, Cea P, Tucci P, Addonizio JC. Multiple penile horns: case report and review. J Urol. 1988;139:1055–6.
10. Zhu JW, Luo D, Li CR, Lu Y, Ji X, Zhu J, Ming YL, Shen CH. A case of penile verrucous carcinoma associated with cutaneous horn. Clin Exp Dermatol. 2007;32:213–4.
11. Solivan GA, Smith KJ, James WD. Cutaneous horn of the penis: its association with squamous cell carcinoma and HPV-16 infection. J Am Acad Dermatol. 1990;23:969–72.
12. Wade TR, Kopf AW, Ackerman AB. Bowenoid papulosis of the penis. Cancer. 1978;42:1890–903.
13. Ikenberg H, Gissmann L, Gross G, Grussendorf-Conen EI, zur Hausen H. Human papillomavirus type-16-related DNA in genital Bowen's disease and in Bowenoid papulosis. Int J Cancer. 1983;32:563–5.
14. Steffen C. Concurrence of condylomata acuminata and bowenoid papulosis: confirmation of the hypothesis that they are related conditions. Am J Dermatopathol. 1982;4:5–8.
15. Patterson JW, Kao GF, Graham JH, Helwig EB. Bowenoid papulosis. A clinicopathologic study with ultrastructural observations. Cancer. 1986;57:823–36.
16. Stühmer A. Balanitis xerotica obliterans (post-operationem) und ihre Beziehungen zur "Kraurosis glandis et praeputii penis". Arch Dermatol Syph. 1928;156:613–23.
17. Velazquez EF, Cubilla AL. Lichen sclerosus in 68 patients with squamous cell carcinoma of the penis: frequent atypias and correlation with special carcinoma variants suggests a precancerous role. Am J Surg Pathol. 2003;27:1448–53.
18. Renaud-Vilmer C, Cavelier-Balloy B, Verola O, Morel P, Servant JM, Desgrandchamps F, Dubertret L. Analysis of alterations adjacent to invasive squamous cell carcinoma of the penis and their relationship with associated carcinoma. J Am Acad Dermatol. 2010;62:284–90.
19. von Krogh G, Horenblas S. Diagnosis and clinical presentation of premalignant lesions of the penis. Scand J Urol Nephrol Suppl. 2000;205:201–14.
20. Pietrzak P, Hadway P, Corbishley CM, Watkin NA. Is the association between balanitis xerotica obliterans and penile carcinoma underestimated? BJU Int. 2006;98:74–6.
21. Nasca MR, Innocenzi D, Micali G. Penile cancer among patients with genital lichen sclerosus. J Am Acad Dermatol. 1999;41:911–4.
22. Lesourd A. Anatomo-pathology of malignant penile tumors. Prog Urol. 2005;15:801–4.
23. Powell JJ, Wojnarowska F. Lichen sclerosus. Lancet. 1999;353:1777–83.
24. Oertell J, Duarte S, Ayala J, Chaux A, Velazquez EF, Cubilla AL. Squamous cell carcinoma (SCC) exclusive of the foreskin: distinctive association with low grade variants, multicentricity and lichen sclerosus. Mod Pathol. 2002;15:175A.
25. Chaux A, Pfannl R, Rodríguez IM, Barreto JE, Velazquez EF, Lezcano C, Piris A, Netto GJ, Cubilla AL. Distinctive immunohistochemical profile of penile intraepithelial lesions: a study of 74 cases. Am J Surg Pathol. 2011;35:553–62.
26. Cubilla AL, Velazquez EF, Young RH. Epithelial lesions associated with invasive penile squamous cell carcinoma: a pathologic study of 288 cases. Int J Surg Pathol. 2004;12:351–64.
27. Velazquez EF, Amin MB, Cubilla AL, Jenkins D, MOCH H, Piris A, Quint WGV. Penile intraepithelial neoplasia. In: Moch H, Humprey PA, Ulbright TM, Reuter VE, editors. WHO Classification of Tumours of the Urinary System and Male Genital Organs. Fourth edition. IARC Lyon; 2016. p. 277–9.
28. Oertel J, Iglesias M, Amat L, Ayala E, Velazquez EF, Barreto JE, Ayala G, Cubilla AL. Squamous hyperplasia (SH), lichen sclerosus (LS), differentiated pein (PeIN) and low grade variants of squamous cell carcinoma (SCC): distinctive preputial lesions in a survey of 99 circumcision specimens from a region of high incidence of penile cancer. Mod Pathol. 2009;22:187A.
29. Chaux A, Pfannl R, Lloveras B, Alejo M, Clavero O, Lezcano C, Muñoz N, de Sanjosé S, Bosch X, Hernández-Pérez M, Velazquez EF, Cubilla AL. Distinctive association of p16INK4a overexpression with penile intraepithelial neoplasia depicting warty and/or basaloid features: a study of 141 cases evaluating a new nomenclature. Am J Surg Pathol. 2010;34:385–92.
30. Chaux A, Velazquez EF, Amin A, Soskin A, Pfannl R, Rodríguez IM, Barreto JE, Lezcano C, Ayala G, Netto GJ, Cubilla AL. Distribution and characterization of subtypes of penile intraepithelial neoplasia and their association with invasive carcinomas: a pathological

study of 139 lesions in 121 patients. Hum Pathol. 2012;43:1020–7.

31. Gregoire L, Cubilla AL, Reuter VE, Haas GP, Lancaster WD. Preferential association of human papillomavirus with high-grade histologic variants of penile-invasive squamous cell carcinoma. J Natl Cancer Inst. 1995;87:1705–9.
32. Soskin A, Vieillefond A, Carlotti A, Plantier F, Chaux A, Ayala G, Velazquez EF, Cubilla AL. Warty/basaloid penile intraepithelial neoplasia is more prevalent than differentiated penile intraepithelial neoplasia in nonendemic regions for penile cancer when compared with endemic areas: a comparative study between pathologic series from Paris and Paraguay. Hum Pathol. 2012;43:190–6.
33. Young RH, Srigley JR, Amin MB, Ulbright TM, Cubilla AL. Tumors of the prostate gland, seminal vesicles, male urethra and penis, vol. 3. 28th ed. Washington, DC: AFIP Fascicle; 2000.
34. Cubilla AL, Reuter V, Velazquez E, Piris A, Saito S, Young RH. Histologic classification of penile carcinoma and its relation to outcome in 61 patients with primary resection. Int J Surg Pathol. 2001;9:111–20.
35. Riggio T. Buschke and Lowenstein condyloma acuminatum. Arch Ital Dermatol Sifilogr Venereol. 1954;26:472–82.
36. Löning T, Riviere A, Henke RP, von Preyss S, Dörner A. Penile/anal condylomas and squamous cell cancer. A HPV DNA hybridization study. Virchows Arch A Pathol Anat Histopathol. 1988;413:491–8.
37. Zhang N, Gong K, Zhang X, Yang Y, Na Y. Extramammary Paget's disease of scrotum–report of 25 cases and literature review. Urol Oncol. 2010;28:28–33.
38. Williamson JD, Colome MI, Sahin A, Ayala AG, Medeiros LJ. Pagetoid bowen disease: a report of 2 cases that express cytokeratin 7. Arch Pathol Lab Med. 2000;124:427–30.
39. Amin A, Griffith RC, Chaux A. Penile intraepithelial neoplasia with pagetoid features: report of an unusual variant mimicking Paget disease. Hum Pathol. 2014;45:889–92.
40. Epstein JH, Cubilla AL, Humphrey PA. Tumors of the prostate gland, seminal vescicles, penis and scrotum. Atlas of tumor pathology. Washington, DC: AFIP; 2011. pp. 405–612.
41. Chang J, Prieto VG, Sangueza M, Plaza JA. Diagnostic utility of p63 expression in the differential diagnosis of pagetoid squamous cell carcinoma in situ and extramammary Paget disease: a histopathologic study of 70 cases. Am J Dermatopathol. 2014;36:49–53.
42. Salamanca J, Benito A, García-Peñalver C, Azorín D, Ballestín C, Rodríguez-Peralto JL. Paget's disease of the glans penis secondary to transitional cell carcinoma of the bladder: a report of two cases and review of the literature. J Cutan Pathol. 2004;31:341–5.
43. Mahto M, Nathan M, O'Mahony C. More than a decade on: review of the use of imiquimod in lower anogenital intraepithelial neoplasia. Int J STD AIDS. 2010;21:8–16.
44. Hadway P, Corbishley CM, Watkin NA. Total glans resurfacing for premalignant lesions of the penis: initial outcome data. BJU Int. 2006;98:532–6.
45. Shindel AW, Mann MW, Lev RY, Sengelmann R, Petersen J, Hruza GJ, Brandes SB. Mohs micrographic surgery for penile cancer: management and long-term followup. J Urol. 2007;178:1980–5.
46. Frimberger D, Hungerhuber E, Zaak D, Waidelich R, Hofstetter A, Schneede P. Penile carcinoma. Is Nd:YAG laser therapy radical enough? J Urol. 2002;168:2418–21.
47. Meijer RP, Boon TA, van Venrooij GE, Wijburg CJ. Long-term follow-up after laser therapy for penile carcinoma. Urology. 2007;69:759–62.
48. Colecchia M, Nicolai N, Secchi P, Bandieramonte G, Paganoni AM, Sangalli LM, Pizzocaro G, Piva L, Salvioni R. pT1 penile squamous cell carcinoma: a clinicopathologic study of 56 cases treated by CO2 laser therapy. Anal Quant Cytol Histol. 2009;31:153–60.
49. Velazquez EF, Barreto JE, Rodriguez I, Piris A, Cubilla AL. Limitations in the interpretation of biopsies in patients with penile squamous cell carcinoma. Int J Surg Pathol. 2004;12:139–46.
50. Minhas S, Kayes O, Hegarty P, Kumar P, Freeman A, Ralph D. What surgical resection margins are required to achieve oncological control in men with primary penile cancer? BJU Int. 2005;96:1040–3.

13 Tumors of the Penis and Scrotum

Maurizio Colecchia, Alessia Bertolotti, Biagio Paolini, and Roberto Salvioni

Squamous Cell Carcinoma: General Features and Pathogenesis

Squamous cell carcinoma (SCC) is the most frequent penile tumor, occurring as usual-type SCC in almost 50 % of cases. It presents most frequently in the sixth to seventh decades of life [1], while it is uncommon in young adults. The different rates among countries and regional differences in prevalence even in the same country are not fully understood; the comparison of subtypes of penile cancer reported from high- and low-incidence regions showed no geographical differences between histologic subtypes and in the frequency of HPV-related tumors [2]. For instance, a similar distribution of penile cancer subtypes was observed in Paraguay and the USA, supporting the notion that previously reported geographical variations may have been the result of staging variation at clinical presentation, probably because lesions tend to be diagnosed early (i.e., in precancerous or in situ stages) in developed countries [2, 3]. The presence of human papillomavirus (HPV) was found to be a risk factor for penile SCC [4]: depending on the population examined, the technique used, and tumor morphology, the HPV detection rate has been estimated to range from 30 to 83 % of cases, while the prevalence is thought to be around 50 % [5]. In a recent immunohistochemical and HPV in situ hybridization (HPV ISH) study in a North American population, a low percentage (27 %) of high-risk HPV-positive cases of penile cancer was found [6]. In the majority of these cases, high-risk HPV subtypes (HPV-16 and HPV-18) were integrated into the genome with a characteristic nuclear ISH reactivity; the same integrated subtype was observed in both primary and metastatic tumors. HPV is most frequently associated with basaloid or warty carcinoma variants, where it has been reported in 75–100 % of cases, while the majority of usual/keratinizing and verrucous carcinomas are not HPV related [1, 2, 6–9].

Similar to what has been described for vulvar lesions, a bimodal pathogenesis for HPV-related and non-HPV-related cancers has been proposed [9–11]. Lichen sclerosus may represent a preneoplastic condition (see Chap. 12) in particular for some non-HPV-related cancers, i.e., verrucous, usual-type, papillary, and pseudohyperplastic

M. Colecchia (✉)
Uropathology Unit, Department of Pathology, Fondazione IRCCS Istituto Nazionale dei Tumori di Milano, Milan, Italy
e-mail: maurizio.colecchia@istitutotumori.mi.it

A. Bertolotti • B. Paolini
Department of Pathology, Fondazione IRCCS Istituto Nazionale dei Tumori di Milano, Milan, Italy

R. Salvioni
Department of Urology, Fondazione IRCCS Istituto Nazionale dei Tumori di Milano, Milan, Italy
e-mail: roberto.salvioni@istitutotumori.mi.it

M. Colecchia (ed.), *Pathology of Testicular and Penile Neoplasms*,
DOI 10.1007/978-3-319-27617-5_13

carcinomas [12]. When we consider carcinomas affecting exclusively the foreskin, the association of lichen sclerosus with penile invasive carcinoma is much higher (69 %) [13]. Several other risk factors have been associated with the development of this cancer, including phimosis, smoking or chewing tobacco, chronic inflammation, tears, abrasions, balanitis, injuries to the penis, and poor hygiene [8, 9, 11]. A rare occurrence is the anaplastic transformation of verrucous carcinoma induced by radiotherapy [14].

Classification

A new morphological and molecular classification of the histologic types of penile SCC based on the presence of HPV has been presented in the latest edition of the WHO classification of urological tumors [15] (Table 13.1). For the aim of this textbook, we will focus on the spectrum of penile squamous cell carcinoma following the classification based on patterns of growth [9] according to an update of the 2004 World Health Organization classification [16].

Patterns of Growth

Superficial Spreading Growth Pattern

This pattern occurs when a slow-growing neoplasm associated with SCC of the usual type widely involves the superficial layers of the glans, sulcus, and/or foreskin. In 60 % of cases, more than one epithelial compartment is involved, while only 25 % of lesions are confined to the glans [9]. In the cut section shown in Fig. 13.1, the specimen consists of band-like white or gray-white tissue with thickening of the surface. There is an extensive in situ component (penile intraepithelial neoplasia, PeIN) intermixed with

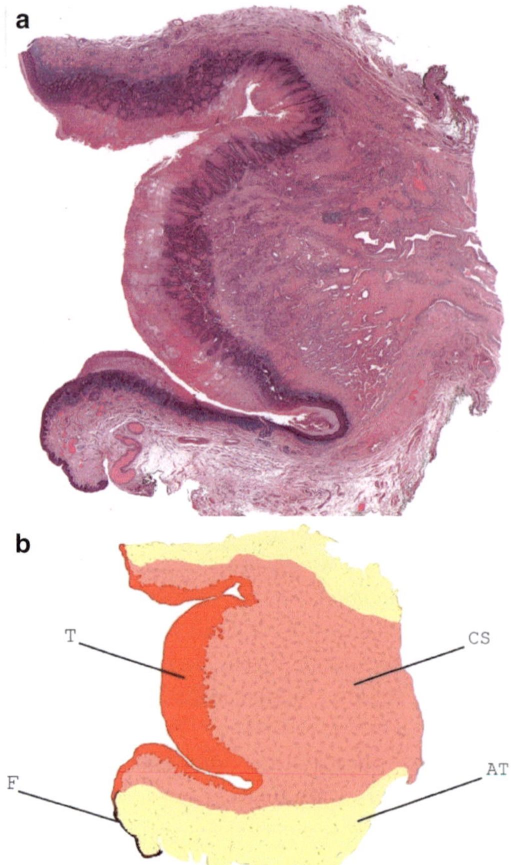

Fig. 13.1 Superficial spreading pattern of growth at low magnification. (**a**) Usual-type SCC involving the glans, sulcus, and foreskin with an in situ component and infiltration of the lamina propria. Careful examination of the surgical margins of the foreskin is mandatory to avoid recurrences. (**b**) Superficially spreading tumor (*T*) involves the glans, foreskin (*F*), and coronal sulcus, affecting the lamina propria and initially the corpus spongiosum (*CS*). *AT* adipose tissue

Table 13.1 Classification of penile squamous cell carcinomas according the HPV status

Non-HPV related	HPV related	Others
1. Usual	1. Basaloid	1. Mixed
2. Verrucous	2. Warty	2. Unclassified
3. Papillary NOS	3. Warty-basaloid	
4. Cuniculatum	4. Papillary basaloid	
5. Pseudoglandular	5. Clear cell	
6. Pseudohyperplastic	6. Lymphoepithelioma-like	
7. Adenosquamous		
8. Sarcomatoid		

minimally invasive carcinoma throughout the epithelium, with infiltration limited to the lamina propria. The superficial growth spreading to the foreskin warrants accurate examination of the surgical margins near the coronal sulcus, which should be examined in its entirety with circumferential sampling.

Vertical Growth Pattern

The cut surface of neoplasms with this pattern of growth shows deeply invasive carcinoma invading the corpus spongiosum with frequent penetration of the tunica albuginea and corpora cavernosa (Fig. 13.2a, b).

Almost 20 % of penile carcinomas are of this type, presenting as a large, fungating, and often ulcerated mass [9]. The more common histologic types associated with this pattern are basaloid, sarcomatoid, and high-grade usual SCC, and they often occur with regional lymph node metastases, carrying a poor prognosis.

Verruciform Growth Pattern

The glans is the most commonly involved site, with slow-growing proliferations that have a large, granular, exophytic surface (Fig. 13.3). Many tumors are low grade, infiltrating only the lamina propria. The most frequently associated histologic types are verrucous, warty (condylomatous), and papillary. Giant condylomata may show a similar pattern of growth (see Chap. 12).

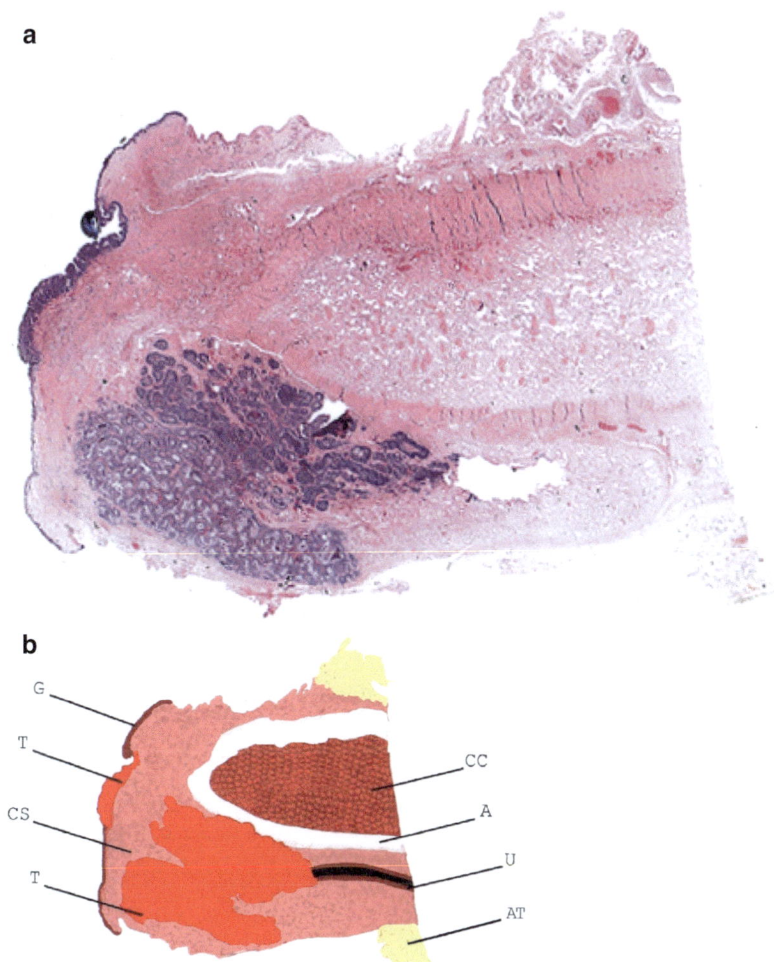

Fig. 13.2 Vertical pattern of growth. (**a**) Cut section showing a deeply invasive nodular ulcerated mass infiltrating the corpus spongiosum and tunica albuginea. (**b**) Vertical growth: tumor *(in red)* infiltrates corpus spongiosum and albuginea. In this section the corpus cavernosum is not infiltrated. *T* tumor, *G* epithelium of the glans, *CS* corpus spongiosum, *CC* corpus cavernosum, *A* tunica albuginea, *AT* adipose tissue, *U* urethra (Published with kind permission of ©Maurizio Colecchia 2015. All Rights Reserved)

Mixed and Multicentric Growth Patterns

Some penile tumors show two or three patterns of growth and are often at an advanced stage (10–30 % of all penile cancers). The most frequently reported histologic types are hybrid/verrucous and usual SCC. Less frequent is the occurrence of two or more independent foci of carcinoma separated by benign foci in a multicentric pattern. This growth pattern has been mostly reported in pseudohyperplastic carcinomas.

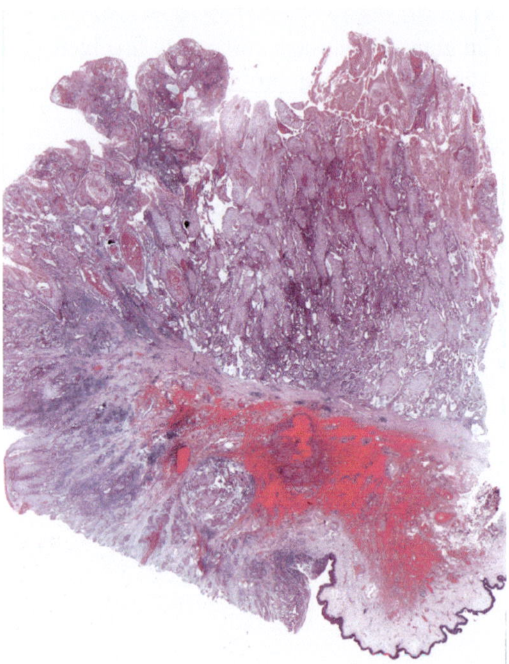

Fig. 13.3 Verruciform pattern of growth. Cut section of a carcinoma of the glans with verruciform pattern of growth

The recognition in penile biopsy specimens of the histologic types occurring with these different patterns of growth can guide the choice of the surgical procedure (i.e., partial versus radical penectomy); however, small biopsies often present objective limitations in their reliability to identify more or less aggressive subtypes and other important prognostic factors [17] (Fig. 13.4).

Squamous Cell Carcinoma, Usual Type

This is the most common histologic subtype of penile SCC (50–60 % of cases). The most frequent patterns of growth are vertical and superficial spreading patterns. Macroscopically, usual SCC presents as an exo- or endophytic, ulcerative, white-gray nodule. Accurate gross examination allows the detection of linear prominences (1–2 mm in thickness) in the mucous membrane adjacent to the invasive tumor, which microscopically appear as squamous hyperplasia or well-differentiated PeIN (Fig. 13.5a, b).

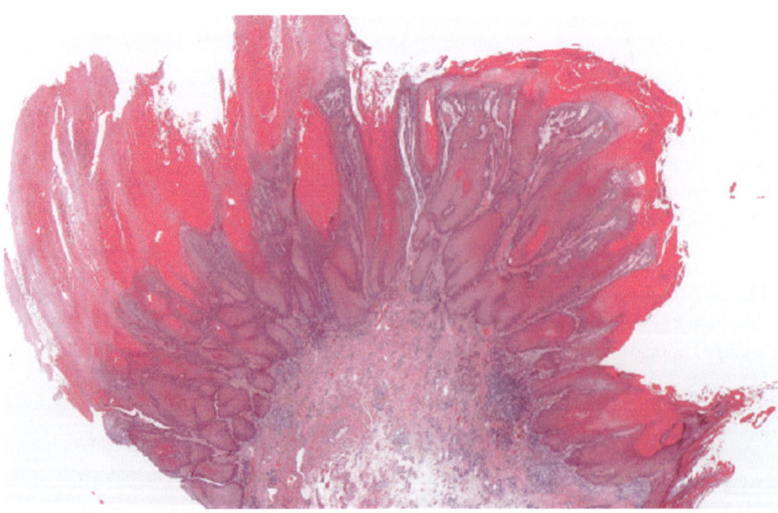

Fig. 13.4 Verruciform pattern of growth. This small biopsy shows a distinctive verruciform pattern of growth in a lesion with a low-grade appearance and microinvasion of the lamina propria. A conservative surgical approach is indicated in this case

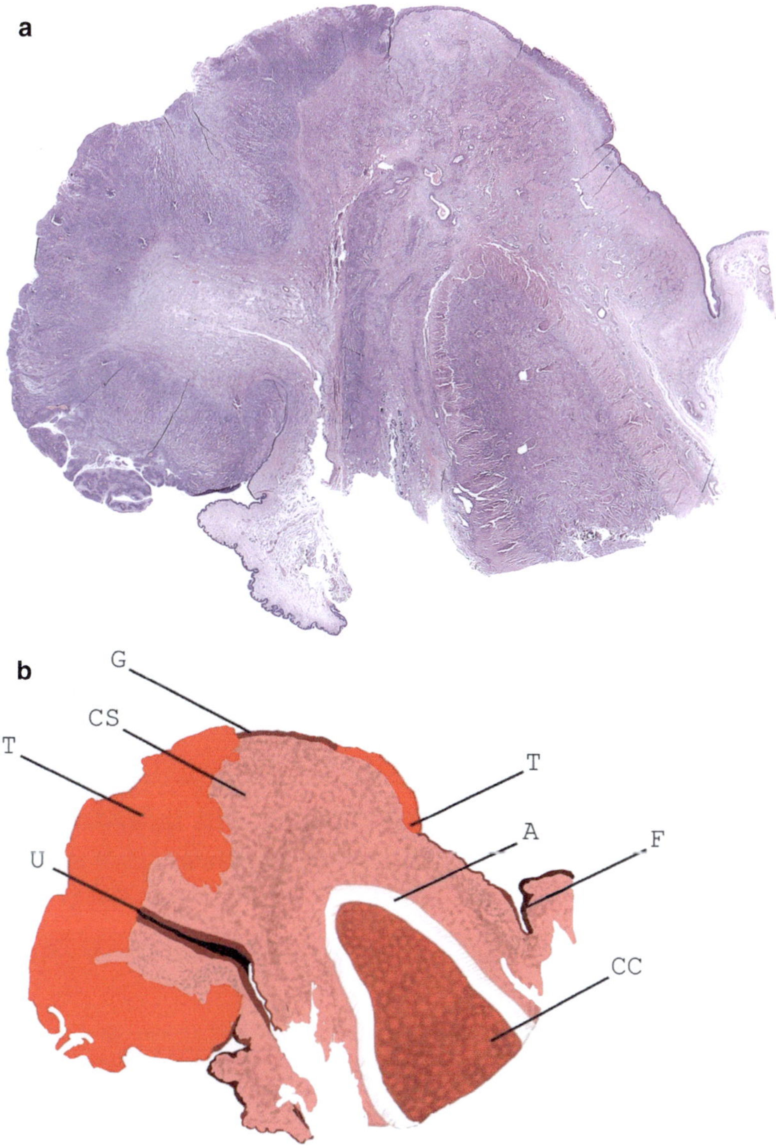

Fig. 13.5 Usual-type SCC. (**a**) Endophytic white-gray tumor infiltrating the corpora spongiosa with adjacent penile intraepithelial neoplasia and squamous hyperplasia in the mucosa of the glans. (**b**) Diagram of **a** *T* tumor, *G* squamous hyperplasia in the epithelium of the glans, *CS* corpus spongiosum, *CC* corpus cavernosum, *A* tunica albuginea, *U* urethra, *F* foreskin (Published with kind permission of ©Maurizio Colecchia 2015. All Rights Reserved)

Grading

Usual SCC is an infiltrating carcinoma that can be classified with a 3-grade system according to the level of keratinization, cellular pleomorphism, and the presence of regular nests or sheets of tumor cells.

Grade 1, well differentiated. The main features are sheets or nests of invasive carcinoma cells with central keratinization and keratin pearls (Fig. 13.6). It is less common than the other 2 grades, and its features sometimes overlap with pseudohyperplastic carcinoma.

Grade 2, moderately differentiated. The main features are smaller nests with scant keratinization and irregular outlines. There is limited pleomorphism; the cell nuclei are monomorphic with abundant cytoplasm. This grade is the most frequently observed, along with focal transition to grade 3 (Fig. 13.7).

Grade 3, poorly differentiated. The main features are nests, cords, and solid sheets of cells with

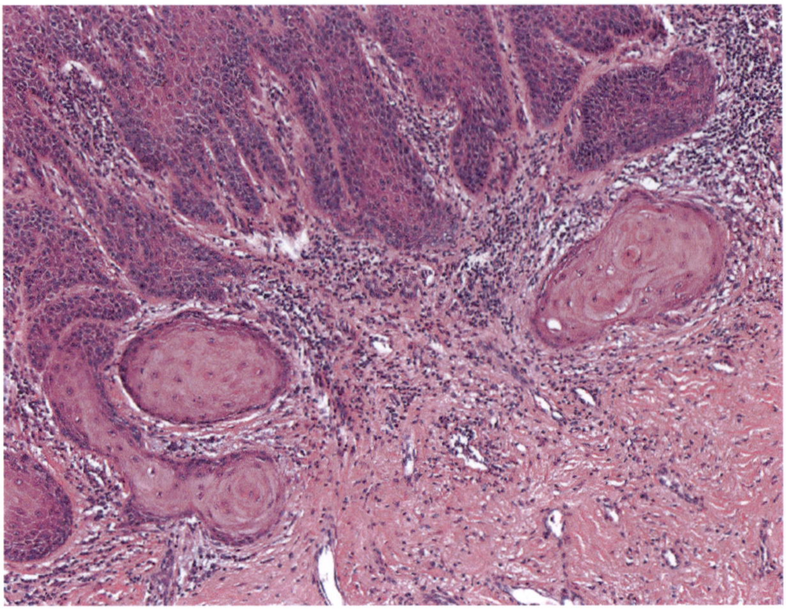

Fig. 13.6 SCC, grade 1. Well-differentiated grade 1 SCC showing extreme differentiation with large nests of tumor cells and keratin pearls

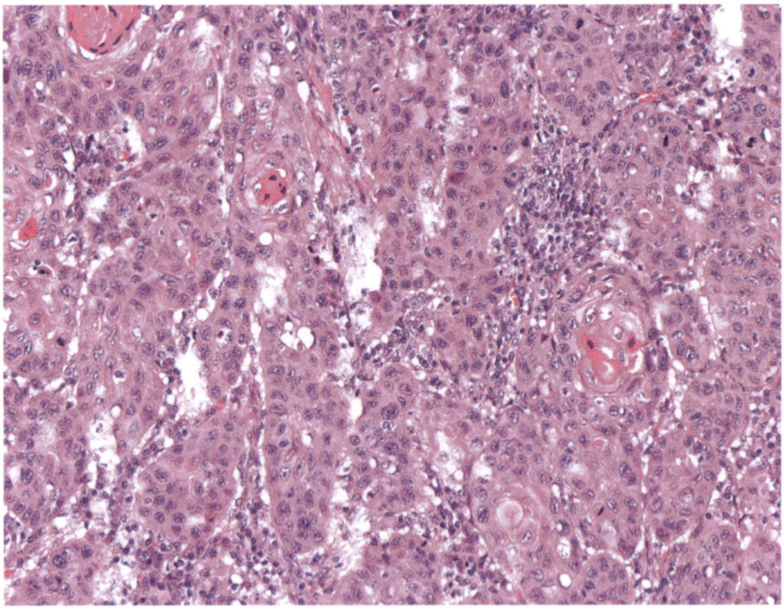

Fig. 13.7 SCC, grade 2. The cell nests are more irregular and smaller than in grade 1 SCC. There is pleomorphism and nuclear atypia. Keratin is commonly present

focal areas containing spindle, trabecular, and clear cells (Fig. 13.8).

Sarcomatoid change is considered a separate category, sometimes designated as grade 4, which often is combined with other tumor types and conveys a very poor prognosis.

The most difficult differential diagnosis is grade 3 SCC, due to its overlapping features with urothelial carcinomas and melanomas. Unusual patterns such as pseudohyperplastic, acantholytic, clear-cell, small-cell, and other patterns may be focally present [11, 16, 18].

A difficult to subclassify group of exophytic papillary lesions is collectively referred to as "verruciform neoplasms" (Table 13.2). Benign lesions such as giant condylomata (see Chap. 12) belong to this group as well as

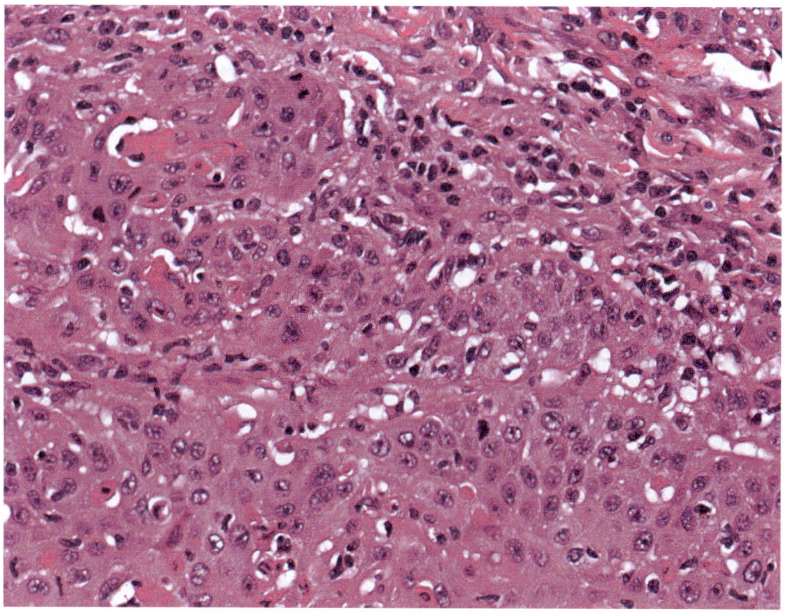

Fig. 13.8 SCC, grade 3. Poorly differentiated grade 3 SCC shows nonkeratinizing carcinoma with a solid pattern. Nuclear pleomorphism and mitoses are common features

Table 13.2 Verruciform penile tumors

1	Verrucous carcinoma	HPV unrelated; broad, pushing base; papillary surface without koilocytosis
2	Warty carcinoma	HPV related (HPV 16–18); irregular infiltrative base; koilocytosis throughout the papillomatous proliferations
3	Papillary carcinoma	HPV infection rarely detected; papillary surface; no koilocytosis
4	Carcinoma cuniculatum	Variant of verrucous carcinoma; deep invaginations
5	Condyloma acuminatum/giant condyloma	HPV related (low risk); koilocytosis limited to the surface

malignant tumors including warty "condylomatous" carcinoma, verrucous carcinoma, and papillary SCC.

Warty Carcinoma

Warty carcinomas are slow-growing lesions that may originate years before their histologic assessment. They are similar to vulvar neoplasms [19], and the first well-reported description in the penis can be found in the series of condylomata acuminata and related malignant lesions published in 1965 by Davies [20], who writes that "malignant condyloma occupies an intermediate position between giant condyloma and squamous cell carcinoma" [20]. Warty carcinoma presents as a large, firm, cauliflower-like mass with a white-gray surface, sometimes affecting multiple anatomical compartments. It has been found to encompass the glans, coronal sulcus, and foreskin as a cobblestone-like, firm mass (Fig. 13.9).

The gross appearance can be quite similar to that of condyloma acuminatum, but the nodularity is asymmetrical and frequently confluent. The cut surface of the penectomy specimen of Fig. 13.10a, b shows a papillomatous growth with penetration into the corpus spongiosum. The epithelium of the papillae appears as a whitish nodular growth with a dark core.

Microscopically there are complex papillae with pointed tips, irregular fibrovascular cores, and parakeratosis (Fig. 13.11). The nuclei are large and wrinkled, with frequent bi- or multinucleation and koilocytotic atypia. The changes are present at the surface of the papillae and also in invasive foci. Keratin-filled cysts are often present [21].

The tumor-stroma interface is usually irregular and infiltrative (Fig. 13.12). Mitoses are frequent and sometimes abnormal. Some warty carcinomas

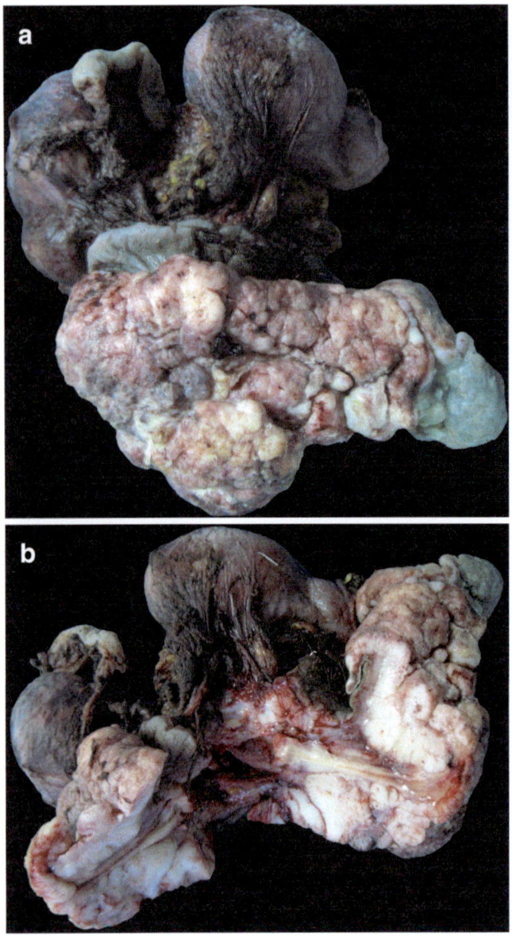

Fig. 13.9 Warty carcinoma. (**a**) Gross penectomy specimens showing an exophytic, cauliflower-like, white-gray mass with a cobblestone appearance. The involvement of the various anatomical levels is easily recognized on the cut section (**b**) in this advanced neoplasm (Published with kind permission of ©Maurizio Colecchia 2015. All Rights Reserved)

show clear-cell features (Fig. 13.13). The main differential diagnosis is with benign condyloma, which lacks the cellular pleomorphism seen in warty carcinoma [22]. In benign lesions the nuclear koilocytosis is confined to the superficial layers, while in warty carcinoma, it extends throughout the tumor. More challenging cases present as noninvasive, flat, papillary lesions in the glans. In this presentation the detection of high-risk HPV (usually subtype 16), which is typical of warty carcinoma, may be necessary to distinguish it from giant condyloma [23]. The reported incidence of HPV in warty carcinoma varies [4, 5, 21, 23–25]. The variability may be explained by different factors, including (a) viral DNA degradation in the preanalytic phase, (b) different sensitivity of the techniques used for HPV detection, and (c) selection of warty carcinomas based on nonuniform histopathologic criteria. Similar to other verruciform tumors, $p16^{INK4a}$ is the best immunohistochemical marker of warty carcinoma [24]. Verrucous and papillary carcinomas are low-grade verruciform neoplasms (see below) that are frequently misdiagnosed as warty carcinoma. Verrucous carcinomas are extremely well-differentiated proliferations without cytoplasmic clearing or koilocytic nuclear atypia. The epithelium-stroma interface lacks the irregular and infiltrative outline seen in warty carcinoma. The greatest diagnostic difficulty is with papillary carcinoma not otherwise specified (NOS), a hyperparakeratotic papillomatous proliferation with an irregular ("jagged") stroma-epithelium interface without koilocytosis. The clinical behavior of warty carcinoma is intermediate between that of the other types of low-grade verruciform tumors (papillary, verrucous) and usual SCC [1, 18, 21]. Local recurrence after penectomy has been reported in 10 % of cases and lymph node metastasis in 17–18 % [21].

Verrucous Carcinoma

Verrucous carcinoma is a slow-growing exophytic neoplasm which in its pure form accounts for 3–7 % of penile cancers [1, 14, 26]. In its classical occurrence, it is a 2–3 cm lesion of the glans, but it can also affect the foreskin or be multicentric. The use of strict microscopic criteria for its diagnosis allows a uniform classification of this unusual carcinoma, which in the past has been classified as Buschke-Löwenstein tumor or giant condyloma acuminatum [26]. The expression of $p16^{INK4a}$ and Ki67 is significantly lower in verrucous carcinoma than in usual-type SCC, while there is overexpression of p53 and Rb [27]. The reported low detection rate of HPV suggests that HPV infection has a limited oncogenic role in this

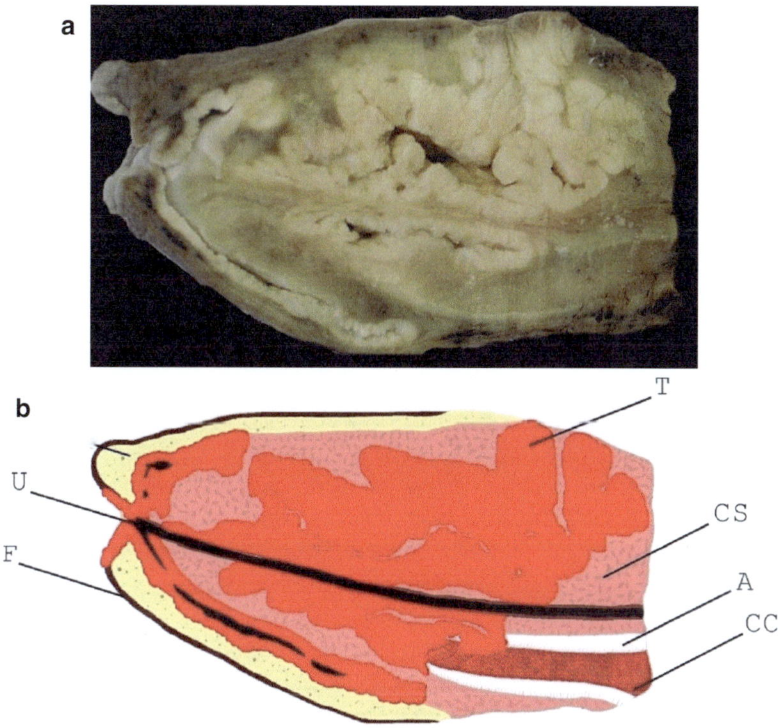

Fig. 13.10 Warty carcinoma. (**a**) Cut surface of penectomy specimen showing a papillomatous growth with an exophytic and endophytic growth pattern. There is irregular infiltration appearing as multiple, rounded lobules of tumor. The lesion extensively involves the foreskin, coronal sulcus, and glans. (**b**) Diagram of **a**. *T* tumor, *CS* corpus spongiosum, *CC* corpus cavernosum, *A* tunica albuginea, *F* foreskin, *U* urethra (Published with kind permission of ©Maurizio Colecchia 2015. All Rights Reserved)

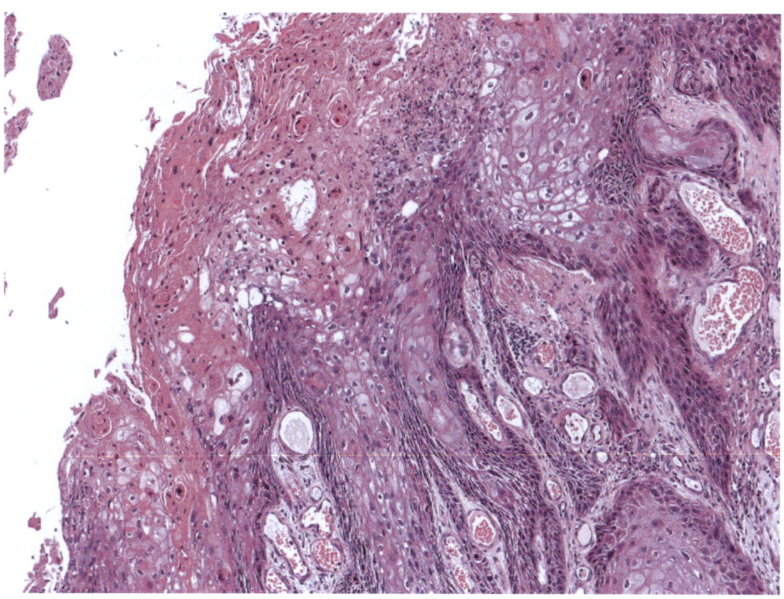

Fig. 13.11 Warty carcinoma. Prominent koilocytosis in the papillomatous growth of the tumor with parakeratosis in the superficial layers

histologic tumor type. Verrucous carcinoma can progress locally, but distant metastases are very infrequent [26, 28]. Macroscopically it presents as an exophytic, white-grayish lesion with a superficial verruciform appearance. Less than one-fourth of cases are deeply invasive into the corpora cavernosa, and the front of invasion shows a sharply delineated interface between the

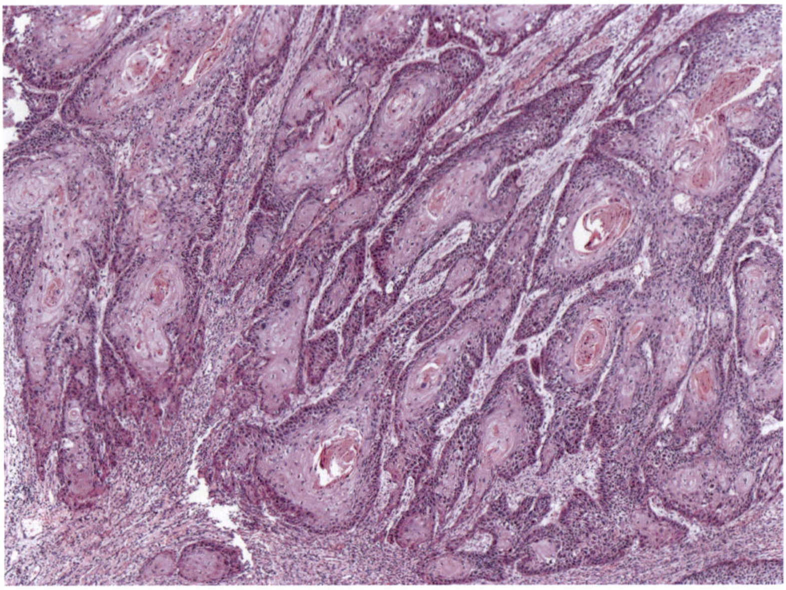

Fig. 13.12 Warty carcinoma. Same case as Fig. 13.11, with an irregular and infiltrative tumor-stroma interface composed of small irregular nests with atypia. Koilocytotic changes are present in the infiltrating cell nests of this well-differentiated carcinoma

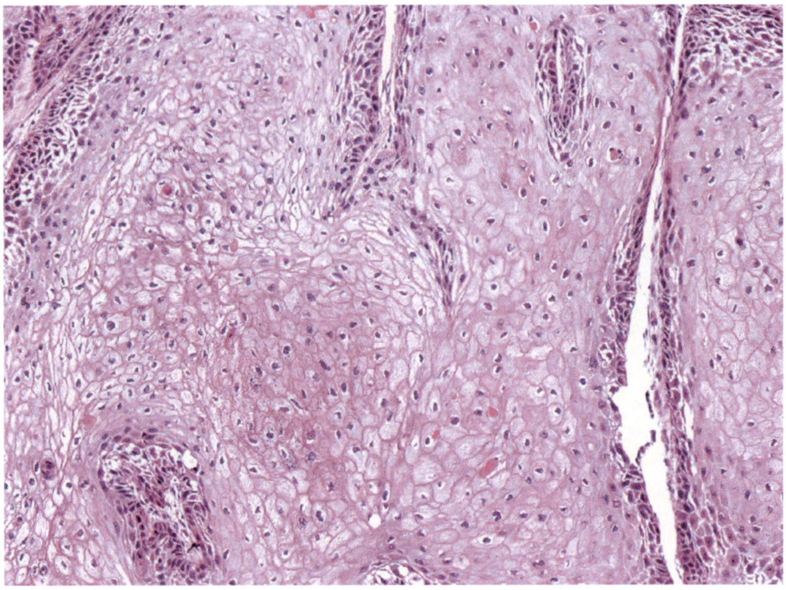

Fig. 13.13 Warty carcinoma. Clear-cell features with some crinkly nuclei

neoplasm and the lamina propria. Microscopically the lesion is well differentiated with hyperkeratosis, papillomatosis, and acanthosis (Figs. 13.14 and 13.15). The tumor cells show prominent intercellular bridges with no atypia. The bases of the squamous tongues are broad, with pushing, regular borders (Fig. 13.16). Few mitoses are present. Unlike condylomatous papillae, the papillae in verrucous carcinoma are not arboriform; they lie close to each other, show keratin plugs in the center, and are without central fibrovascular cores (Fig. 13.15). In the adjacent mucosa, there is squamous hyperplasia, lichen sclerosus, or well-differentiated PeIN [12]. The main differential diagnoses are verrucous hyperplasia and mixed SCC; hyperplastic lesions are smaller and the broad base lacks the downward growth of the bulbous squamous projections

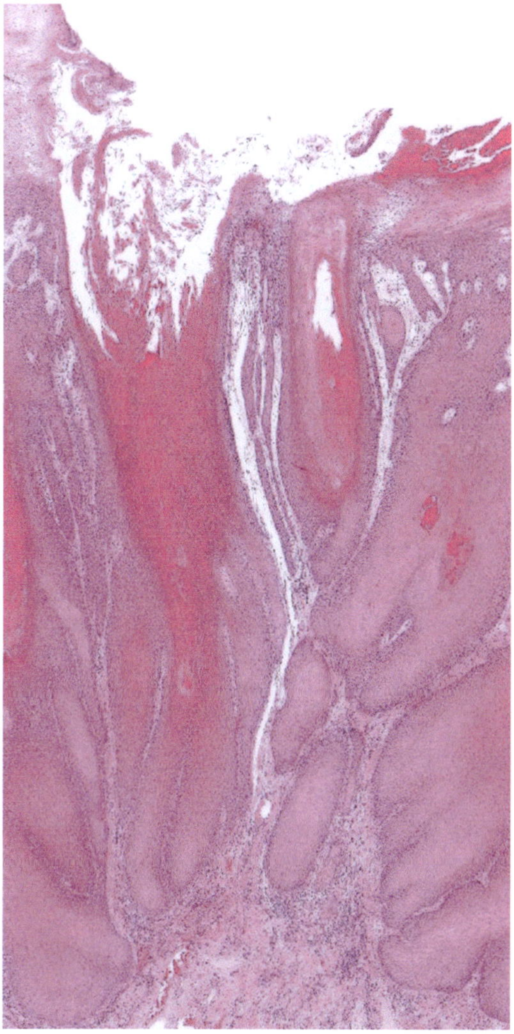

Fig. 13.14 Verrucous carcinoma. Hyperkeratosis, papillomatosis, and acanthosis with a broad base on the corpus spongiosum

observed in the carcinomatous counterpart. Mixed SCCs consist of usual-type areas intermingled with verrucous carcinoma. Papillary SCC has more cellular atypia and has an irregular front of invasion that is easy to distinguish. Regional lymph node or distant metastasis does not occur in typical cases of verrucous carcinoma [9], and given its low malignant potential, partial or local excision is the treatment of choice. The mortality rate of pure verrucous carcinoma is zero [1, 9, 18]. On the basis of a preoperative biopsy that is diagnostic of verrucous carcinoma, prophylactic lymphadenectomy is not recommended [29].

Papillary Squamous Cell Carcinoma

Papillary SCC NOS is the third distinctive type of low-grade verruciform neoplasms of the penis [30]. The macroscopic presentation in the penectomy specimen shows an exophytic papillomatous tumor with extensive superficial involvement of the glans, coronal sulcus, and foreskin. The most common microscopic distinguishing features compared with verrucous SCC are the complex papillae with irregular fibrovascular cores; typically the tips of the papillae are polymorphic (straight, blunt, rounded, spiky, etc.) (Fig. 13.17). Papillary SCC lacks the viral changes seen in warty carcinoma, while there is more nuclear atypia than in verrucous SCC; the HPV detection rate is very low or even zero [4, 16, 30, 31]. The tumor-stroma interface is jagged and the frequency of deeper infiltration into the corpora cavernosa is higher (25–33 %) than in verrucous carcinomas [9, 11, 16, 30]. Many associated lesions have been reported, with a prevalent occurrence of squamous hyperplasia with differentiated PeIN.

Papillary carcinoma has low-grade histology and a metastatic rate similar to warty carcinoma, but it generally has a good prognosis: the recurrence rate is about 12 %, and the rates of inguinal lymph node metastases and mortality both range from 0 to 12 % [9]. Unlike other verruciform tumors (warty, verrucous, and cuniculatum carcinomas), the papillary pattern may superficially be part of basaloid or warty-basaloid invasive carcinoma. This unusual tumor, similar to urothelial carcinoma (see Fig. 12.13), is composed of papillae with fibrovascular cores lined by poorly differentiated cells and, being an HPV-related neoplasm of the family of basaloid carcinomas, shows characteristic p16-positive immunostaining that lacks in papillary carcinoma [32] (Table 13.2).

Carcinoma Cuniculatum

This very unusual tumor is similar to verrucous carcinoma at the surface, but its hallmark is the presence of extensive infiltration of erectile tissues with the formation of sinuses and cyst-like tracts (Fig. 13.18) [33]. Fistulae opening to the foreskin or penile shaft are frequently observed and are comparable to those in plantar epithelioma cuniculatum

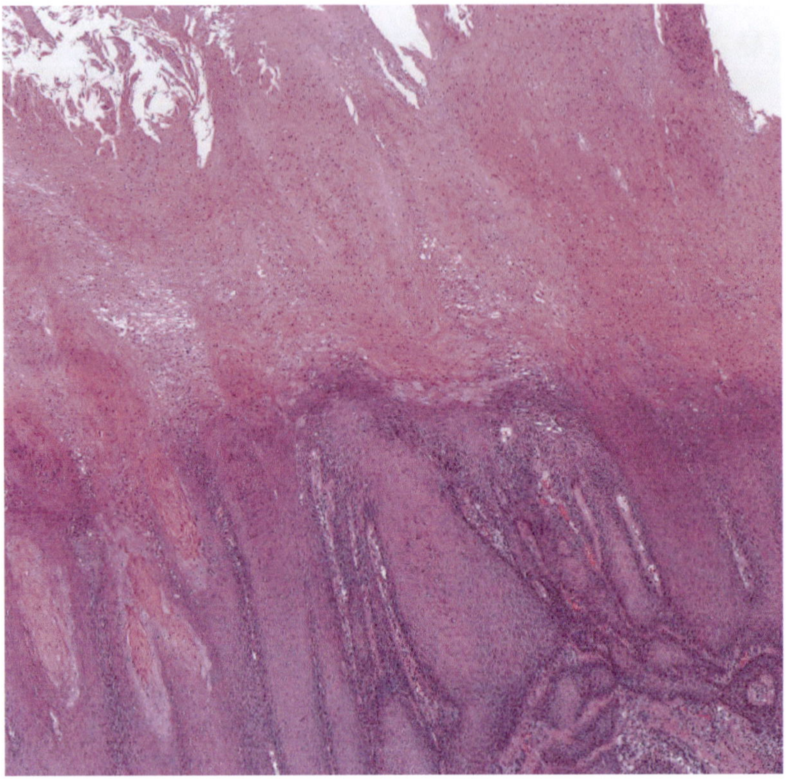

Fig. 13.15 Verrucous carcinoma. The papillae are not arboriform, and they lack fibrovascular cores. There are keratin plugs in the center. The tips of the papillae show hyperkeratosis

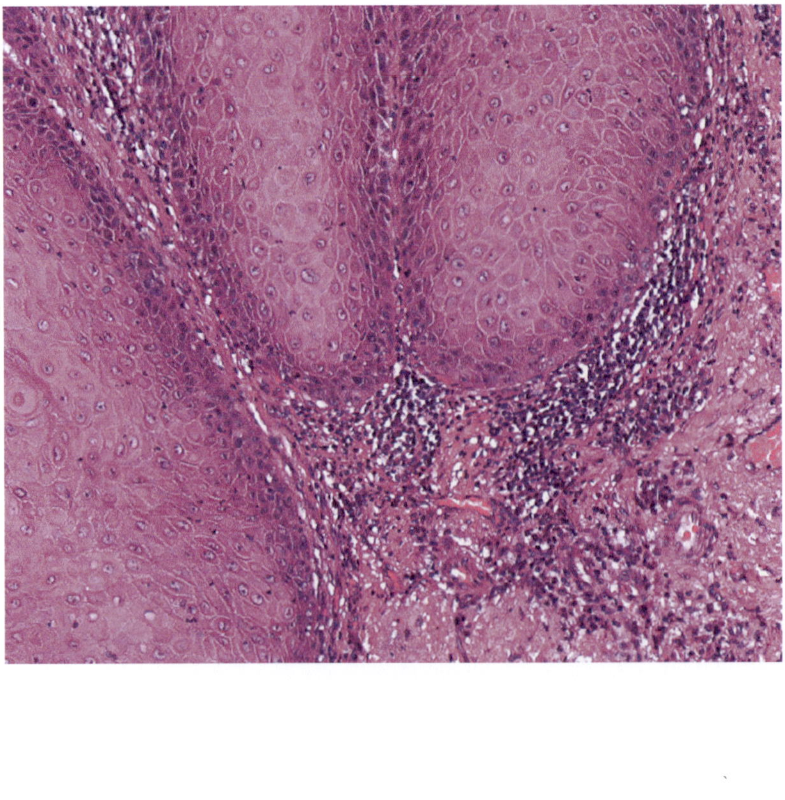

Fig. 13.16 Verrucous carcinoma. The tumor base has broad bulbous fronds of extremely well-differentiated squamous cells with broad pushing margins. The dermal-tumor interface shows an apparently intact basement membrane and absence of an active basal layer

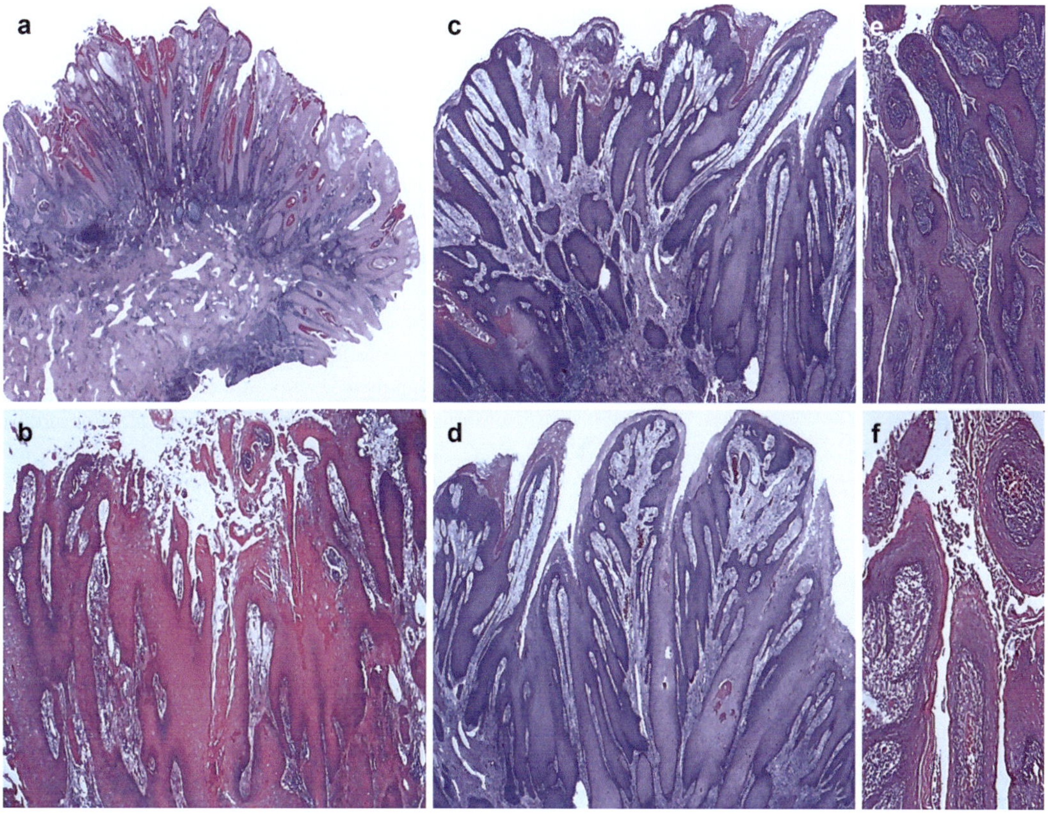

Fig. 13.17 (a–f) Papillary carcinoma. Complex papillae lacking viral changes and with absent atypia in a papillary carcinoma (Courtesy Prof. Antonio Cubilla)

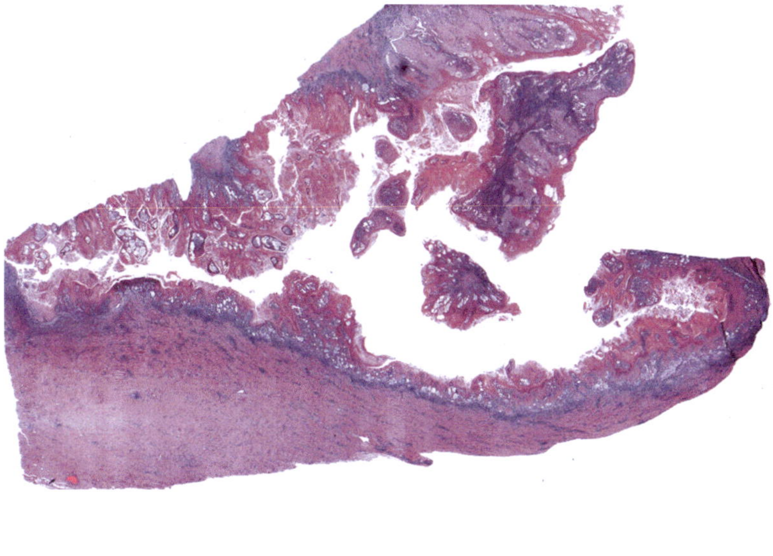

Fig. 13.18 Carcinoma cuniculatum. Low power view of a cut-section. Note the endophytic burrowing channels, the pseudocystic space and interanastomotic and complex pattern of the lesion

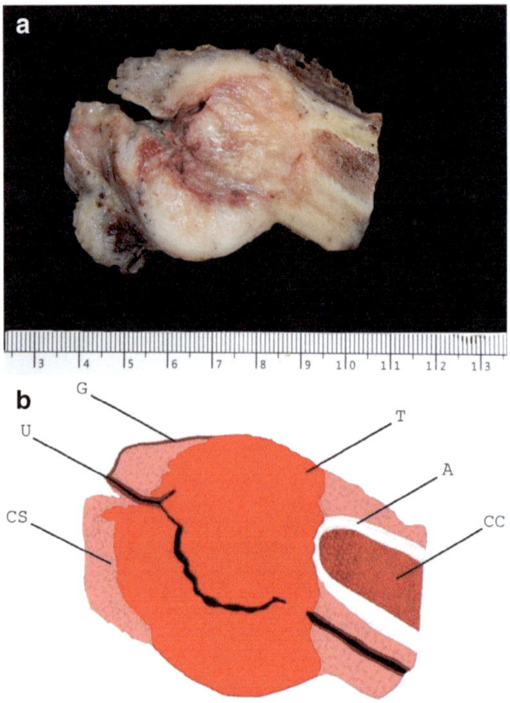

Fig. 13.19 Sarcomatoid carcinoma, gross specimen. (**a**) A polypoid solid mass ulcerates the surface of the glans, extensively involving the corpus cavernosum. (**b**) Diagram of **a**. *T* tumor, *G* epithelium of the glans, *CS* corpus spongiosum, *CC* corpus cavernosum, *A* tunica albuginea, *U* urethra (Published with kind permission of ©Maurizio Colecchia 2015. All Rights Reserved)

[34, 35]. The prognosis is similar to that of verrucous carcinoma; of the cases reported in the literature, none metastasized.

Sarcomatoid Carcinoma

The relatively uncommon occurrence of sarcomatoid carcinoma in the genitourinary tract [36] is confirmed by its low prevalence among penile tumors. Sarcomatoid carcinomas account for approximately 4 % of penile carcinomas. They are a high-grade, most likely HPV-unrelated variant of SCC characterized by biphasic neoplasia predominantly composed of spindle cells (>50 %) [9]. The gross appearance of most tumors is a large, polypoid, fungating, and frequently ulcerated mass affecting the glans, with a vertical pattern of growth deeply infiltrating the corpora cavernosa (Fig. 13.19a, b); also the foreskin is frequently infiltrated. The presence of corporal intrapenile metastasis (so-called satellitosis), an unusual type of cancer progression [37], has been identified in the corpora cavernosa and the skin. Poorly differentiated spindle cell proliferation arising from the epithelium of the distal penis most likely represents a sarcomatoid carcinoma (Fig. 13.20), although the connection with the lining epithelium

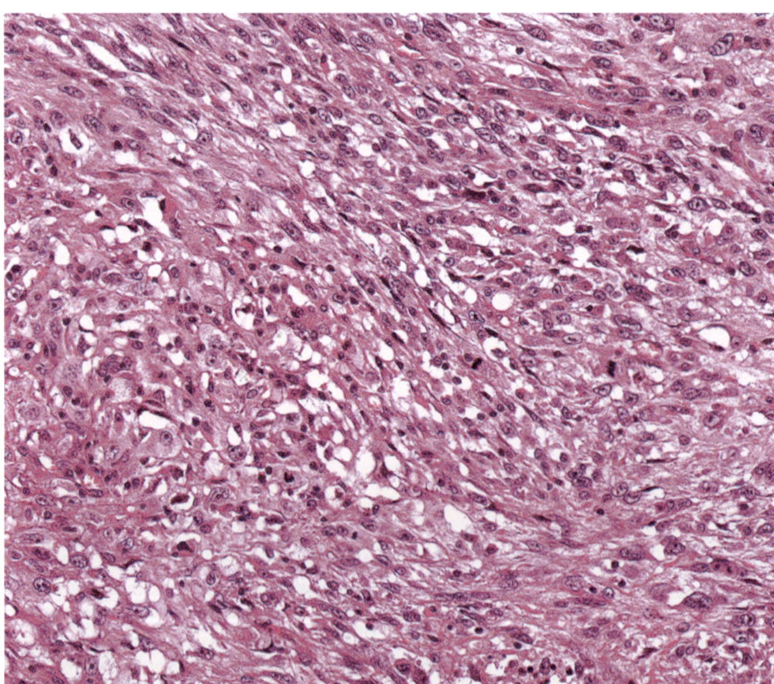

Fig. 13.20 Sarcomatoid carcinoma. Spindle cell features are present. This tumor area simulates a leiomyosarcoma

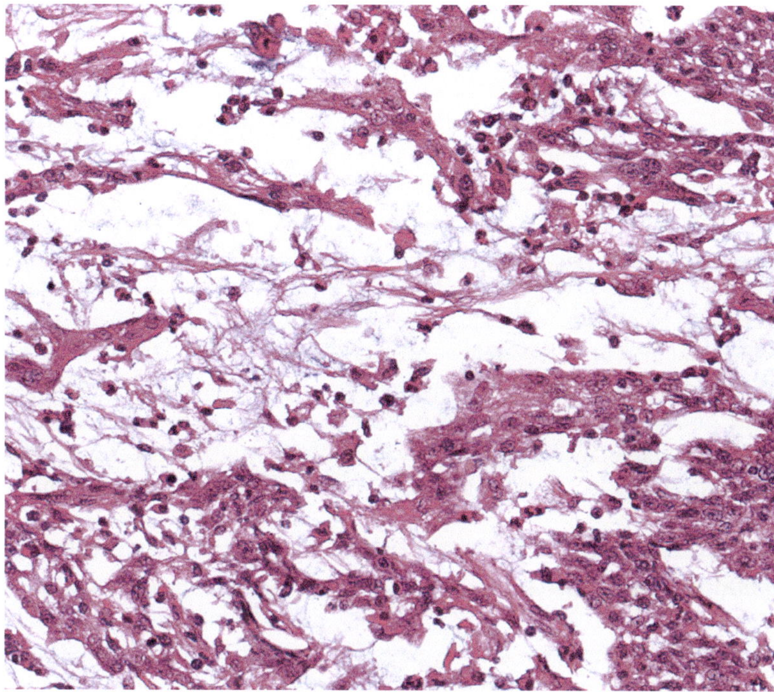

Fig. 13.21 Sarcomatoid carcinoma, microscopic appearance. Spindle cell proliferation in myxoid stroma simulating a myxoid sarcoma

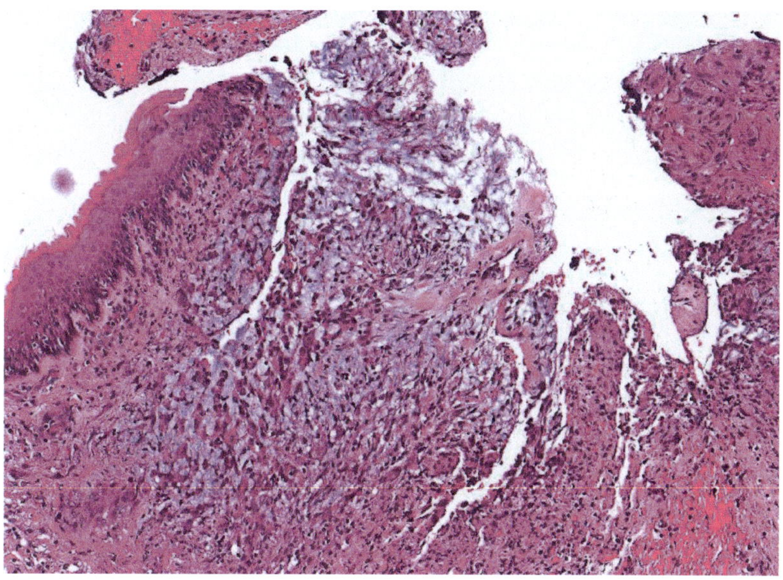

Fig. 13.22 Sarcomatoid carcinoma, microscopic appearance. Sarcomatoid carcinoma in myxoid matrix ulcerating the epithelium of the foreskin

may be difficult to assess even after extensive sampling. For this reason, despite the lack of a connection with the epithelium of the glans or the absence of high-grade PeIN, a large spindle cell tumor ulcerating the distal penis represents in the majority of cases sarcomatoid differentiation in an SCC. The spindle cell component is frequently disposed in interlacing bundles or embedded in a loose myxoid stroma resembling fibrosarcoma or leiomyosarcoma (Figs. 13.21 and 13.22). Other areas may have angiosarcomatoid features, while heterologous elements (cartilaginous tissue, bone, strap cells corresponding to striated muscle with rhabdomyomatous features) have rarely been reported. Instead, pleomorphic giant cells and multinucleated cells are frequent. The differential diagnosis includes different kinds of sarcomas and melanomas, but penile sarcomas are located in the deep penile shaft, an uncommon site for penile carcinoma. Squamous differentiation and immunohistochemical positivity for p63 cytokeratins and 34βE12 are specific markers to categorize these tumors as epithelial (Fig. 13.23).

Patients with sarcomatoid carcinomas have a poor prognosis, and the survival is usually short (less than 1 year) [38]. The lymph node metastasis rate is very high (75–89 %) and local and systemic recurrence is common (67 %) [9]. The spindle cell component may be observed in a recurrent tumor with previous nonsarcomatoid differentiation, as in the case of verrucous carcinoma with anaplastic transformation following radiotherapy [14]. These tumors convey a very poor prognosis.

Basaloid Carcinoma

Basaloid carcinoma (BC) is an aggressive tumor occurring as a large, ulcerated mass with endophytic, vertical growth deeply penetrating the corpora cavernosa. It is generally composed of a monotonous population of small- to medium-sized cells with basophilic cytoplasm [9, 39]. The pattern of solid nests of small cells is predominant, while focal basaloid features may be seen in association with other penile tumor subtypes [40]. The solid pattern of growth with small, poorly differentiated cells with scant cytoplasm resembles basal cell carcinoma (BCC) of the vulva [19]. The preferred site of origin of BC is the glans. The most frequent pattern is vertical growth (nodular) (Fig. 13.24), but some cases with a superficial spreading pattern have been reported. The nests are composed of anaplastic and small cells with round to oval nuclei, and mitoses are frequently observed (Figs. 13.25 and 13.26); high-power magnification shows uniform ovoid basaloid cells with inconspicuous nucleoli and central comedonecrosis with a mixture of necrotic debris and keratin material. Other, more unusual, microscopic features are spindle cell features, a "starry sky" appearance due to individual cell necrosis, and interstitial hyalinization. In the majority of BC cases, carcinoma in situ (CIS) is present adjacent to invasive carcinoma [39] (Figs. 13.24 and 13.27). The 16^{INK4a} immunostain is usually positive in intraepithelial and invasive BC (Fig. 13.28) [41]. A common finding is lymphovascular and perineural invasion, while a large-cell pattern with more pleomorphic nuclei is observed rarely. Another uncommon occurrence is papillary BC, a superficial papillary tumor composed of papillae with small basophilic cells resembling papil-

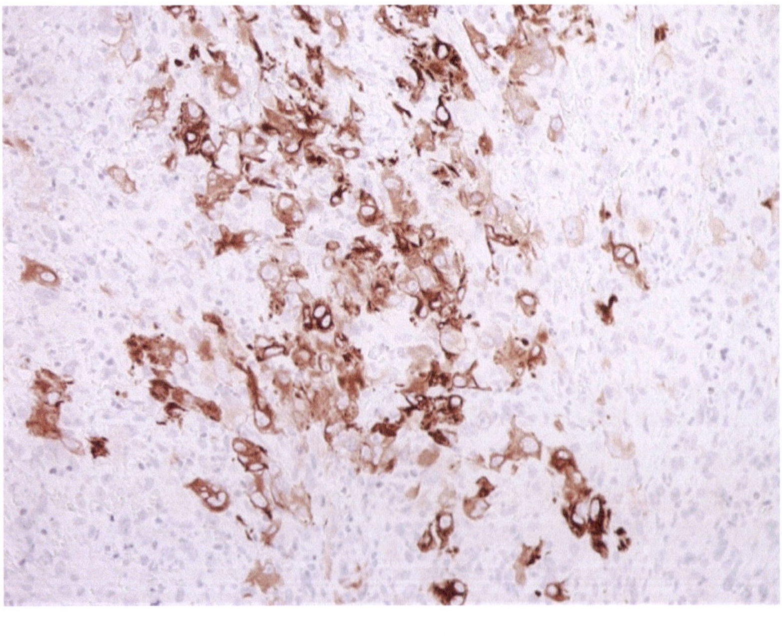

Fig. 13.23 Sarcomatoid carcinoma. Rare spindle cells immunostained by cytokeratin pool

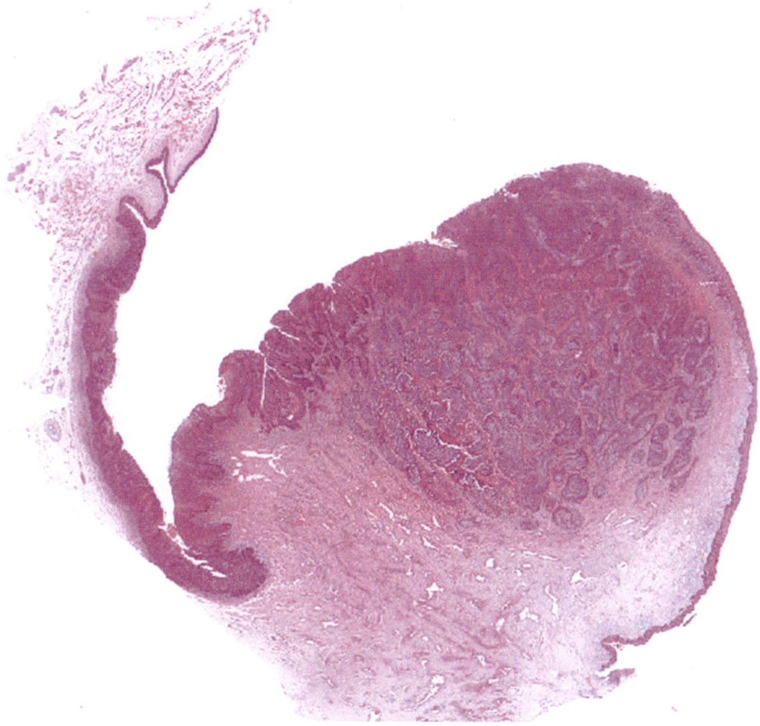

Fig. 13.24 Basaloid carcinoma. Neoplasm with a prevalent basaloid component with vertical growth pattern and in situ component (Published with kind permission of ©Maurizio Colecchia 2015. All Rights Reserved)

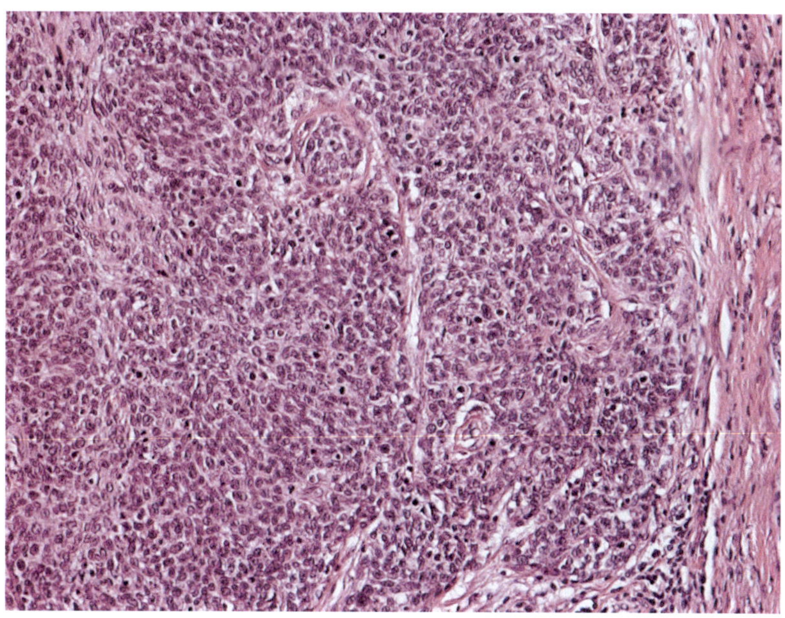

Fig. 13.25 Basaloid carcinoma. Solid nests consisting of basophilic small ovoid basaloid cells with small nucleoli and numerous mitoses

lary urothelial carcinoma [42]; this neoplasm is usually HPV related and immunoreactive to p16. HPV positivity has been reported in a high percentage of BCs, ranging from 71 to 80 % [4, 24, 43]. The presence of squamous cell differentiation in less than 20 % of the tumor is reported in the mixed subtype classified as mixed squamous-basaloid carcinoma.

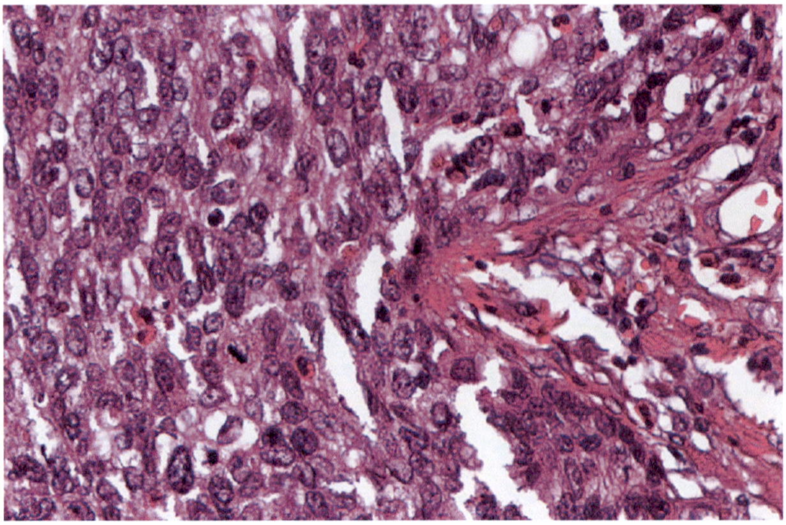

Fig. 13.26 Basaloid carcinoma. Basophilia in a poorly differentiated basaloid carcinoma with numerous mitoses

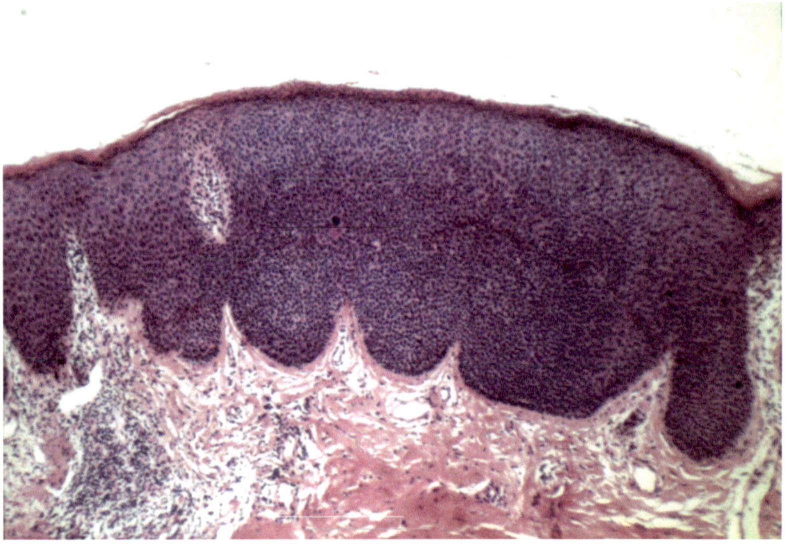

Fig. 13.27 In situ basaloid carcinoma. Most of the carcinoma in situ is uniformly composed of small immature cells

BC has a high incidence of nodal metastasis, with more than 50 % of cases showing regional metastasis at presentation [18, 39]. Recurrences have been reported in one-third of cases [39]. The mortality rate due to systemic spread is very high (>60 %), and particularly tumors deeply infiltrating the corpora cavernosa with a >10 mm diameter carry a bad prognosis [39].

The main differential diagnoses are (a) high-grade usual-type SCC, (b) BCC of the skin, (c) urothelial urethral carcinoma, and (d) small cell neuroendocrine carcinoma. Usual-type SCC shows pleomorphic cells with abundant keratinized cytoplasm, while BC shows uniform nests of small cells throughout the tumor and keratinization is confined to the central area. BCCs usually originate in the skin of the shaft and are more frequently observed in the scrotum. Urothelial urethral carcinoma most frequently occurs adjacent to CIS or papillary carcinoma in the urothelial mucosa, and absence of p16 immunostaining and positivity for GATA3 support the urothelial origin. Neuroendocrine carcinoma, in particular metastasis of Merkel cell carcinoma, has organoid, ribbon/trabecular features that are absent in BC. Immunohistochemical staining for

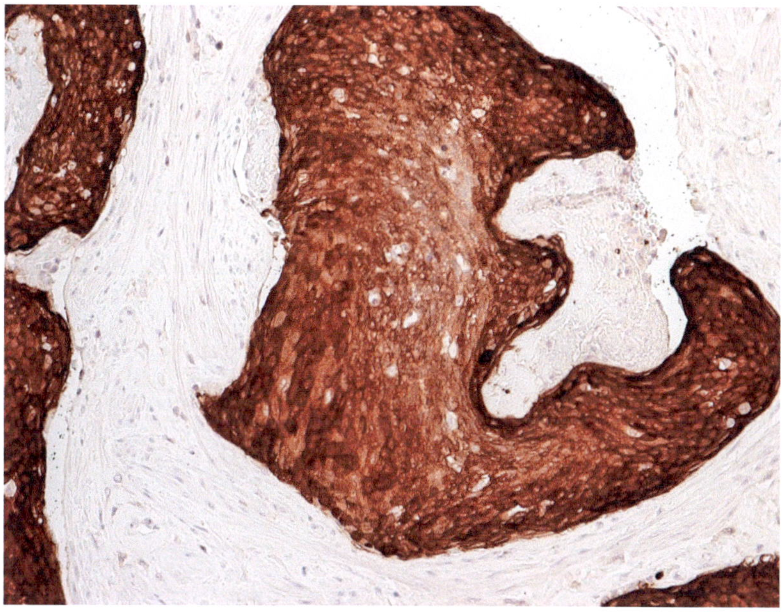

Fig. 13.28 p16 immunostaining in basaloid carcinoma. Solid aggregate of cells in basaloid carcinoma showing p16 immunostaining

CK20 and neuroendocrine markers is sometimes necessary for a definitive diagnosis.

Pseudohyperplastic Carcinoma

This is a recently described variant of low-grade SCC, preferentially affecting the foreskin and occurring at a more advanced age than usual-type SCC. It is an extremely well-differentiated, nonverruciform neoplasm strongly associated with the occurrence of lichen sclerosus in a similar way to other variants of SCC exclusive to the foreskin and characterized by low grade and multicentricity [13]. In a series of ten cases reported by Cubilla et al. [44], the authors named this unusual variant "pseudohyperplastic SCC." The name emphasizes the difficulty in distinguishing it from pseudoepitheliomatous hyperplasia, especially in small biopsies. In partial penectomies the infiltration of the corpus spongiosum or dartos is a distinguishing feature of carcinoma, which shows a stromal reaction around the infiltrative nests. Macroscopically, pseudohyperplastic carcinoma is flat or slightly elevated, often multicentric, restricted to the mucosa, and measuring less than cm 3 in diameter. Microscopically, the downward proliferation of well-differentiated carcinoma shows superficial infiltration of the lamina propria and preputial dartos (Fig. 13.29). The nests rarely show keratinization; the absence of papillomatous growth, observed in papillary carcinoma, and the irregular interface with the underlying stroma allow the differentiation from verrucous carcinoma. The good prognosis of this variant is related to its low-grade and superficial invasion of the corpora spongiosa. Other noninfiltrative lesions commonly observed in the adjacent mucosa are squamous hyperplasia, flat hyperplasia, and – less commonly – verrucous hyperplasia. No inguinal node metastases are reported in this entity.

Pseudoglandular Carcinoma

This is a highly unusual variant of SCC characterized by pseudoglandular spaces partially filled with eosinophilic debris containing squamous cells, keratin, and microabscesses (Fig. 13.30) [45]. At low magnification a multicystic or honeycomb appearance is the predominant feature with amorphous material in the lumen (Fig. 13.31). Synonyms are acantholytic SCC and adenoid SCC, used for neoplasms with more than 30 % of the tumor volume showing pseudoglandular features. Recently, an unusual pseudoangiomatoid variant was described in a

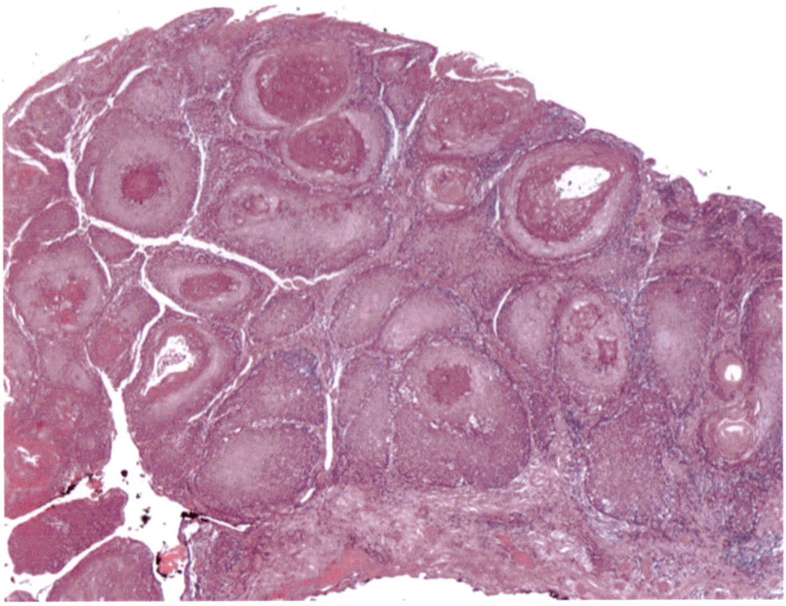

Fig. 13.29 Pseudohyperplastic carcinoma. Downward proliferation of well-differentiated carcinoma showing nests infiltrating the lamina propria

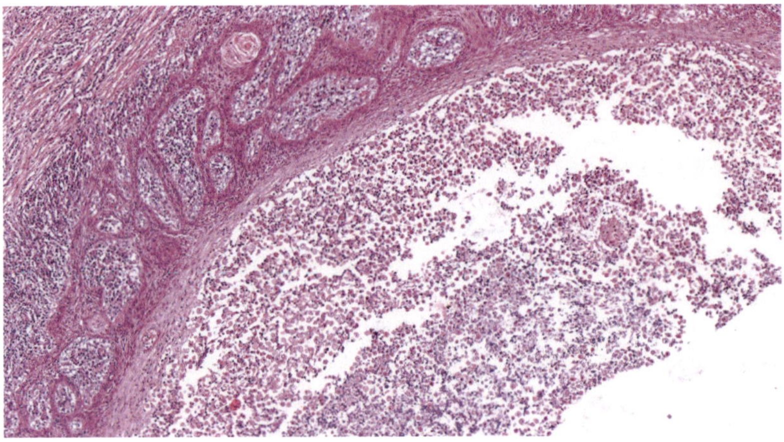

Fig. 13.30 Pseudoglandular SCC. Pseudoglandular spaces filled with eosinophilic debris, squamous cells, keratin, and inflammatory cells

middle-aged patient who died 6 months after penectomy with widespread lung metastases (Fig. 13.32a, b) [46]. Poor prognosis of pseudoglandular SCC is common to all reported series, with a mortality rate higher than 70 % [45].

Adenosquamous Carcinoma

This unusual neoplasm, probably originating in the penile surface epithelium, has the macroscopic appearance of an exophytic, yellow-gray, firm, granular mass. Microscopically it shows glands of small to medium size containing intraluminal secretory material. Often there is mucinous, alcian-positive material in the lumen. The remainder of the mass shows squamous differentiation, contributing to the biphasic appearance of this tumor. The preferential site is the perimeatal glans, but extension to the coronal sulcus and foreskin has been reported [47]. CEA immunostaining is typically observed in the glandular component. Local recurrence has been observed in up to 25 % of cases and inguinal node metastases in 43–50 % [48].

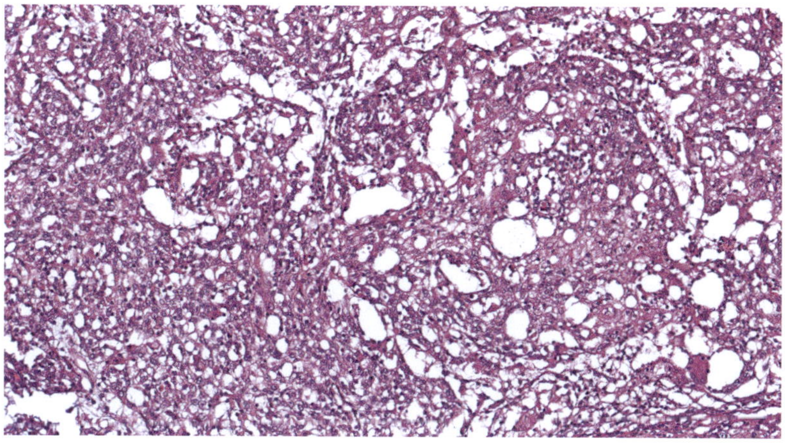

Fig. 13.31 Pseudoglandular SCC. Predominant multicystic microscopic feature corresponding to the acantholytic appearance of the tumor

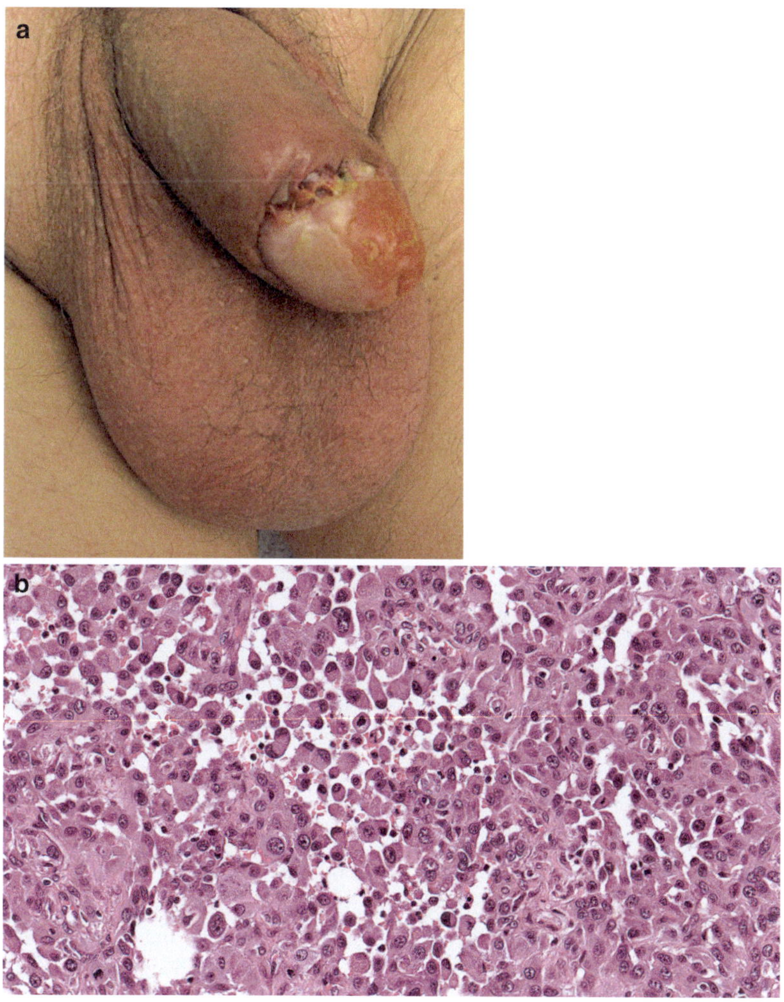

Fig. 13.32 Pseudoglandular carcinoma, pseudoangiomatoid variant. Unusual presentation of pseudoangiomatous pattern in a pseudoglandular (acantholytic) carcinoma. The lesion occurred in the glans (**a**) as a crusted, flat lesion that metastasized to the lung after radical penectomy. (**b**) Neoplastic cells with epithelioid cell features are dispersed in a pseudovascular space

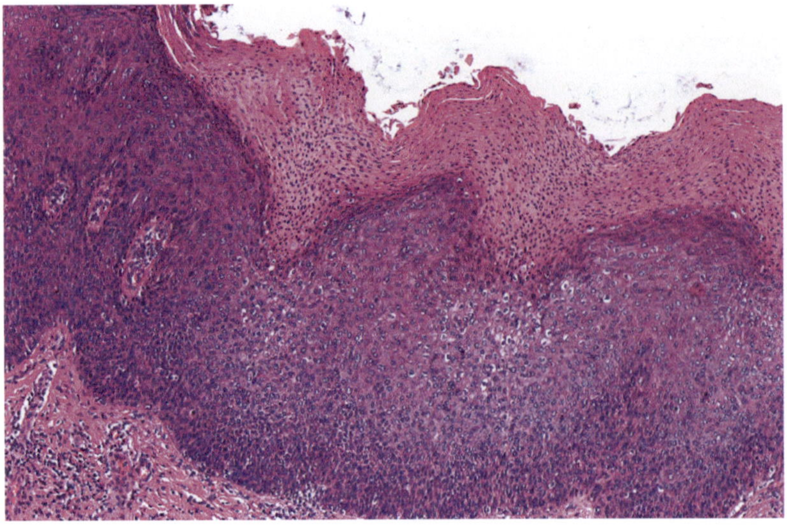

Fig. 13.33 Warty-basaloid PeIN. Penile intraepithelial neoplasia showing warty-basaloid features (Published with kind permission of ©Maurizio Colecchia 2015. All Rights Reserved)

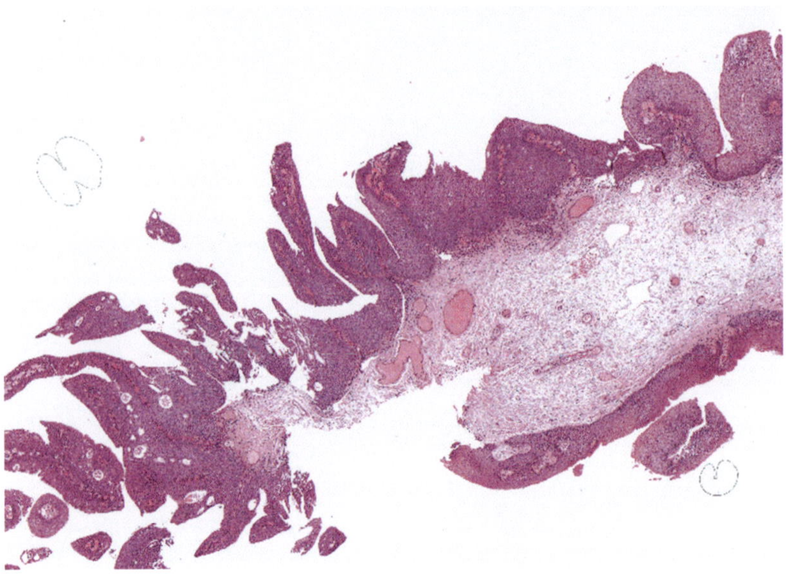

Fig. 13.34 Mixed carcinoma. Papillary growth in a tumor with prominent condylomatous changes

Mixed Carcinomas

Mixed penile tumors harbor more than one histologic subtype and each of the subtypes should make up at least 20 % of the tumor mass [2, 9]. Their frequency ranges between 20 and 33 % of all penile carcinomas. Most of these tumors are located in the glans. Macroscopically the superficial verruciform neoplasm is often admixed with a vertical pattern as observed in the basaloid subtype or in poorly differentiated SCC and in the most common mixed carcinoma: warty-basaloid SCC [49, 50]. This tumor has more than 10 % of basaloid cells that are located in superficial papillae or the deep front of invasion or in both areas. The same histologic type shows koilocytosis and other characteristic features of warty carcinoma in more than 10 % of the tumor mass, even in the intraepithelial variant (Fig. 13.33). Microscopically the presence of papillomatous tumor with long, rounded papillae showing fibrovascular cores and conspicuous koilocytosis is a very frequent finding (Fig. 13.34) and the papillary-warty variant typically overexpresses p16

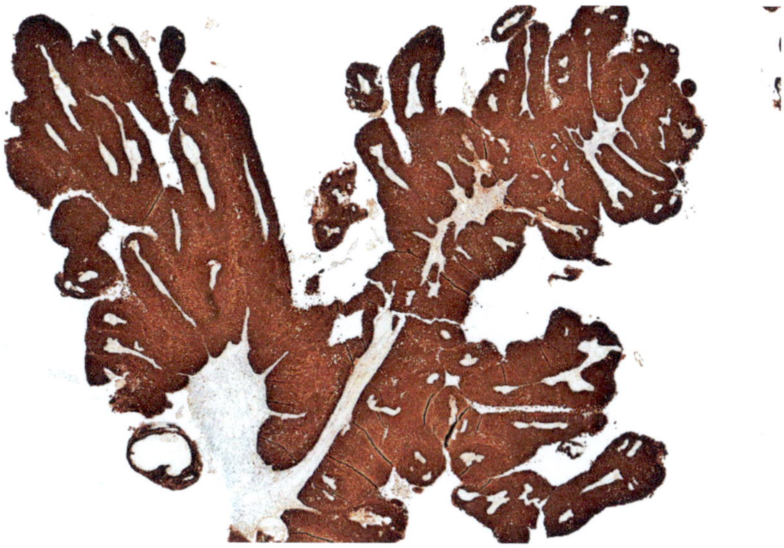

Fig. 13.35 p16 immunostaining in the papillary-warty variant. p16 immunostaining is diffusely positive in this PeIN with papillomatous growth

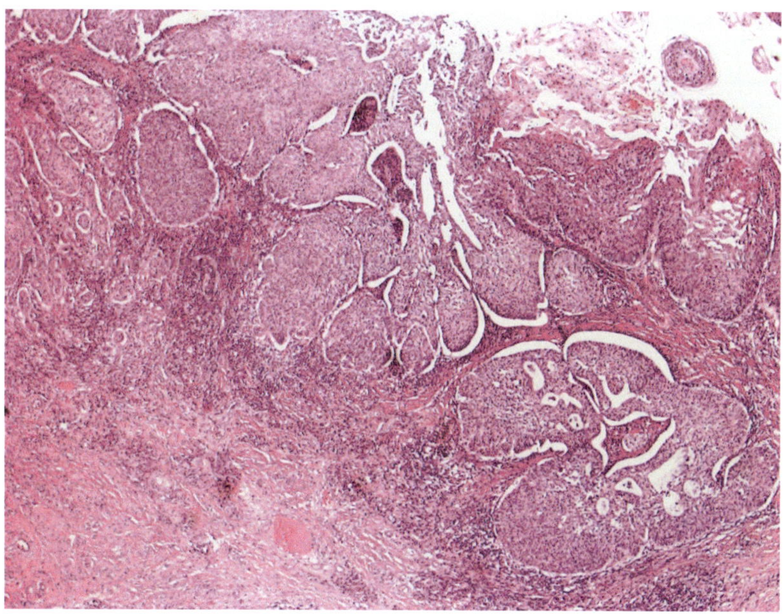

Fig. 13.36 Mixed carcinoma. Occurrence of pseudoglandular (acantholytic) carcinoma (on the right) adjacent to a well-differentiated SCC

(Fig. 13.35). Warty-basaloid carcinomas show a higher rate of metastasis (52 %) than warty carcinomas (33 %) [49], as the clinical behavior is related to the histologic grade, tumor thickness, and presence of vascular/perineural invasion (see Sect. "Prognostic Factors for SCC of the Penis"). Another classical example of mixed SCC is verrucous carcinoma with higher-grade foci consisting of usual SCC, so-called hybrid carcinoma [51]. Other less frequent combinations include usual-warty, mixed usual-basaloid, and occasionally observed cases of pseudoglandular carcinoma adjacent to a well-differentiated SCC (Fig. 13.36). Hybrid carcinoma occasionally presents lymph node metastases, which explains the presence of metastatic cases otherwise never reported in true verrucous carcinoma. The mortality rate is low and the selection of treatment

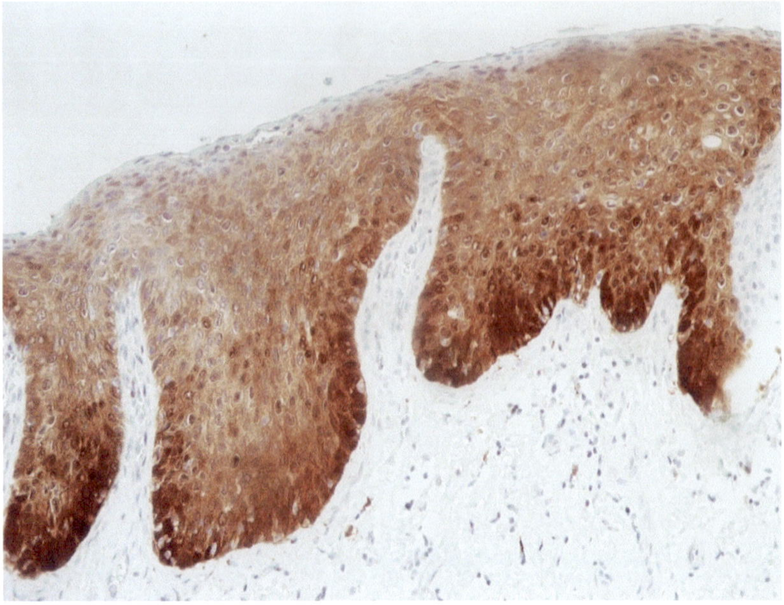

Fig. 13.37 p16 immunostaining in HPV-related (undifferentiated) penile intraepithelial neoplasia. Overexpression of p16 protein is associated with HPV

(conservative versus radical with or without groin dissection) requires careful histologic grading and assessment of perineural invasion [52].

Molecular Changes in Penile Carcinoma: Role of HPV Infection

The critical role of HPV infection in cancers of the lower genital tract has been delineated during the last several decades, and particularly the presence of high-risk HPV subtypes in a subset of around half of penile carcinomas is widely accepted [5].

The oncogenic role of HPV-16 in tumors of the mucosal epithelium of the glans has been reported in a review of human carcinogens [53]. HPV-16 infection appears to influence p16 protein and Rb gene expression, with the virus typically presenting in the nucleus of tumor cells in an episomal or integrated form. It is the most common viral type in penile carcinoma, accounting for 60–70 % of high-risk HPV-positive cancers [5, 43, 54]. Two mechanisms of dysregulated cell cycle control and apoptosis have been reported in penile carcinoma: one is HPV mediated and targets the $p16^{INK4a}$-cyclin D-Rb pathway [55], while the other is not HPV mediated, with p14 gene mutation, MDM amplification, and altered p53 expression (sometimes with mutation of the p53 gene). Both mechanisms bring about cell cycle arrest with altered apoptosis, while inactivation of the Rb gene results in loss of negative control of p16 with overexpression of p16 protein. The altered expression of p16 protein was first associated with HPV's oncogenic potential in cervical and genital lesions [24, 56].

Integrated HPV produces the E7 oncoprotein, which induces inactivation of the Rb gene and overexpression of the p16 protein, as can be detected by immunohistochemical staining (Fig. 13.37). In addition to p16 immunohistochemistry, the detection of HPV in clinical specimens is based on nucleic acid probe technology, using hybridization procedures (Southern blot, Northern blot, ISH, hybrid capture) and DNA/RNA detection by means of the more accurate and expensive real-time polymerase chain reaction (PCR). An HPV ISH reaction is the in situ detection of the integrated virus in the infected nucleus: a case is considered positive when unequivocal punctuated blue nuclear staining is observed in tumor cells (Fig. 13.38).

In a series of 48 penile carcinomas studied by tissue microarrays, Chaux et al. reported a combined methodology using p16 immunohistochemistry, routine morphology, and ISH [57].

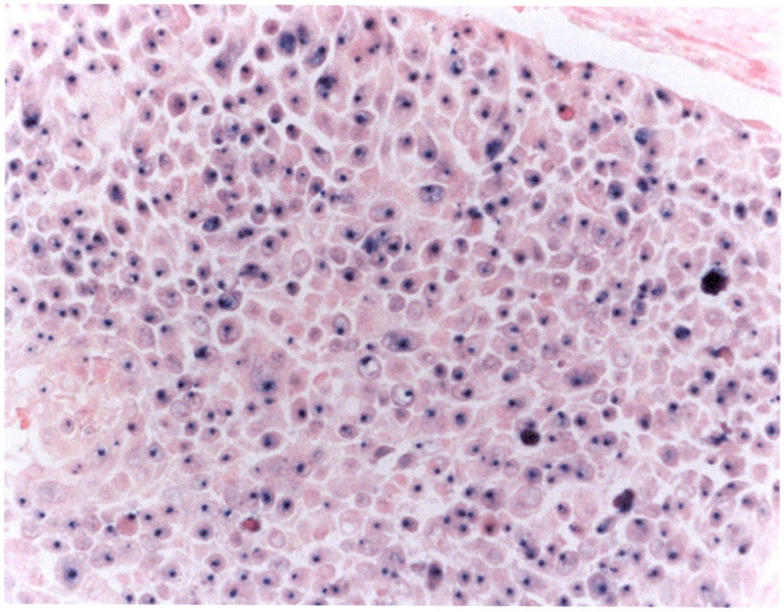

Fig. 13.38 Human papillomavirus ISH reaction. Blue nuclear staining is observed in tumor cells by chromogenic in situ hybridization (Courtesy of Dr A. Gloghini, Istituto Nazionale dei Tumori, Milan, Italy)

The gold standard technique was PCR, but according to the authors, the technical requirements and elevated costs preclude the routine use of PCR assays. They recommend combining the two techniques (p16 immunohistochemical staining and ISH) with routine morphology to enhance the sensitivity (88 % when this approach is applied) with sufficient specificity [57].

Alternative mechanisms targeting the $p^{16INK4a}$-cyclin D-Rb pathway have been investigated: the pathway can be disrupted by silencing the gene through promoter methylation and expression of the BMI-1 PcG gene, which has a critical downstream target involving $p16^{INK4a}$ and p14 [55].

The possible influence of HPV infection on the clinical outcome of penile cancer is debated. Some studies claim that the presence of high-risk HPV DNA in penile carcinoma predicts a favorable survival outcome [54], while other authors reported no survival differences [58]. Two studies showing the association of HPV infection and $p16^{INK4a}$ overexpression found overexpression of p16 to be associated with a favorable prognosis [59, 60], while in another recent tissue microarray study, the authors reported that neither HPV infection nor $p16^{INK4a}$ overexpression significantly predicted overall survival or cancer-specific survival [61]. A larger series of patients with long follow-up is required for the adequate definition of this prognostic factor.

Among the HPV-unrelated subtypes of SCC, verrucous carcinoma showed HPV DNA in 13 % of cases, while overexpression of p53 and Rb proteins was reported along with a low incidence of p16 expression in the large series studied by Stankiewicz [27]. This observation and the presence of altered expression of p21 and EGFR as well as AKT inactivation in HPV-positive and HPV-negative tumors have contributed to the dilemma that, although penile cancer arises by two separate mechanisms, one virus related and the other virus unrelated, there is a possible final common pathway to penile carcinogenesis.

One study investigated the human epidermal growth factor receptor (HER) family composed of the transmembrane tyrosine kinase receptors EGFR, HER2, HER3, and HER4 [62]. These receptors are activated by extracellular ligands stimulating intracellular signaling pathways, including the PI3K/AKT pathway, which regulate cell differentiation, migration, and survival. EGFR, HER3, and HER4 but not HER2 are associated with penile carcinogenesis. HPV-negative tumors tend to express significantly more phosphorylated EGFR (pEGFR) than HPV-positive tumors, and pEGFR expression correlates with activated AKT protein, indicating that EGFR is an upstream regulator of AKT signaling in penile cancer. HER3 is inversely expressed, with significant overstaining in HPV-positive tumors, and its expression correlates positively with cytoplasmic AKT expression. HER4 and PTEN expression are not related to HPV infection. These molecular assessments have opened the way to targeted treatment with anti-EGFR agents. However, the results are still preliminary, and treated patients have been found to relapse after initial partial remissions [63].

Many other molecular markers have been investigated, but how high-risk HPV types impact on the expression of key cell cycle proteins such as p53, p21, p16, and others is far from being fully understood. Lam and Chan [64] analyzed the expression of p21 and p53 in 42 penile carcinomas and found p21 in 40 % of invasive cancers with an inverse relationship to p53. p53 immunostaining was found in all HPV-positive cases, but other authors reported an inverse or negative relation between these 2 factors, showing p53 expression in less differentiated tumors and in lymph node metastases, which would support the concept that p53 is a marker of worse prognosis [65]. Recent studies have demonstrated the implication of the PTEN/PI3K/AKT pathway in penile carcinogenesis [62, 66], but the suggested role of the mammalian target of rapamycin (mTOR) pathway in the development of lymph node metastasis deserves further investigation.

There have been few attempts to link chromosomal abnormalities to the biologic behavior of penile cancer. Genetic imbalances have been reported in penile cancer, and DNA sequence copy number gains were found in 8q24, 16p11-12, 20q11-13, 22q, 19q13, and 5p15 in one study [67]. Other candidate genes in the genomic map of penile cancer that might prove to be targets for rare metastatic cases include PRKCI, PI3K, DCUN1D1, LAMP3, and others associated with gains in 3p12.3 and S-phase kinase-associated protein 2, which is associated with gain and/or amplification of the 5p15.33–p11 region [68]. Although other cytogenetic changes have been described, none of these are characteristic. As with all malignant tumors, penile tumor progression involves the loss of cell-to-cell interaction and invasion of the extracellular matrix. A study by Campos et al. [69] showed that low expression of E-cadherin, an epithelial cell adhesion molecule, and increased immunoreactivity of the matrix metalloproteinases MMP-2 and MMP-9 were correlated with a higher risk of metastases; moreover, MMP-9 expression was an independent risk factor for recurrence.

As other genes are currently under investigation including COX-2, MYC, SOX2, and AT-rich interactive domain 1A (ARID1A), a clearer picture of the molecular changes in penile carcinomas is slowly emerging. The presence of a final common pathway to penile carcinogenesis with similar molecular mechanisms seems a possibility, although penile cancer arises by two separate mechanisms, one involving p53 and the other mediated by HPV in the subset of HPV-positive penile carcinomas.

Prognostic Factors for SCC of the Penis

The use of heterogeneous pathologic methodologies and the studies regarding variable patient populations without uniform treatment and follow-up have led to contradictory results and limitations in the pathologic evaluation of prognostic factors. In Table 13.3 the main prognostic factors for SCC of the penis are reported.

Table 13.3 Prognostic factors for squamous cell carcinoma of the penis. References in parentheses

Nodal status [70–74]
Histologic grade [75, 76]
Depth of infiltration [77]
Anatomical levels [78–80]
Perineural invasion [52]
Lymphatic [81] and vascular embolization [82]
Modality of growth, front pattern of invasion [1, 83]
Proliferative index [84]
Molecular factors [85]

Nodal Status

The single most important prognostic factor for overall outcome in penile carcinoma is the nodal status. Such is its importance that the 5-year and 10-year survival rates for patients with lymph node involvement are 48 % and 46 %, respectively, versus 91 and 88 % for patients with pathologically negative lymph nodes [80]. Prophylactic lymphadenectomy has a better 5-year survival rate than deferred lymphadenectomy, and indications for extended pelvic lymph node dissection are the number of metastatic inguinal lymph nodes, their maximum diameter, and the presence of extranodal spread [74]. Nomograms predictive of pathologic inguinal node involvement in patients with SCC have enough accuracy to evaluate the real incidence of metastases (on the basis of the clinical stage of the involved lymph nodes, grade, vascular invasion, and anatomical levels of invasion) [86] and to estimate predictions of survival at 5 years [87].

Histologic Grade

Histologic grade shows a highly accurate correlation with prognosis. A study in the Netherlands using the 3-tier grading system for SCC found in well-differentiated (grade 1) SCC 24 % of metastatic inguinal lymph nodes, compared with 46 % in moderately differentiated (grade 2) and 82 % in poorly differentiated (grade 3) SCC [75]. Any proportion of grade 3 SCC carries a poor prognosis [76].

Depth of Infiltration and Anatomical Levels of Invasion

The depth of infiltration has prognostic value and accurate measurement of tumor invasion in millimeters is required particularly in surgical specimens, both penectomy and circumcision, while the evaluation in small biopsies is generally unaccurate, given that only 9 % of biopsy results are confirmed in penectomies [17]. Measurement may be performed from the basement membrane to the deepest point of invasion [77]; the risk of metastases is especially high in tumors invading more than 10 mm and with infiltration of the corpora cavernosa in the glans or deep preputial dartos in the foreskin [78]. The invasion of anatomical levels is subject to error in pathology reports due to confusion of the anatomical location with the site of the tumor. The importance of this information is confirmed by the stage of penile cancer being based on the anatomical levels of invasion in the current TNM system [88] (Table 13.3). The anatomical levels of invasion, 1, 2, and 3, in the glans correspond to the lamina propria, corpus spongiosum, and corpora cavernosa, while levels 2 and 3 in the foreskin correspond to the dartos and skin [79]. They are evaluated with a scoring system referred to as "Prognostic Index" by Chaux et al. [80], which consists of the addition of numerical values given to histologic grade (1–3), deepest anatomical level involved by cancer (1–3), and presence of perineural invasion (0 or 1). According to the Prognostic Index, scores of 5 and 6 are associated with a high mortality rate [80].

Perineural Invasion, Lymphatic and Vascular Embolization

Perineural invasion is easily observed but it is not frequently reported in the diagnosis. It is an independent prognostic parameter associated with regional metastasis in tumors with 5–10 mm depth of invasion [52]. Lymphatic embolization and vascular embolization have been reported as independent predictive variables of inguinal lymph node involvement in patients with SCC of the penis according to a multicenter Italian study [82].

Modality of Growth, Front of Invasion, and Histologic Subtypes

The correlation between tumor growth pattern and presence of regional metastases and survival has been studied [1, 75]: high mortality was found for patients having tumors with a vertical growth pattern (67 %), while the mortality dropped to 10 % in superficially spreading carcinomas [1]. Another factor affecting prognosis is the modality of growth of the deepest invasive tumor component in relation to the stroma: the infiltrative pattern of invasion was reported to be an independent risk factor for regional node metastasis [83].

According to their histologic subtype, penile carcinomas are subdivided into three risk groups for regional or systemic spread: verruciform tumors belong to the low-risk group, while about half of all penile cancers (including usual SCC and pleomorphic warty carcinomas) belong to the intermediate-risk group; the high-risk group comprises high-grade, deeply invasive tumors that are frequently metastatic at the onset, including basaloid, sarcomatoid, and adenosquamous carcinomas and poorly differentiated SCC.

Among the prognostic factors, histologic subtype was found to be less important than perineural invasion, histologic grade, and vascular invasion in multivariate analysis [18].

Proliferative Index and Molecular Prognostic Factors

Conflicting results have been reported in the literature about the relative risk of tumor metastasis according to different Ki67 values. Several recent series reported no correlation between proliferative index and survival, but two studies estimated a higher risk of lymph node metastasis in tumors with a high proportion of Ki67-positive tumor cells [89, 90].

Many different molecular prognostic factors have been investigated, but the enthusiasm for this research has dwindled because they lacked the levels of evidence for inclusion with a grade of recommendation in clinical practice guidelines [90, 91].

Among other factors, epithelial cadherin and MMP-9 [90], metastasis suppressor protein KAI1/CD82 [92], SOD2 [93], telomerase activity [94], squamous cell carcinoma antigen [95], cyclooxygenase expression (COX-1 and COX-2) [96], and genetic imbalances and ploidy status [97] have been investigated; they were reported to have different degrees of involvement in the pathogenesis of penile cancer and to be potential prognostic factors in this disease. Accumulation of p53 protein was found to be an independent predictor of lymph node metastases, with a significant correlation with poor outcome [54, 65].

Among oncologists dedicated to this pathology, the conviction is that "more research is needed to identify molecular markers which could lead to advances in personalized medicine" [91].

Local, Regional, and Systemic Spread

Local spread of the superficial spreading pattern of growth of penile cancers originating in the glans frequently shows extension to the coronal sulcus and foreskin, while foreskin carcinomas spread to the skin of the shaft, coronal sulcus, or glans. Similar growth features have been reported in intraepithelial pagetoid spread simulating Paget's disease [98]. The vertical growth pattern is associated with infiltration of anatomical levels and extension to the lamina propria, corpus spongiosum, albuginea, and corpora cavernosa. Extension to the penile fascia in cancer of the coronal sulcus involves deep penetration of the corpora cavernosa through the feeding vessels of the tunica albuginea, and rounded nodules of carcinoma ("satellite nodules") are sometimes observed separately from the main tumor mass in surgical samples. The importance of vascular (Fig. 13.39) and perineural invasion has been mentioned in the paragraph about prognostic factors.

Regional lymph node spread of penile cancer is common, while metastases to the pelvic nodes are less frequent and are mostly associated with inguinal lymph node involvement [74]. Anatomical variation of the sentinel lymph node, the first site of metastasis [99, 100], may interfere with the standardized protocol of lymph node dissection. Preoperative lymphoscintigraphy and dynamic sentinel node biopsy allow earlier detection of clinically negative metastatic lymph nodes, resulting in improved survival [70, 72, 73]. Systemic spread of penile cancer may involve the retroperitoneal nodes, periscrotal area, and subcutis of the abdomen (Fig. 13.40), heart, lung, bone, and liver.

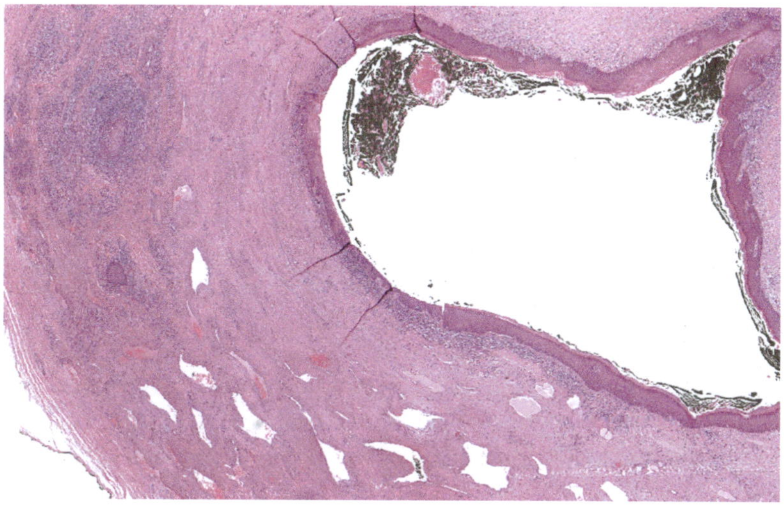

Fig. 13.39 Spread of penile cancer through the vessels of the urethral margin in a penectomy specimen

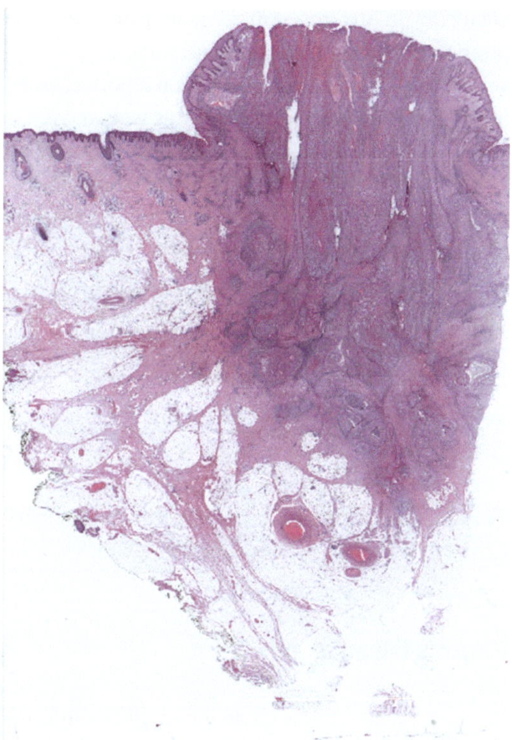

Fig. 13.40 Systemic spread of penile cancer. Squamous cell carcinoma located in the cutis of the abdomen

Positive Resection Margins and Recurrence

The prognosis of patients with recurrence after excision of penile carcinoma is dismal, with higher mortality in the subgroup of patients with recurrent tumors compared with the nonrecurrent subgroup [101]. This is the most important clinical consequence regarding the assessment of resection margins performed after penectomy or penile-preserving surgery [102]. It is still debated if local control can be obtained with margins measuring less than 10–15 mm in partial penectomies [103].

Accurate margin sampling in partial penectomies requires at least three sections: (1) urethra and periurethral tissue, (2) a section including both corpora cavernosa, and (3) the skin (foreskin or shaft with underlying dartos) [9]. In a series of 80 partial penectomies, 14 positive margins were observed [37]. Also other studies reported that local recurrences after limited surgical excision or partial penectomy are not uncommon [102]. Velazquez et al. reported involvement of the urethra and periurethral tissue including the penile fascia by carcinoma. They recommend frozen section examination of the urethral margin, which can be useful to detect tumor emboli within the lymphovascular spaces of the lamina propria and in the blood vessels of the periurethral corpus spongiosum [37]. Another common site of invasion of the glans is the coronal sulcus in cancers arising in the foreskin; a section of the sulcus has to be provided as margin. An uncommon site of positive resection margins is the corpus cavernosum, because of the barrier to tumor spread provided by the tunica albuginea. Leijte et al. analyzed the recurrence patterns in 700 patients from two referral centers for penile carcinoma

[104]. Patients receiving a penile-preserving procedure, those subjected to a wait-and-see policy for nodal status, and those with pN+ disease were at high risk of developing a recurrence, with an overall local recurrence rate after penile-preserving treatment of 27.7 %, of which 74.1 % occurring during the first 2 years [104].

Local recurrence increases the risk of regional inguinal and pelvic lymph node metastases [101]. Comparison of recurrent and nonrecurrent tumors showed that higher-grade tumors (i.e., basaloid and sarcomatoid) tended to be associated with recurrences, a finding that would dissuade clinicians from performing partial penectomies or local excisions in these aggressive variants [101].

Staging

The TNM classification of carcinomas of the penis is reported in Table 13.4. The classification is based on anatomical levels [79, 80], but it is known that the risk of metastases increases in tumors infiltrating more than 5 mm and is high when the corpora cavernosa in the glans and the dermis in the foreskin are affected. Further studies need to evaluate substaging of stage T2 to differentiate between superficial and deep corpus spongiosum infiltration and to take into account carcinomas of the penis limited to the foreskin, which are absent from the latest TNM classification.

Table 13.4 TNM staging system for penile carcinomas (UICC [88])

Primary tumor (T)
Tx primary tumor cannot be assessed
T0 no evidence of primary tumor
Tis carcinoma in situ; *Ta* noninvasive verrucous carcinoma
T1a tumor invades subepithelial connective tissue without lymphovascular invasion and is not poorly differentiated; *T1b* tumor invades subepithelial connective tissue with lymphovascular invasion or is poorly differentiated
T2 tumor invades corpus spongiosum or cavernosum
T3 tumor invades urethra
T4 tumor invades other adjacent structures (perineum, scrotum, prostate)
Regional lymph nodes (N)
N0 no regional lymph node metastasis
N1 metastasis in a single inguinal lymph node
N2 metastasis in multiple or bilateral inguinal lymph nodes
N3 extranodal extension of lymph node metastasis or metastasis in pelvic lymph nodes (unilateral or bilateral)
Distant metastasis (M)
M0 no distant metastasis
M1 distant metastasis

Other Tumors

Clear-Cell Carcinoma

The unusual clear-cell histologic type is a cancer occurring in the foreskin as a proliferation with prominent clear-cell changes and sometimes extensive necrosis. A few cases have been reported showing periodic acid-Schiff positivity as well as MUC1 and EMA immunostaining of the clear cells [105]. The clear-cell changes resemble the histologic features of renal cell carcinoma and are focally observed in some warty carcinomas of the penis. Clear-cell carcinoma is an HPV-related tumor with aggressive behavior which warrants radical treatment, i.e., total penectomy with groin dissection.

Giant Condyloma

This tumor, sometimes referred to as Buschke-Löwenstein tumor, is described in Chap. 12.

Paget's Disease

Primary Paget's disease is an intraepithelial growth of uncertain origin, sometimes originating from the apocrine ducts or sweat glands in the foreskin. It is characterized by basally located large atypical cells with abundant mucin-rich cytoplasm (Fig. 13.41).

Secondary Paget's disease is pagetoid intraepithelial spread of typical penile SCC [98] or – less frequently – of bladder or urethral carcinoma. This extension of adjacent tumors tends to affect the glans in the perimeatal region, extending to the perineum and scrotum.

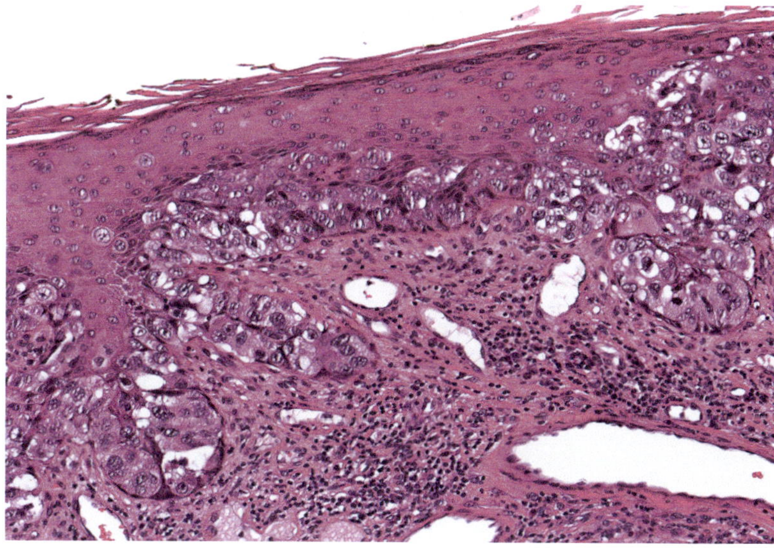

Fig. 13.41 Paget's disease. Large round atypical Paget's cells in the epithelium of the glans

Table 13.5 Immunohistochemistry of Paget's disease

Antibody	Paget's disease	Squamous cell CIS	Melanoma in situ	Urothelial carcinoma
CEA	+	–	–	–
CK7	+	–	–	+
CK20	–	–	–	+
GCDFP-15	+	–	–	–
S100	–	–	+	–
p63	±	+	–	+

Partially reported in Lopez-Beltran [106]

The immunohistochemical findings are quite peculiar: in Table 13.5 the immunostainings of extramammary Paget's disease and different penile tumors are presented.

Among these entities the most common is pagetoid urothelial carcinoma of the penis, where CK20 in addition to CK7 and p63 are useful immunohistochemical markers [107, 108]. A less frequent and less problematic lesion is clear-cell papulosis of the foreskin [109].

Melanoma of the Penis

Since the first description in the mid-nineteenth century, fewer than 100 cases of penile melanoma have been reported, accounting for approximately 1.4 % of all primary penile tumors [110]. Primary melanomas are mainly localized in the glans (Fig. 13.42) and have similar behavior to cutaneous melanoma, with comparable tumor thickness [111]. The adverse prognostic factors these tumors have in common are ulceration, tumor depth of 3.5 mm or more, and tumor diameter of >15 mm. The presence of lymph node metastasis at presentation carries a poor prognosis. Sometimes the presence of an in situ component may complicate the differential diagnosis with Paget's disease (Fig. 13.43). In such cases the expression of melanocytic markers (S100 protein, HMB45 protein, melan-A) can be helpful. A common presentation is mucous lentiginous melanoma, characterized by the proliferation of atypical melanocytes in the basal layer of the epidermis and by lengthening of the rete ridges as often seen in lentiginous tumors [112] (Fig. 13.44). Clinically it is easy to differentiate from penile melanosis, which is characterized by large pigmented macules affecting the glans and foreskin, and at the microscopic level by basal cell hyperpigmentation, stromal melanophages, and melanocytic hyperpla-

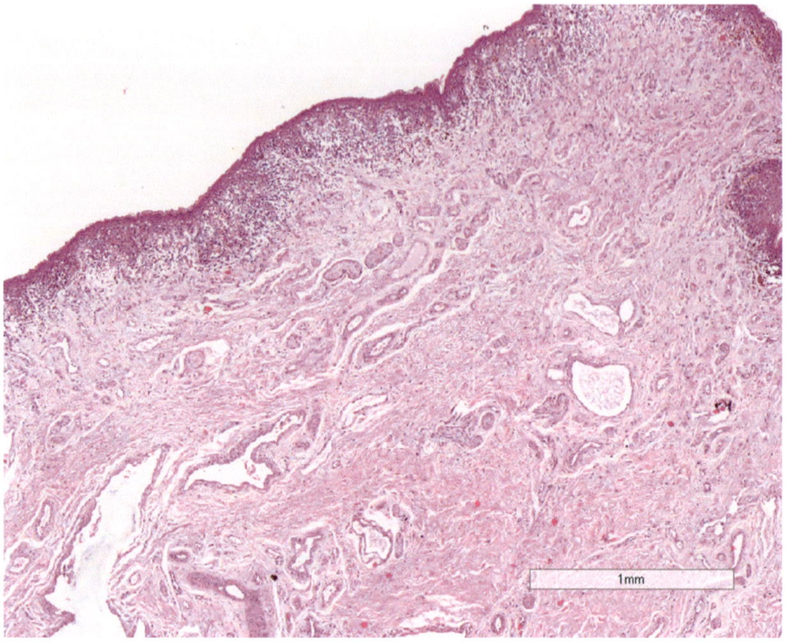

Fig. 13.42 Melanoma of the glans. Common presentation of melanoma in the glans as mucous lentiginous melanoma with marked inflammatory reaction in the dermis

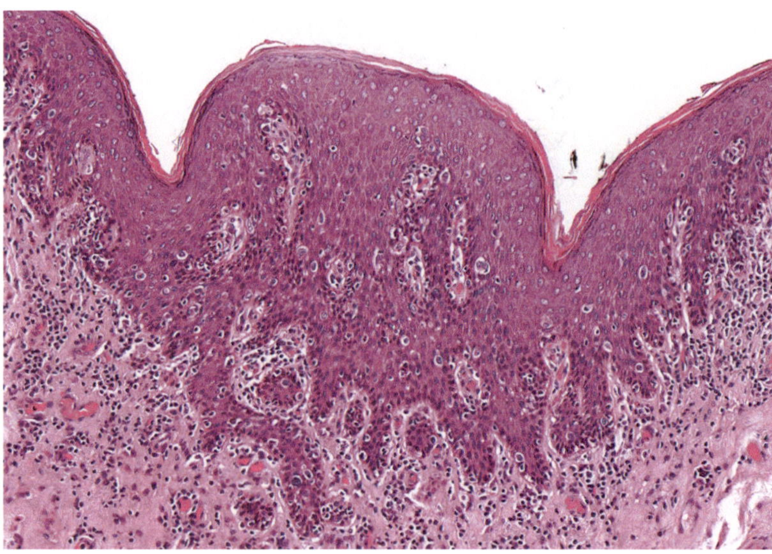

Fig. 13.43 Melanoma in situ. The presence of single, small nests of melanoma cells in the superficial layers of the glandular epithelium provides compelling evidence for in situ melanoma (Published with kind permission of ©Maurizio Colecchia 2015. All Rights Reserved)

sia [113]. The absence of cytologic atypia is a distinctive feature of this benign condition.

Soft Tissue Tumors

The most common sarcomas of the penis are those of vascular origin, including benign variants such as hemangioma, epithelioid hemangioma, angiokeratoma, and lymphangioma as well as malignant variants such as angiosarcoma, epithelioid hemangioendothelioma, and Kaposi sarcoma. Malignant tumors of myoid, fibrous, and neural etiology have also been described. It is particularly important for surgical pathologists, who rarely encounter these tumors, to distinguish sarcomas from sarcomatoid carcinomas [114].

Benign Soft Tissue Tumors

The majority of benign mesenchymal penile neoplasms including hemangiomas, lymphangiomas,

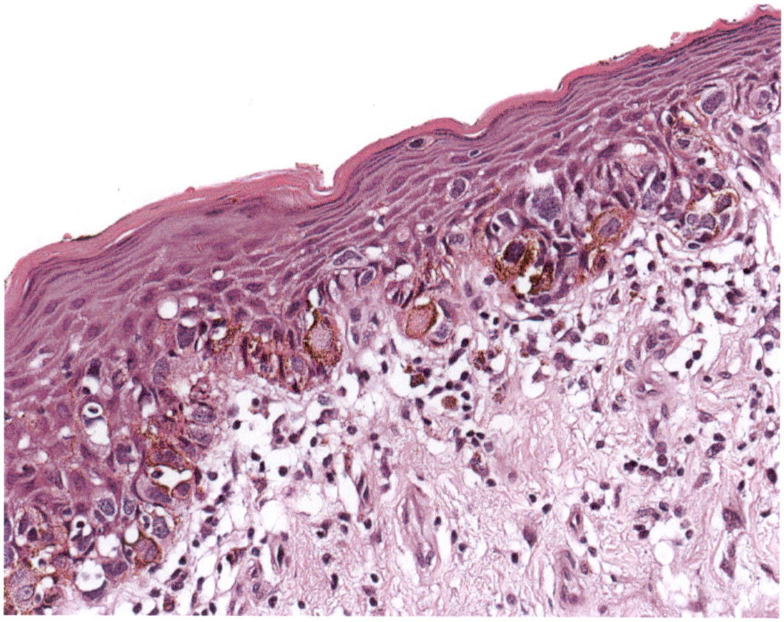

Fig. 13.44 Mucous lentiginous malignant melanoma of the penis. Basilar proliferation of atypical melanocytes in the basal layer

and epithelioid hemangiomas have been reported in case reports; the latter tumors are sometimes confused with epithelioid hemangioendothelioma or epithelioid angiosarcoma [115]. Other less common tumors are neurofibromas, schwannomas, granular cell tumors, leiomyomas, glomus tumors, dermatofibromas, myofibromas, and juvenile xanthogranulomas. Less commonly reported types are lipoma, angiolipoma, and nodular fasciitis [114]. Myointimoma is an unusual but distinct vascular benign tumor affecting the corpus spongiosum and originating from the vascular intima in young adults [116]. Microscopically the lesion is a myointimal intravascular plexiform lesion showing uniform myoid cells with minimal atypia [116, 117]. It can be managed with conservative surgery.

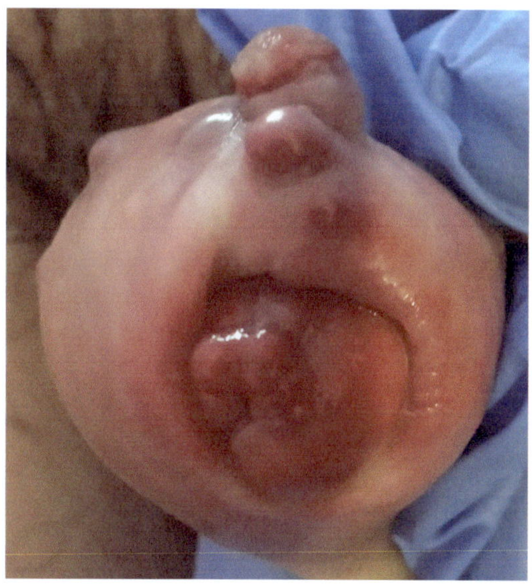

Fig. 13.45 Kaposi sarcoma. Multiple reddish nodules in the glans and foreskin of the penis (Courtesy of Dr T. Torelli, Istituto Nazionale dei Tumori, Milan, Italy. Published with kind permission of ©Maurizio Colecchia 2015. All Rights Reserved)

Malignant Soft Tissue Tumors

Kaposi sarcoma is by far the most common malignant soft tissue tumor affecting the penis [9]. It exists in several different clinical subtypes, all displaying similar microscopic features. Kaposi sarcoma in young adults affects individuals with underlying immunodeficiency caused by HIV infection, immunosuppressive or chemotherapeutic medication, lymphomas, or inherited syndromes. The most common location is the glans, where Kaposi sarcoma presents as purple papules or nodules (Fig. 13.45), which, in well-established lesions, show extravasated erythrocytes, vessels encircling vessels, and the characteristic spindle cell proliferation admixed

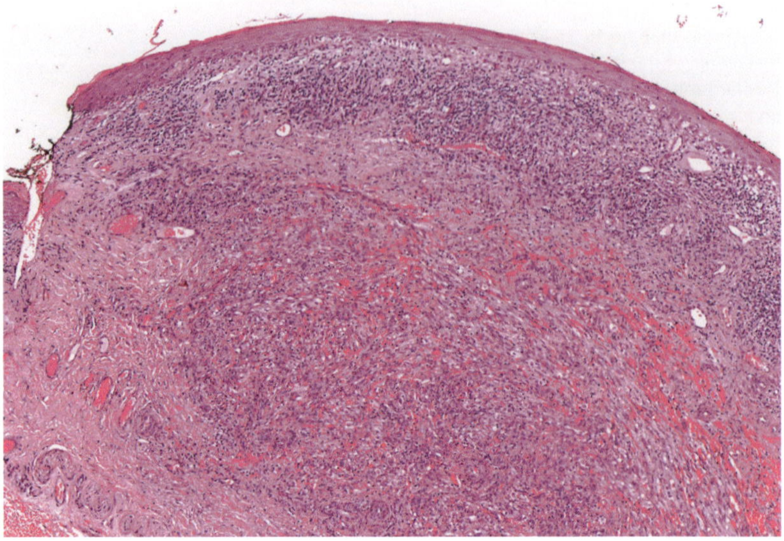

Fig. 13.46 Kaposi sarcoma. Microscopic appearance of the case of Fig. 13.45 showing multiple nodules of Kaposi sarcoma with spindle cell proliferation admixed with slit-like vessels

with slit-like vessels (Fig. 13.46). Tumor cells show nuclear positivity for human herpes virus 8 (HHV-8) staining, which is confirmative of the diagnosis [118, 119].

Leiomyosarcoma

Leiomyosarcoma of the penis is a very rare disease of mid and late adult life [120], arising from both superficial and deep smooth muscle elements. All deep-seated tumors are presumed to be of vascular (corpus cavernosum and corpus spongiosum) origin, while the superficial tumors occur as circumscribed nodules probably derived from the superficial vasculature of the penis or as infiltrative lesions probably derived from the dartos [121].

The most accurate predictors of outcome are tumor depth [122] and size, but only well-demarcated deep-seated tumors require partial or total penectomy, while superficial leiomyosarcomas can be treated with conservative surgery. All tumors contain smooth muscle cells with blunt-ended sometimes pleomorphic nuclei that form fascicles. Tumor growth pattern, mitotic count, and grading are the distinguishing microscopic features. The main differential diagnoses are leiomyoma, myointimoma, nodular Kaposi sarcoma, malignant fibrous histiocytoma, and sarcomatoid carcinoma. Kaposi sarcoma is more frequent than leiomyosarcoma (2:1), and its diagnostic clues (see paragraph on Kaposi sarcoma) in superficial lesions can resemble the fascicular architecture of leiomyosarcoma. Strong reactivity for CD34 and CD31 and the absence of desmin and factor VIII immunostains distinguish nodular Kaposi sarcoma from leiomyosarcoma, which shows alpha muscle actin-positive and HHF35-positive immunostains as well.

Epithelioid Sarcoma

This highly unusual entity occurs either as single or multiple superficial penile nodules or urethral stenosis, symptoms that epithelioid sarcoma shares with Peyronie's disease [123]. Progressive growth should suggest a malignancy and warrant biopsy, because epithelioid sarcoma requires prompt and aggressive intervention. Histologically, epithelioid sarcoma is characterized by spindle and epithelioid cells with eosinophilic cytoplasm, often surrounding an area of central necrosis with a pseudogranulomatous appearance. The epithelioid cells have moderate atypia with vesicular nuclei and prominent nucleoli [124] (Fig. 13.47).

Positive immunostaining for vimentin, EMA, CD99, and CD34 (in 70 % of cases) allows the differential diagnosis with other soft tissue tumors

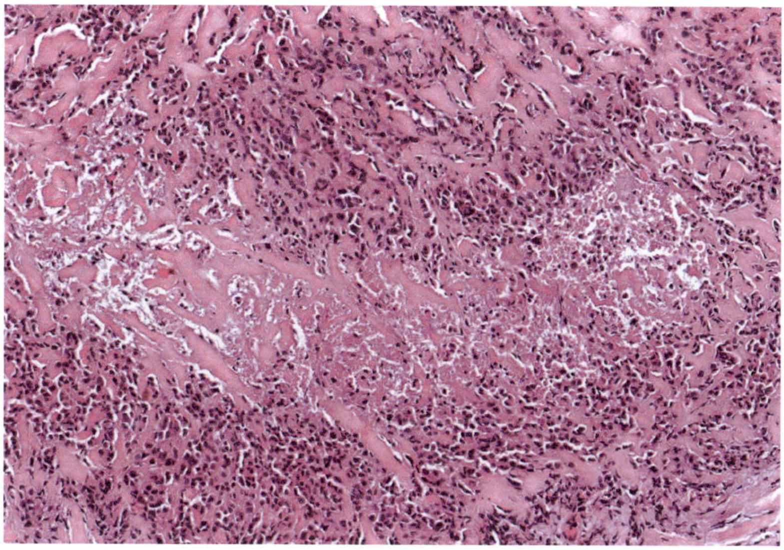

Fig. 13.47 Epithelioid sarcoma. Epithelioid cells with eosinophilic cytoplasm surrounding an area of necrosis

Table 13.6 Typical immunohistochemical staining profile of soft tissue tumors

Neoplasm	Typical immunohistochemical staining profile
Sarcomatoid squamous cell carcinoma	
Sarcomatoid urothelial carcinoma	AE1/AE3 +, EMA +, vimentin +, p53 *variable*, actin -, desmin -, S100 -, CD34 -
Leiomyosarcoma	Desmin +, MSA (HHF35) +, may show keratin *focal*, EMA *focal*, CD34 *focal*, S100 *focal*
Kaposi sarcoma	CD31 +, CD34 +, HHV-8 +, factor VIII -, desmin -
Spindle cell melanoma	S100 +, HMB45 +, melan-A/MART-1 +, microphthalmia transcription factor +, tyrosinase +
Desmoplastic melanoma	S100 +, MSA (HHF35) + (58 % of cases), HMB45 -, melan-A/MART-1 -, microphthalmia transcription factor -, tyrosinase -, may show NSE +, EMA +, NKI/C-3 +, alpha-SMA +
Dermatofibrosarcoma protuberans	CD34 +, factor XIIIa -, t(17;22) by FISH
Rhabdomyosarcoma	Myogenin +, desmin +, MSA (HHF35) +, t(2;13), or t(1;13) in alveolar variant
Myointimoma (not typically a spindle cell neoplasm)	MSA (HHF35) +, alpha-SMA +, calponin +, desmin *minimal reactivity*

(see Table 13.6). A case of pediatric epithelioid sarcoma has been reported [125]. Most recurrences and metastases develop within 3 years of treatment, but late metastases may occur.

Lymphomas

Lymphomas are very infrequently observed as primary penile tumors or secondary localizations of systemic disease. Histiocytic tumors are rare. Priapism has been reported secondary to leukemia in a highly uncommon case [126]. When penile lymphomas do occur, they are mostly non-Hodgkin B-cell lymphomas of the diffuse large-cell type (Fig. 13.48), although other infrequent subtypes may occur including mucosa-associated lymphoid tissue (MALT) lymphoma and T-cell, anaplastic large-cell, and CD30-positive lymphomas. Chemotherapy is generally effective [127].

Metastatic Tumors of the Penis

Metastases to the penis from any kind of tumor are rare. The most common sites of origin are the urinary bladder and prostate, followed by the kidney, gastrointestinal tract, and testis

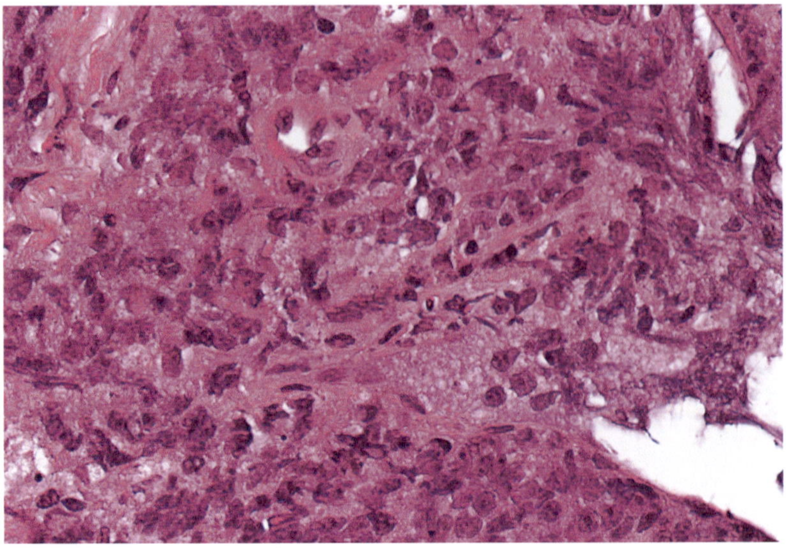

Fig. 13.48 B-cell non-Hodgkin lymphoma. Biopsy of the glans with artifacts showing diffuse large B-cell-type non-Hodgkin lymphoma

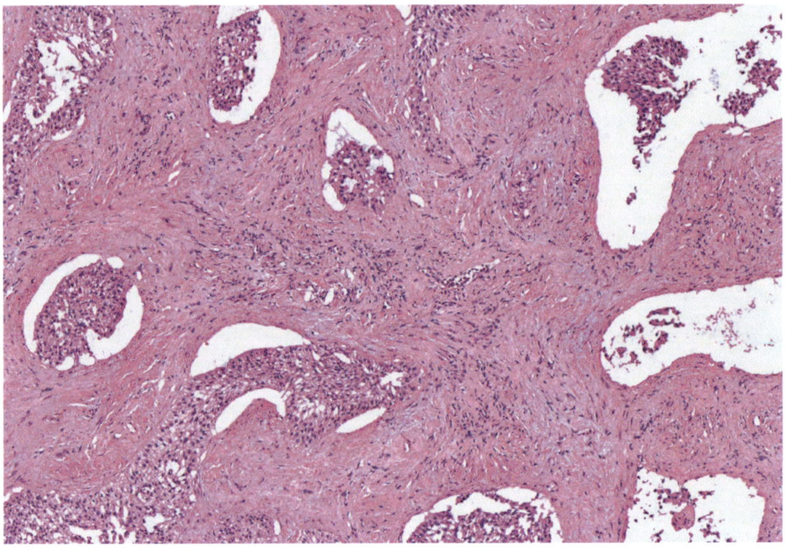

Fig. 13.49 Urothelial carcinoma metastatic to the glans. Angioinvasion in the corpus cavernosum with urothelial aggregates from a metastatic bladder carcinoma

(seminomatous germ cell tumors as well as embryonal carcinomas). Nonpelvic organs have been less frequently reported as primary sites, e.g., the lung, stomach, and pancreas [128, 129]. Commonly the metastasis occurs in the corpus cavernosum of the shaft [129]. Presentation with multiple palpable nodules is frequent, but in almost half of the cases, a prominent clinical finding is priapism ("malignant priapism") [130]. A frequent observation is extension to the glans of urethral urothelial carcinoma (Fig. 13.49).

Tumorlike Lesions

Peyronie's Disease

Peyronie's disease is characterized by a fibrous plaque or scar within the tunica albuginea of the penile shaft, producing an abnormal curvature of the penis [131]. Its pathogenesis appears to be multifactorial, but from a histologic point of view, Peyronie's disease seems strictly related to superficial fibromatosis [9] and persistent chronic inflammation, probably as a result of repetitive stress microtrauma to the penis [132], urethral instrumentation, hypertension, and other factors [9]. The hallmark of the disease, that is to say the fibrous plaque, involves fibroblasts and myofibroblasts, but frequently the lesion is sclerotic with hypocellular areas and in rare cases calcification or ossification admixed with some inflammatory cells. Increased levels of transforming growth factor β1 seem to play a role in the development of the fibrotic plaques [133]. Treatment is mainly surgical, but rare spontaneous regression has been reported.

Lichen Sclerosus et Atrophicus

See Chap. 12.

Melanosis (Lentiginosis)

Melanosis is characterized by large pigmented macules, often multifocal and with irregular borders, affecting the glans and foreskin. Histology shows basal layer hyperpigmentation, epithelial and melanocytic hyperplasia, and stromal melanophages. The lesion has the potential to enlarge, and the absence of melanocytic atypia is a hallmark of this benign condition [113].

Frozen Section

The main indications for frozen sections in penile cancer are examination of the surgical margins and assessment of the nodal status; microscopic tumor is present in 5–30 % of partial penectomies, and frozen section examination of resection margins can lead to a reduction of the incidence of positive surgical margins and recurrence in SCC [103]. Intraoperative examination of the surgical margins includes the skin, corpora cavernosa, corpus spongiosum, urethra, and periurethral tissue. In the majority of surgical margins examined during partial or total penectomies, shaved margins are taken [134].

The most frequent sites of involvement by carcinoma are the periurethral corpus spongiosum, lamina propria, and urethra. Frozen sections are not commonly done in total penectomies, but in superficial spreading carcinoma, possible extension to the skin of the shaft requires surgical margin evaluation. The use of frozen section examination for sentinel lymph node biopsies is controversial [135]. Clinical examination and imaging techniques remain inaccurate for detecting micrometastases. In some centers frozen section is performed in sentinel node biopsy for patients with poorly differentiated, high-grade SCC [134]. Cytologic imprint preparation could be useful to detect metastases [136]. Other details about the pathological assessment of frozen section examination in penile specimens are reported in Chap. 14.

Malignant Lesions of the Scrotum

Squamous Cell Carcinoma

Improved hygiene conditions have led to a marked decrease in the incidence of scrotal carcinoma [9]. This tumor is linked to numerous occupational carcinogens, but nowadays the incidence is 5–10 cases per 10 million population in the USA [9]. The historical importance of occupational carcinogens is exemplified by Percivall Pott's investigation into the incidence of scrotal carcinoma in chimney sweeps, as mentioned in the 2011 Pulitzer Prize winning book by Siddhartha Mukherjee [137]. Most scrotal carcinomas are well to moderately differentiated keratinizing SCCs. SCC of the scrotum is considered and staged as skin carcinoma [9]. Unusual variants (basaloid, papillary, verrucous) are exceptional occurrences in this rare tumor. The presence of dysplastic changes in the epithelium adjacent to the tumor and possible analogies with precancerous conditions of the penis suggest that the HPV-related variant and differentiated squamous intraepithelial lesions have an analogous appearance to penile precursor lesions [11].

Extramammary Paget's Disease

The male genitalia were the first extramammary site described by Crocker as the site of Paget's disease [138]. It is a very unusual neoplasm with

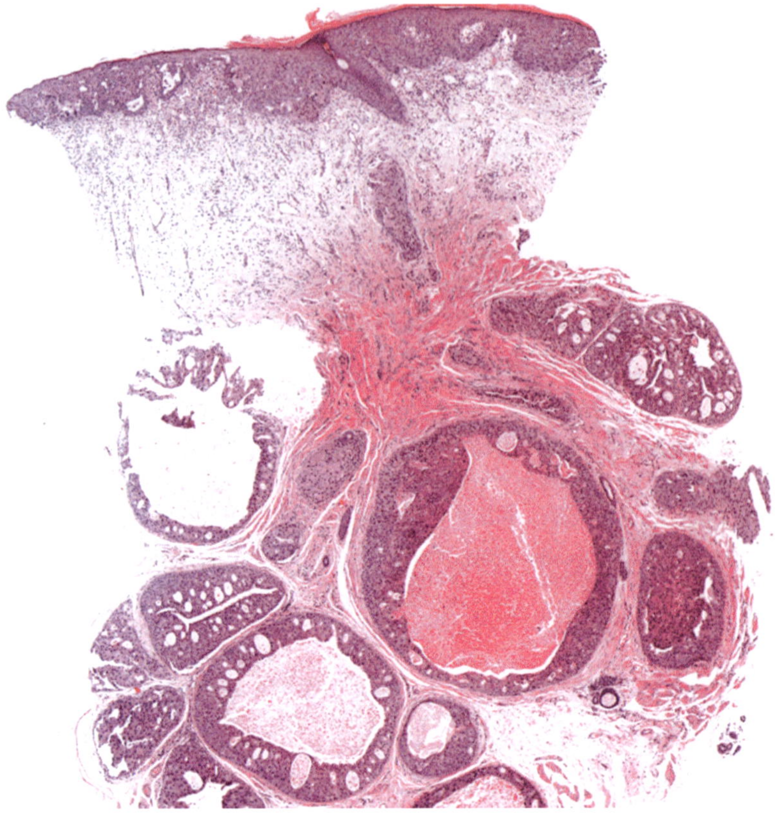

Fig. 13.50 Paget's disease of the scrotum. The epidermis of the scrotum colonized by a population of large, round, or oval atypical cells (Paget's cells) with clear cytoplasm and vesicular nuclei; there are gland-like neoplastic foci with the appearance of tubular glands in the reticular dermis (Published with kind permission of ©Maurizio Colecchia 2015. All Rights Reserved)

fewer than 30 cases reported at the beginning of this century [139].

On physical examination scrotal Paget's disease manifests as an erythematous, eczematoid lesion that is difficult to distinguish from Bowen's disease or in situ carcinoma. Pathognomonic Paget's cells (atypical large, clear, round cells) are observed with intraepidermal localization, rarely involving the dermis. This tumor is presumed to be an intraepidermal adenocarcinoma. Like mammary Paget's disease, scrotal lesions may be the result of epidermotropic spread from an underlying adnexal malignancy (Fig. 13.50) [140], also when secondary involvement of acrosyringeal structures can be observed. Other uncommon sites of extraepidermal origin are the colon-rectum and the urogenital tract [9]. Immunohistochemical findings include the expression of CEA, low-molecular-weight cytokeratins (CK7), CAM 5.2, EMA (Fig. 13.51), mucicarmine, MUC1, and gross cystic disease fluid protein 15 (GCDFP-15) [108]. Local excision may be useful with intraoperative examination of the margins. When radical surgery is difficult to accomplish due to the size of the lesion, topical chemotherapy followed by wide excision and a reconstructive procedure is the treatment of choice.

Basal Cell Carcinoma

Fewer than 50 cases of scrotal BCC have been reported to date [141], even if in terms of incidence it is the third most common malignant scrotal tumor. The differential diagnosis with basaloid SCC is important because of the dismal prognosis of the latter. While scrotal BCC shows the same histopathologic features as its nongenital cutaneous counterpart, it appears to be more aggressive.

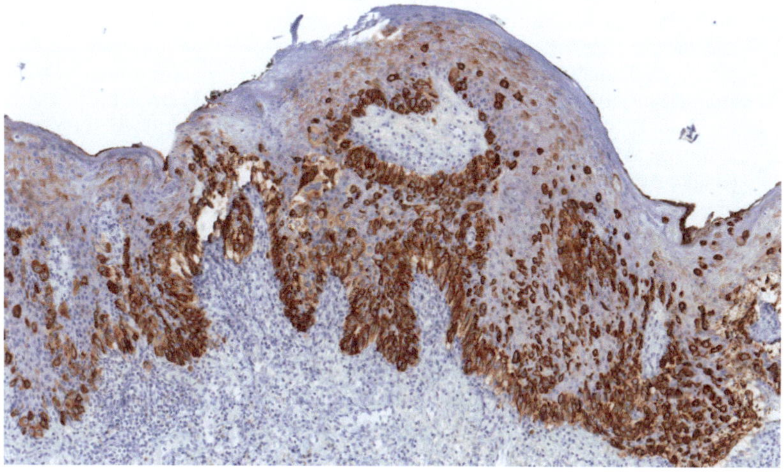

Fig. 13.51 EMA immunostaining in Paget's disease of the scrotum. Immunohistochemical stain of Paget's disease of the scrotum reported in Fig. 13.50 shows diffuse reactivity with epithelial membrane antigen (EMA)

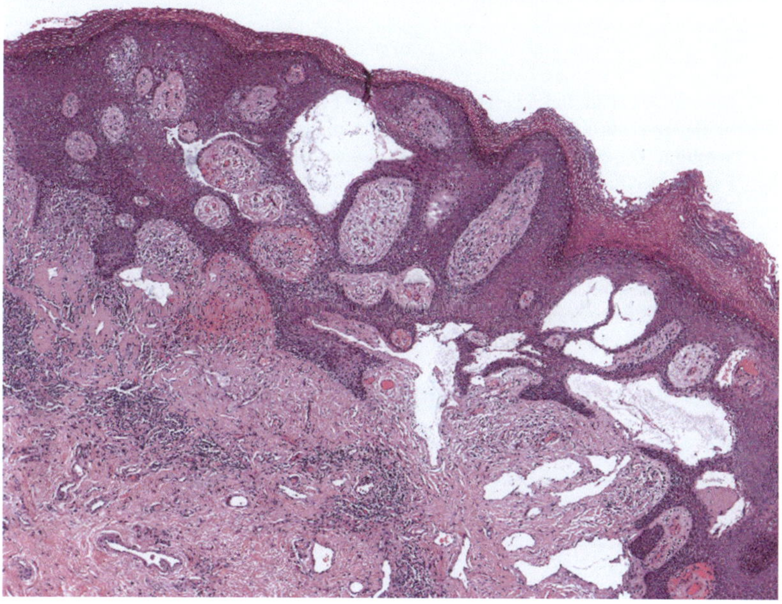

Fig. 13.52 Lymphangioma. Scrotal lymphangioma occurring with scrotal discomfort: the empty spaces devoid of blood have delicate valves. A thin smooth muscle wall is present

Other Lesions

Anecdotal examples of other benign and malignant lesions of the scrotum have been reported mostly as case reports. They included hemangiomas, lymphangiomas (Fig. 13.52), lipomas, granular cell tumors, schwannomas, solitary fibrous tumors, angiomyxomas, and very rare scrotal sarcomas (leiomyosarcoma, liposarcoma, epithelioid sarcoma, rhabdomyosarcoma) [142]. Tumor histology is one of the most important independent prognostic factors [143].

References

1. Cubilla AL, Reuter V, Velazquez E, Piris A, Saito S, Young RH. Histologic classification of penile carcinoma and its relation to outcome in 61 patients with primary resection. Int J Surg Pathol. 2001;9:111–20.
2. Chaux A, Lezcano C, Cubilla AL, Tamboli P, Ro J, Ayala A. Comparison of subtypes of penile squamous cell carcinoma from high and low incidence geographical regions. Int J Surg Pathol. 2010;18:268–77.
3. Chaux A, Velazquez EF, Amin A, Soskin A, Pfannl R, Rodríguez IM, Barreto JE, Lezcano C, Ayala G,

Netto GJ, Cubilla AL. Distribution and characterization of subtypes of penile intraepithelial neoplasia and their association with invasive carcinomas: a pathological study of 139 lesions in 121 patients. Hum Pathol. 2012;43:1020–7.
4. Gregoire L, Cubilla AL, Reuter VE, Haas GP, Lancaster WD. Preferential association of human papillomavirus with high-grade histologic variants of penile-invasive squamous cell carcinoma. J Natl Cancer Inst. 1995;87:1705–9.
5. Miralles-Guri C, Bruni L, Cubilla AL, Castellsagué X, Bosch FX, de Sanjosé S. Human papillomavirus prevalence and type distribution in penile carcinoma. J Clin Pathol. 2009;62:870–8.
6. Mentrikoski MJ, Stelow EB, Culp S, Frierson Jr HF, Cathro HP. Histologic and immunohistochemical assessment of penile carcinomas in a North American population. Am J Surg Pathol. 2014;38:1340–8.
7. Chaux A, Cubilla AL. The role of human papillomavirus infection in the pathogenesis of penile squamous cell carcinomas. Semin Diagn Pathol. 2012;29:67–71.
8. Chaux A, Velazquez EF, Algaba F, Ayala G, Cubilla AL. Developments in the pathology of penile squamous cell carcinomas. Urology. 2010;76:S7–14.
9. Epstein JH, Cubilla AL, Humphrey PA. Tumors of the prostate gland, seminal vesicles, penis and scrotum. Washington, DC: American Registry of Pathology AFIP Atlas of tumor pathology 3rd series, 2011. Fascicle 14, p. 405–612.
10. Longpre MJ, Lange PH, Kwon JS, Black PC. Penile carcinoma: lessons learned from vulvar carcinoma. J Urol. 2013;189:17–24.
11. Velazquez EF, Amin MB, Cubilla AL. Penis and scrotum. Chapter 14. In: Amin MB, Eble JN, Grignon DJ, Srigley JR, editors. Urologic pathology. Philadelphia: Lippincott Williams and Wilkins; 2014.
12. Velazquez EF, Cubilla AL. Lichen sclerosus in 68 patients with squamous cell carcinoma of the penis: frequent atypias and correlation with special carcinoma variants suggests a precancerous role. Am J Surg Pathol. 2003;27:1448–53.
13. Oertell J, Duarte S, Ayala J, Chaux A, Velazquez EF, Cubilla AL. Squamous cell carcinoma (SCC) exclusive of the foreskin: distinctive association with low grade variants, multicentricity and lichen sclerosus. Mod Pathol. 2002;15:175A.
14. Fukunaga M, Yokoi K, Miyazawa Y, Harada T, Ushigome S. Penile verrucous carcinoma with anaplastic transformation following radiotherapy. A case report with human papillomavirus typing and flow cytometric DNA studies. Am J Surg Pathol. 1994;18:501–5.
15. Sanchez DF, Canete S, Fernandez-Nestosa MJ, Lezcano C, Rodriguez I, Barreto J, Alvarado-Cabreo I, Cubilla AL. HPV- and non-HPV-related subtypes of penile squamous cell carcinoma (SCC): morphological features and differential diagnosis according to the new WHO classification (2015). Semin Diagn Pathol. 2015;32:198–221.
16. Chaux A, Velazquez EF, Barreto JE, Ayala E, Cubilla AL. New pathologic entities in penile carcinomas: an update of the 2004 World Health Organization classification. Semin Diagn Pathol. 2012;29:59–66.
17. Velazquez EF, Barreto JE, Rodriguez I, Piris A, Cubilla AL. Limitations in the interpretation of biopsies in patients with penile squamous cell carcinoma. Int J Surg Pathol. 2004;12:139–46.
18. Guimarães GC, Cunha IW, Soares FA, Lopes A, Torres J, Chaux A, Velazquez EF, Ayala G, Cubilla AL. Penile squamous cell carcinoma clinicopathological features, nodal metastasis and outcome in 333 cases. J Urol. 2009;182:528–34.
19. Kurman RJ, Toki T, Schiffman MH. Basaloid and warty carcinomas of the vulva. Distinctive types of squamous cell carcinoma frequently associated with human papillomaviruses. Am J Surg Pathol. 1993;17:133–45.
20. Davies SW. Giant condyloma acuminata: incidence among cases diagnosed as carcinoma of the penis. J Clin Pathol. 1965;18:142–9.
21. Cubilla AL, Velazques EF, Reuter VE, Oliva E, Mihm Jr MC, Young RH. Warty (condylomatous) squamous cell carcinoma of the penis: a report of 11 cases and proposed classification of 'verruciform' penile tumors. Am J Surg Pathol. 2000;24:505–12.
22. Epstein JI, Netto GJ. Differential diagnosis in surgical pathology: genitourinary system. Chapter 5: penis/scrotum. Philadelphia: Lippincott Williams and Wilkins; 2014.
23. Bezerra AL, Lopes A, Landman G, Alencar GN, Torloni H, Villa LL. Clinicopathologic features and human papillomavirus dna prevalence of warty and squamous cell carcinoma of the penis. Am J Surg Pathol. 2001;25:673–8.
24. Cubilla AL, Lloveras B, Alejo M, Clavero O, Chaux A, Kasamatsu E, Monfulleda N, Tous S, Alemany L, Klaustermeier J, Muñoz N, Quint W, de Sanjose S, Bosch FX. Value of p16(INK)[4](a) in the pathology of invasive penile squamous cell carcinomas: A report of 202 cases. Am J Surg Pathol. 2011;35: 253–61.
25. Chan KW, Lam KY, Chan AC, Lau P, Srivastava G. Prevalence of human papillomavirus types 16 and 18 in penile carcinoma: a study of 41 cases using PCR. J Clin Pathol. 1994;47:823–6.
26. Johnson DE, Lo RK, Srigley J, Ayala AG. Verrucous carcinoma of the penis. J Urol. 1985;133:216–8.
27. Stankiewicz E, Kudahetti SC, Prowse DM, Ktori E, Cuzick J, Ambroisine L, Zhang X, Watkin N, Corbishley C, Berney DM. HPV infection and immunochemical detection of cell-cycle markers in verrucous carcinoma of the penis. Mod Pathol. 2009;22:1160–8.
28. Masih AS, Stoler MH, Farrow GM, Wooldridge TN, Johansson SL. Penile verrucous carcinoma: a clinicopathologic, human papillomavirus typing and flow cytometric analysis. Mod Pathol. 1992;5:48–55.
29. Mukai S, Nakahara K, Nagai T, Kamibeppu T, Sugie S, Tsukino H, Kamimura T, Wakeda H, Kamoto

T. Pure verrucous carcinoma of the penis: two cases. Med Surg Urol. 2014;3:125–7.

30. Chaux A, Soares F, Rodríguez I, Barreto J, Lezcano C, Torres J, Velazquez EF, Cubilla AL. Papillary squamous cell carcinoma, not otherwise specified (NOS) of the penis: clinicopathologic features, differential diagnosis, and outcome of 35 cases. Am J Surg Pathol. 2010;34:223–30.
31. Cubilla AL, Lloveras B, Alejo M, Clavero O, Chaux A, Kasamatsu E, Velazquez EF, Lezcano C, Monfulleda N, Tous S, Alemany L, Klaustermeier J, Muñoz N, Quint W, de Sanjose S, Bosch FX. The basaloid cell is the best tissue marker for human papillomavirus in invasive penile squamous cell carcinoma: a study of 202 cases from Paraguay. Am J Surg Pathol. 2010;34:104–14.
32. Cubilla AL, Velazquez EF, Ayala GE, Chaux A, Torres J, Reuter V. Identification of prognostic pathologic parameters in squamous cell carcinoma of the penis: significance and difficulties. Pathol Case Rev. 2005;10:3–13.
33. Barreto JE, Velazquez EF, Ayala E, Torres J, Cubilla AL. Carcinoma cuniculatum: a distinctive variant of penile squamous cell carcinoma: report of 7 cases. Am J Surg Pathol. 2007;31:71–5.
34. Seehafer JR, Rahman D, Soderstrom CW. Epithelioma cuniculatum: verrucous carcinoma of the foot. Cutis. 1979;23:287–90.
35. Kathuria S, Rieker J, Jablokow VR, Van den Broek H. Plantar verrucous carcinoma (epithelioma cuniculatum): case report with review of the literature. J Surg Oncol. 1986;31:71–5.
36. Reuter VE. Sarcomatoid lesions of the urogenital tract. Semin Diagn Pathol. 1993;10:188–201.
37. Velazquez EF, Soskin A, Bock A, Codas R, Barreto JE, Cubilla AL. Positive resection margins in partial penectomies: sites of involvement and proposal of local routes of spread of penile squamous cell carcinoma. Am J Surg Pathol. 2004;28:384–9.
38. Velazquez EF, Melamed J, Barreto JE, Aguero F, Cubilla AL. Sarcomatoid carcinoma of the penis: a clinicopathologic study of 15 cases. Am J Surg Pathol. 2005;29:1152–8.
39. Cubilla AL, Reuter VE, Gregoire L, Ayala G, Ocampos S, Lancaster WD, Fair W. Basaloid squamous cell carcinoma: a distinctive human papilloma virus-related penile neoplasm: a report of 20 cases. Am J Surg Pathol. 1998;22:755–61.
40. Soskin A, Vieillefond A, Carlotti A, Plantier F, Chaux A, Ayala G, Velazquez EF, Cubilla AL. Warty/basaloid penile intraepithelial neoplasia is more prevalent than differentiated penile intraepithelial neoplasia in nonendemic regions for penile cancer when compared with endemic areas: a comparative study between pathologic series from Paris and Paraguay. Hum Pathol. 2012;43:190–6.
41. Winters R, Trotman W, Adamson CS, Rajendran V, Tang A, Elhosseiny A, Evans MF. Screening for human papillomavirus in basaloid squamous carcinoma: utility of p16(INK4a), CISH, and PCR. Int J Surg Pathol. 2011;19:309–14.
42. Cubilla AL, Lloveras B, Alemany L, Alejo M, Vidal A, Kasamatsu E, Clavero O, Alvarado-Cabrero I, Lynch C, Velasco-Alonso J, Ferrera A, Chaux A, Klaustermeier J, Quint W, de Sanjosé S, Muñoz N, Bosch FX. Basaloid squamous cell carcinoma of the penis with papillary features: a clinicopathologic study of 12 cases. Am J Surg Pathol. 2012;36:869–75.
43. Rubin MA, Kleter B, Zhou M, Ayala G, Cubilla AL, Quint WG, Pirog EC. Detection and typing of human papillomavirus DNA in penile carcinoma: evidence for multiple independent pathways of penile carcinogenesis. Am J Pathol. 2001;159:1211–8.
44. Cubilla AL, Velazquez EF, Young RH. Pseudohyperplastic squamous cell carcinoma of the penis associated with lichen sclerosus. An extremely well-differentiated, nonverruciform neoplasm that preferentially affects the foreskin and is frequently misdiagnosed: a report of 10 cases of a distinctive clinicopathologic entity. Am J Surg Pathol. 2004;28:895–900.
45. Cunha IW, Guimaraes GC, Soares F, Velazquez E, Torres JJ, Chaux A, Ayala G, Cubilla AL. Pseudoglandular (adenoid, acantholytic) penile squamous cell carcinoma: a clinicopathologic and outcome study of 7 patients. Am J Surg Pathol. 2009;33:551–5.
46. Colecchia M, Insabato L. Pseudoglandular (adenoid, acantholytic) penile squamous cell carcinoma. Am J Surg Pathol. 2009;33:1421–2.
47. Cubilla AL, Ayala MT, Barreto JE, Bellasai JG, Nöel JC. Surface adenosquamous carcinoma of the penis. A report of three cases. Am J Surg Pathol. 1996;20:156–60.
48. Masera A, Ovcak Z, Volavsek M, Bracko M. Adenosquamous carcinoma of the penis. J Urol. 1997;157:2261.
49. Chaux A, Tamboli P, Ayala A, Soares F, Rodríguez I, Barreto J, Cubilla AL. Warty-basaloid carcinoma: clinicopathological features of a distinctive penile neoplasm. Report of 45 cases. Mod Pathol. 2010;23:896–904.
50. Chaux A, Pfannl R, Lloveras B, Alejo M, Clavero O, Lezcano C, Muñoz N, de Sanjosé S, Bosch X, Hernández-Pérez M, Velazquez EF, Cubilla AL. Distinctive association of p16INK4a overexpression with penile intraepithelial neoplasia depicting warty and/or basaloid features: a study of 141 cases evaluating a new nomenclature. Am J Surg Pathol. 2010;34:385–92.
51. Kato N, Onozuka T, Yasukawa K, Kimura K, Sasaki K. Penile hybrid verrucous-squamous carcinoma associated with a superficial inguinal lymph node metastasis. Am J Dermatopathol. 2000;22:339–43.
52. Velazquez EF, Ayala G, Liu H, Chaux A, Zanotti M, Torres J, Cho SI, Barreto JE, Soares F, Cubilla AL. Histologic grade and perineural invasion are more important than tumor thickness as predictor

of nodal metastasis in penile squamous cell carcinoma invading 5 to 10 mm. Am J Surg Pathol. 2008;32:974–9.
53. IARC Monograph Working Group. A review of human carcinogens-Part B: biological agents. Lancet Oncol. 2009;10:321–2.
54. Lont AP, Kroon BK, Horenblas S, Gallee MP, Berkhof J, Meijer CJ, Snijders PJ. Presence of high-risk human papillomavirus DNA in penile carcinoma predicts favorable outcome in survival. Int J Cancer. 2006;119:1078–81.
55. Ferreux E, Lont AP, Horenblas S, Gallee MP, Raaphorst FM, von Knebel Doeberitz M, Meijer CJ, Snijders PJ. Evidence for at least three alternative mechanisms targeting the p16INK4A/cyclin D/Rb pathway in penile carcinoma, one of which is mediated by high-risk human papillomavirus. J Pathol. 2003;201:109–18.
56. Sano T, Oyama T, Kashiwabara K, Fukuda T, Nakajima T. Expression status of p16 protein is associated with human papillomavirus oncogenic potential in cervical and genital lesions. Am J Pathol. 1998;153:1741–8.
57. Chaux A, Cubilla AL, Haffner MC, Lecksell KL, Sharma R, Burnett AL, Netto GJ. Combining routine morphology, p16(INK4a) immunohistochemistry, and in situ hybridization for the detection of human papillomavirus infection in penile carcinomas: a tissue microarray study using classifier performance analyses. Urol Oncol. 2014;32:171–7.
58. Bezerra AL, Lopes A, Santiago GH, Ribeiro KC, Latorre MR, Villa LL. Human papillomavirus as a prognostic factor in carcinoma of the penis: analysis of 82 patients treated with amputation and bilateral lymphadenectomy. Cancer. 2001;91:2315–21.
59. Gunia S, Erbersdobler A, Hakenberg OW, Koch S, May M. p16(INK4a) is a marker of good prognosis for primary invasive penile squamous cell carcinoma: a multi-institutional study. J Urol. 2012;187:899–907.
60. Djajadiningrat RS, Jordanova ES, Kroon BK, van Werkhoven E, de Jong J, Pronk DT, Snijders PJ, Horenblas S, Heideman DA. Human papillomavirus prevalence in invasive penile cancer and association with clinical outcome. J Urol. 2015;193:526–31.
61. Bezerra SM, Chaux A, Ball MW, Faraj SF, Munari E, Gonzalez-Roibon N, Sharma R, Bivalacqua TJ, Burnett AL, Netto GJ. Human papillomavirus infection and immunohistochemical p16(INK4a) expression as predictors of outcome in penile squamous cell carcinomas. Hum Pathol. 2015;46:532–40.
62. Stankiewicz E, Prowse DM, Ng M, Cuzick J, Mesher D, Hiscock F, Lu YJ, Watkin N, Corbishley C, Lam W, Berney DM. Alternative HER/PTEN/Akt pathway activation in HPV positive and negative penile carcinomas. PLoS One. 2011;6:e17517.
63. Necchi A, Nicolai N, Colecchia M, Catanzaro M, Torelli T, Piva L, Salvioni R. Proof of activity of anti-epidermal growth factor receptor-targeted therapy for relapsed squamous cell carcinoma of the penis. J Clin Oncol. 2011;29:e650–2.
64. Lam KY, Chan KW. Molecular pathology and clinicopathologic features of penile tumors: with special reference to analyses of p21 and p53 expression and unusual histologic features. Arch Pathol Lab Med. 1999;123:895–904.
65. Lopes A, Bezerra AL, Pinto CA, Serrano SV, de MellO CA, Villa LL. p53 as a new prognostic factor for lymph node metastasis in penile carcinoma: analysis of 82 patients treated with amputation and bilateral lymphadenectomy. J Urol. 2002;168:81–6.
66. Chaux A, Munari E, Cubilla AL, Hicks J, Lecksell K, Burnett AL, Netto GJ. Immunohistochemical expression of the mammalian target of rapamycin pathway in penile squamous cell carcinomas: a tissue microarray study of 112 cases. Histopathology. 2014;64:863–71.
67. Alves G, Heller A, Fiedler W, Campos MM, Claussen U, Ornellas AA, Liehr T. Genetic imbalances in 26 cases of penile squamous cell carcinoma. Genes Chromosomes Cancer. 2001;31:48–53.
68. Berney D. Molecular aspects of carcinoma of the penis. The science. Abstract SC-03-002 26 European Congress of Pathology. London, 2014.
69. Campos RS, Lopes A, Guimarães GC, Carvalho AL, Soares FA. E-cadherin, MMP-2, and MMP-9 as prognostic markers in penile cancer: analysis of 125 patients. Urology. 2006;67:797–802.
70. Graafland NM, Lam W, Leijte JA, Yap T, Gallee MP, Corbishley C, van Werkhoven E, Watkin N, Horenblas S. Prognostic factors for occult inguinal lymph node involvement in penile carcinoma and assessment of the high-risk EAU subgroup: a two-institution analysis of 342 clinically node-negative patients. Eur Urol. 2010;58:742–7.
71. Novara G, Galfano A, De Marco V, Artibani W, Ficarra V. Prognostic factors in squamous cell carcinoma of the penis. Nat Clin Pract Urol. 2007;4:140–6.
72. Lont AP, Kroon BK, Gallee MP, van Tinteren H, Moonen LM, Horenblas S. Pelvic lymph node dissection for penile carcinoma: extent of inguinal lymph node involvement as an indicator for pelvic lymph node involvement and survival. J Urol. 2007;177:947–52.
73. Johnson TV, Hsiao W, Delman KA, Jani AB, Brawley OW, Master VA. Extensive inguinal lymphadenectomy improves overall 5-year survival in penile cancer patients: results from the Surveillance, Epidemiology, and End Results program. Cancer. 2010;116:2960–6.
74. Lughezzani G, Catanzaro M, Torelli T, Piva L, Biasoni D, Stagni S, Crestani A, Guttilla A, Raggi D, Giannatempo P, Necchi A, Pizzocaro G, Colecchia M, Salvioni R, Nicolai N. The relationship between characteristics of inguinal lymph nodes and pelvic lymph node involvement in penile squamous cell carcinoma: a single institution experience. J Urol. 2014;191:977–82.
75. Horenblas S, van Tinteren H. Squamous cell carcinoma of the penis. IV. Prognostic factors of survival:

analysis of tumor, nodes and metastasis classification system. J Urol. 1994;151:1239–43.

76. Chaux A, Torres J, Pfannl R, Barreto J, Rodriguez I, Velazquez EF, Cubilla AL. Histologic grade in penile squamous cell carcinoma: visual estimation versus digital measurement of proportions of grades, adverse prognosis with any proportion of grade 3 and correlation of a Gleason-like system with nodal metastasis. Am J Surg Pathol. 2009;33: 1042–8.
77. Emerson RE, Ulbright TM, Eble JN, Geary WA, Eckert GJ, Cheng L. Predicting cancer progression in patients with penile squamous cell carcinoma: the importance of depth of invasion and vascular invasion. Mod Pathol. 2001;14:963–8.
78. Cubilla AL. The role of pathologic prognostic factors in squamous cell carcinoma of the penis. World J Urol. 2009;27:169–77.
79. Cubilla AL, Piris A, Pfannl R, Rodriguez I, Agüero F, Young RH. Anatomic levels: important landmarks in penectomy specimens: a detailed anatomic and histologic study based on examination of 44 cases. Am J Surg Pathol. 2001;25:1091–4.
80. Chaux A, Caballero C, Soares F, Guimarães GC, Cunha IW, Reuter V, Barreto J, Rodríguez I, Cubilla AL. The prognostic index: a useful pathologic guide for prediction of nodal metastases and survival in penile squamous cell carcinoma. Am J Surg Pathol. 2009;33:1049–57.
81. Slaton JW, Morgenstern N, Levy DA, Santos Jr MW, Tamboli P, Ro JY, Ayala AG, Pettaway CA. Tumor stage, vascular invasion and the percentage of poorly differentiated cancer: independent prognosticators for inguinal lymph node metastasis in penile squamous cancer. J Urol. 2001;165:1138–42.
82. Ficarra V, Zattoni F, Cunico SC, Galetti TP, Luciani L, Fandella A, Guazzieri S, Maruzzi D, Sava T, Siracusano S, Pilloni S, Tasca A, Martignoni G, Gardiman M, Tardanico R, Zambolin T, Cisternino A, Artibani W, Gruppo Uro-Oncologico del Nord Est (Northeast Uro-Oncological Group) Penile Cancer Project. Lymphatic and vascular embolizations are independent predictive variables of inguinal lymph node involvement in patients with squamous cell carcinoma of the penis: Gruppo Uro-Oncologico del Nord Est (Northeast Uro-Oncological Group) Penile Cancer data base data. Cancer. 2005;103:2507–16.
83. Guimarães GC, Lopes A, Campos RS, Zequi Sde C, Leal ML, Carvalho AL, da Cunha IW, Soares FA. Front pattern of invasion in squamous cell carcinoma of the penis: new prognostic factor for predicting risk of lymph node metastases. Urology. 2006;68:148–53.
84. Guimarães GC, Leal ML, Campos RS, Zequi Sde C, da Fonseca FP, da Cunha IW, Soares FA, Lopes A. Do proliferating cell nuclear antigen and MIB-1/Ki-67 have prognostic value in penile squamous cell carcinoma? Urology. 2007;70:137–42.
85. Kroon BK, Leijte JA, van Boven H, Wessels LF, Velds A, Horenblas S, van't Veer LJ. Microarray gene-expression profiling to predict lymph node metastasis in penile carcinoma. BJU Int. 2008;102:510–5.
86. Ficarra V, Zattoni F, Artibani W, Fandella A, Martignoni G, Novara G, Galetti TP, Zambolin T, Kattan MW, G.U.O.N.E. Penile Cancer Project Members. Nomogram predictive of pathological inguinal lymph node involvement in patients with squamous cell carcinoma of the penis. J Urol. 2006;175:1700–4.
87. Kattan MW, Ficarra V, Artibani W, Cunico SC, Fandella A, Martignoni G, Fandella A, Novara G, Galetti TP, Zattoni F, GUONE Penile Cancer Project Members. Nomogram predictive of cancer specific survival in patients undergoing partial or total amputation for squamous cell carcinoma of the penis. J Urol. 2006;175:2103–8.
88. UICC. TNM classification of malignant tumours. 7th ed. New York: Wiley & Sons; 2009.
89. Protzel C, Knoedel J, Zimmermann U, Woenckhaus C, Poetsch M, Giebel J. Expression of proliferation marker Ki67 correlates to occurrence of metastasis and prognosis, histological subtypes and HPV DNA detection in penile carcinomas. Histol Histopathol. 2007;22:1197–204.
90. Zhu Y, Zhou XY, Yao XD, Dai B, Ye DW. The prognostic significance of p53, Ki-67, epithelial cadherin and matrix metalloproteinase-9 in penile squamous cell carcinoma treated with surgery. BJU Int. 2007;100:204–8.
91. Van Poppel H, Watkin NA, Osanto S, Moonen L, Horwich A, Kataja V, ESMO Guidelines Working Group. Penile cancer: ESMO Clinical Practice Guidelines for diagnosis, treatment and follow-up. Ann Oncol. 2013;24:vi115–24.
92. Protzel C, Kakies C, Kleist B, Poetsch M, Giebel J. Down-regulation of the metastasis suppressor protein KAI1/CD82 correlates with occurrence of metastasis, prognosis and presence of HPV DNA in human penile squamous cell carcinoma. Virchows Arch. 2008;452:369–75.
93. Termini L, Fregnani JH, Boccardo E, da Costa WH, Longatto-Filho A, Andreoli MA, Costa MC, Lopes A, da Cunha IW, Soares FA, Villa LL, Guimarães GC. SOD2 immunoexpression predicts lymph node metastasis in penile cancer. BMC Clin Pathol. 2015;15:3–8.
94. Alves G, Fiedler W, Guenther E, Nascimento P, Campos MM, Ornellas AA. Determination of telomerase activity in squamous cell carcinoma of the penis. Int J Oncol. 2001;18:67–70.
95. Hungerhuber E, Schlenker B, Schneede P, Stief CG, Karl A. Squamous cell carcinoma antigen correlates with tumor burden but lacks prognostic potential for occult lymph node metastases in penile cancer. Urology. 2007;70:975–9.
96. Golijanin D, Tan JY, Kazior A, Cohen EG, Russo P, Dalbagni G, Auborn KJ, Subbaramaiah K, Dannenberg AJ. Cyclooxygenase-2 and microsomal prostaglandin E synthase-1 are overexpressed in

squamous cell carcinoma of the penis. Clin Cancer Res. 2004;10:1024–31.
97. Muneer A, Kayes O, Ahmed HU, Arya M, Minhas S. Molecular prognostic factors in penile cancer. World J Urol. 2009;27:161–7.
98. Amin A, Griffith RC, Chaux A. Penile intraepithelial neoplasia with pagetoid features: report of an unusual variant mimicking Paget disease. Hum Pathol. 2014;45:889–92.
99. Leijte JA, Kroon BK, Valdés Olmos RA, Nieweg OE, Horenblas S. Reliability and safety of current dynamic sentinel node biopsy for penile carcinoma. Eur Urol. 2007;52:170–7.
100. Leijte JA, Hughes B, Graafland NM, Kroon BK, Olmos RA, Nieweg OE, Corbishley C, Heenan S, Watkin N, Horenblas S. Two-center evaluation of dynamic sentinel node biopsy for squamous cell carcinoma of the penis. J Clin Oncol. 2009;27:3325–9.
101. Chaux A, Reuter V, Lezcano C, Velazquez EF, Torres J, Cubilla AL. Comparison of morphologic features and outcome of resected recurrent and nonrecurrent squamous cell carcinoma of the penis: a study of 81 cases. Am J Surg Pathol. 2009;33:1299–306.
102. Lont AP, Gallee MP, Meinhardt W, van Tinteren H, Horenblas S. Penis conserving treatment for T1 and T2 penile carcinoma: clinical implications of a local recurrence. J Urol. 2006;176:575–80.
103. Hoffman MA, Renshaw AA, Loughlin KR. Squamous cell carcinoma of the penis and microscopic pathologic margins: how much margin is needed for local cure? Cancer. 1999;85:1565–8.
104. Leijte JA, Kirrander P, Antonini N, Windahl T, Horenblas S. Recurrence patterns of squamous cell carcinoma of the penis: recommendations for follow-up based on a two-centre analysis of 700 patients. Eur Urol. 2008;54:161–9.
105. Liegl B, Regauer S. Penile clear cell carcinoma: a report of 5 cases of a distinct entity. Am J Surg Pathol. 2004;28:1513–7.
106. Lopez-Beltran A, Menendez CL, Montironi R, Cheng L. Rare tumors and tumor-like conditions in urological pathology. Switzerland: Springer International Publishing; 2015. p. 410.
107. Smith KJ, Tuur S, Corvette D, Lupton GP, Skelton HG. Cytokeratin 7 staining in mammary and extramammary Paget's disease. Mod Pathol. 1997;10:1069–74.
108. Liegl B, Leibl S, Gogg-Kamerer M, Tessaro B, Horn LC, Moinfar F. Mammary and extramammary Paget's disease: an immunohistochemical study of 83 cases. Histopathology. 2007;50:439–47.
109. Lee JY. Clear cell papulosis: a unique disorder in early childhood characterized by white macules in milk-line distribution. Pediatr Dermatol. 1998;15:328–9.
110. Sánchez-Ortiz R, Huang SF, Tamboli P, Prieto VG, Hester G, Pettaway CA. Melanoma of the penis, scrotum and male urethra: a 40-year single institution experience. J Urol. 2005;173:1958–65.
111. van Geel AN, den Bakker MA, Kirkels W, Horenblas S, Kroon BB, de Wilt JH, Eggermont AM, Mooi WJ, van der Aa MN. Prognosis of primary mucosal penile melanoma: a series of 19 Dutch patients and 47 patients from the literature. Urology. 2007;70:143–7.
112. Zurrida S, Bartoli C, Clemente C, De Palo G. Malignant melanoma of the penis. A report of four cases. Tumori. 1990;76:599–602.
113. Barnhill RL, Albert LS, Shama SK, Goldenhersh MA, Rhodes AR, Sober AJ. Genital lentiginosis: a clinical and histopathologic study. J Am Acad Dermatol. 1990;22:453–60.
114. Katona TM, Lopez-Beltran A, MacLennan GT, Cheng L, Montironi R, Cheng L. Soft tissue tumors of the penis: a review. Anal Quant Cytol Histol. 2006;28:193–206.
115. Fetsch JF, Sesterhenn IA, Miettinen M, Davis Jr CJ. Epithelioid hemangioma of the penis: a clinicopathologic and immunohistochemical analysis of 19 cases, with special reference to exuberant examples often confused with epithelioid hemangioendothelioma and epithelioid angiosarcoma. Am J Surg Pathol. 2004;28:523–33.
116. Fetsch JF, Brinsko RW, Davis Jr CJ, Mostofi FK, Sesterhenn IA. A distinctive myointimal proliferation ('myointimoma') involving the corpus spongiosum of the glans penis: a clinicopathologic and immunohistochemical analysis of 10 cases. Am J Surg Pathol. 2000;24:1524–30.
117. McKenney JK, Collins MH, Carretero AP, Boyd TK, Redman JF, Parham DM. Penile myointimoma in children and adolescents: a clinicopathologic study of 5 cases supporting a distinct entity. Am J Surg Pathol. 2007;31:1622–6.
118. Lowe FC, Lattimer DG, Metroka CE. Kaposi's sarcoma of the penis in patients with acquired immunodeficiency syndrome. J Urol. 1989;142:1475–7.
119. Micali G, Nasca MR, De Pasquale R, Innocenzi D. Primary classic Kaposi's sarcoma of the penis: report of a case and review. J Eur Acad Dermatol Venereol. 2003;17:320–3.
120. Dehner LP, Smith BH. Soft tissue tumors of the penis. A clinicopathologic study of 46 cases. Cancer. 1970;25:1431–47.
121. Fetsch JF, Davis Jr CJ, Miettinen M, Sesterhenn IA. Leiomyosarcoma of the penis: a clinicopathologic study of 14 cases with review of the literature and discussion of the differential diagnosis. Am J Surg Pathol. 2004;28:115–25.
122. Antunes AA, Nesrallah LJ, Goncalves PD, Ferreira YA, Campagnari JC, Srougi M. Deep-seated sarcomas of the penis. Int Braz J Urol. 2005;31:245–50.
123. Usta MF, Adams DM, Zhang JW, Davis R, Hellstrom WJ. Penile epithelioid sarcoma and the case for a histopathological diagnosis in Peyronie's disease. BJU Int. 2003;91:519–21.
124. Rossi G, Ferrari G, Longo L, Trentini GP. Epithelioid sarcoma of the penis: a case report and review of the literature. Pathol Int. 2000;50:579–85.
125. Lowentritt B, Parsons JK, Argani P, Gearhart JP. Pediatric epithelioid sarcoma of the penis. J Urol. 2004;172:296–7.

126. Ponniah A, Brown CT, Taylor P. Priapism secondary to leukemia: effective management with prompt leukapheresis. Int J Urol. 2004;11:809–10.
127. Arena F, di Stefano C, Peracchia G, Barbieri A, Cortellini P. Primary lymphoma of the penis: diagnosis and treatment. Eur Urol. 2001;39:232–5.
128. Hizli F, Berkmen F. Penile metastasis from other malignancies. A study of ten cases and review of the literature. Urol Int. 2006;76:118–21.
129. Chaux A, Amin M, Cubilla AL, Young RH. Metastatic tumors to the penis: a report of 17 cases and review of the literature. Int J Surg Pathol. 2011;19:597–606.
130. Celma Doménech A, Planas Morin J, de Torres Ramírez I, Bestard Vallejo J, Mir Marisma C, Morote Robles J. Priapism secondary to penis infiltration of bladder cancer. Actas Urol Esp. 2008;32:749–51.
131. Gelbard MK, Dorey F, James K. The natural history of Peyronie's disease. J Urol. 1990;144:1376–9.
132. Leopardi O, Colombo F, Frigo B, Zucchi A, Patelli E, Colecchia M, Mantovani F, Naughten W, Pisani E. Immunohistochemical and quantitative study of mast cells in La Peyronie's disease. Eur Urol. 2000;37:176–82.
133. Abdel-Hamid IA, Anis T. Peyronie's disease: perspectives on therapeutic targets. Expert Opin Ther Targets. 2011;15:913–29.
134. Shen S, Truong LD, Ro JY. Frozen section library: genitourinary tract. Chapter 3. London/New York: Springer; 2009.
135. Cabanas RM. The concept of the sentinel lymph node. Recent Results Cancer Res. 2000;157:109–20.
136. Algaba F, Arce Y, López-Beltrán A, Montironi R, Mikuz G, Bono AV, European Society of Uropathology; Uropathology Working Group. Intraoperative frozen section diagnosis in urological oncology. Eur Urol. 2005;47:129–36.
137. Mukherjee S. The emperor of all maladies. A biography of cancer. New York: Simon and Shuster; 2010.
138. Crocker HR. Paget's disease affecting the scrotum and penis. Trans Pathol Soc Lond. 1889;40:187–91.
139. Park S, Grossfeld GD, McAninch JW, Santucci R. Extramammary Paget's disease of the penis and scrotum: excision, reconstruction and evaluation of occult malignancy. J Urol. 2001;166:2112–7.
140. Terada T, Kamo M, Sugiura M. Apocrine carcinoma of the scrotum with extramammary Paget's disease. Int J Dermatol. 2013;52:504–6.
141. Wright JL, Morgan TM, Lin DW. Primary scrotal cancer: disease characteristics and increasing incidence. Urology. 2008;72:1139–43.
142. Froehner M, Koch R, Lossnitzer A, Schober RR, Schuler M, Wirth MP. Adult inguinoscrotal sarcomas: outcome analysis of 21 cases, systematic review of the literature and meta-analysis. World J Urol. 2014;32:445–51.
143. Johnson TV, Hsiao W, Delman KA, Canter DJ, Master VA. Scrotal cancer survival is influenced by histology: a SEER study. World J Urol. 2013;31:585–90.

Handling of the Surgical Specimen and Pathology Reporting of Penile Neoplasms

14

Rodolfo Montironi, Roberta Mazzucchelli, Matteo Santoni, Valeria Sotte, Antonio Lopez-Beltran, Liang Cheng, and Marina Scarpelli

Introduction

Penile neoplastic disease mostly affects men aged between 50 and 70, with incidence variations depending on histological types [1]. Accounting for less than 1 % of male malignancies, penile cancer is a rare tumor in Western countries. However, if referred to only some countries in South America, Africa, and Asia, the relative frequency rises to 20 % [2].

Risk factors for penile neoplasm are the absence of circumcision, phimosis, chronic inflammation, lichen sclerosus, smoking, radiotherapy, and ultraviolet A photochemotherapy in patients with psoriasis [1, 3, 4]. The pathogenesis of penile cancer can be high-risk HPV related or HPV unrelated. In contrast with the slow decrease in penile carcinoma incidence reported in some countries, HPV-related forms are increasing in others, including the United States [5].

R. Montironi (✉) • R. Mazzucchelli • M. Scarpelli
Pathological Anatomy, Polytechnic University of the Marche Region, School of Medicine, United Hospitals, Ancona, Italy
e-mail: r.montironi@univpm.it; r.mazzucchelli@univpm.it; m.scarpelli@univpm.it

M. Santoni • V. Sotte
Medical Oncology, Polytechnic University of the Marche Region, School of Medicine, United Hospitals, Ancona, Italy
e-mail: mattymo@alice.it; valeria.sotte@gmail.it

A. Lopez-Beltran
Department of Pathology and Surgery, Faculty of Medicine, University of Cordoba, Cordoba, Spain
e-mail: em1lobea@uco.es

L. Cheng
Department of Pathology and Laboratory Medicine, Indiana University School of Medicine, Indianapolis, IN, USA
e-mail: lcheng@iupui.edu

Anatomy

Penile tumors mostly originate from any of the mucosal districts of the distal penis: glans, coronal sulcus, and foreskin. Penile mucosal tissue extends from the preputial orifice to the fossa navicularis. In a section, different anatomical layers can be distinguished. The glans, from surface to depth, consists of the lamina propria, corpus spongiosum, tunica albuginea, and corpora cavernosa. The foreskin is constituted of an internal mucosal stratum and an external cutaneous layer with different histological characteristics. The two strata are separated (from mucosal to skin level) by the lamina propria, dartos, dermis, and epidermis. The penile fascia surrounds the shaft inserting into the lamina propria of the coronal sulcus. The fossa navicularis constitutes the distal 5–6 mm of the penile urethra, even though its squamous epithelium is continuous with that of the perimeatal glans.

M. Colecchia (ed.), *Pathology of Testicular and Penile Neoplasms*,
DOI 10.1007/978-3-319-27617-5_14

The penile urethra runs in the ventral part of the shaft enclosed in the lamina propria, corpus spongiosum, and penile fascia [6].

Handling of the Surgical Specimen

Circumcision can be used in the case of small lesions of the foreskin, even though a high recurrence rate should be taken into account. Partial penectomy is preferable when the tumor involves the glans or the shaft, whereas total penectomy, associated to perineal urethrotomy, with or without lymphadenectomy, represents the best approach in bulky tumors [7, 8]. A possible choice, in order to stage the cancer, is the technique of sentinel lymph nodes. Finally, whole mounting is a reasonable procedure in the case of penectomy, improving the staging with a negligible increase in costs and turnaround time.

Circumcision

In circumcision, after identification, both the mucosal and the cutaneous margin are stained with different colors to allow them to be distinguished. Special attention should be paid to the coronal sulcus margin, considering that the majority of squamous neoplasms derive from the mucosal surface of the foreskin. Afterward the lightly stretched specimen is pinned to cardboard and set for several hours in formalin. Once the specimen is fixed, the entire block should be cut vertically and each section labeled from 1 to 12. After this process, it is possible to examine the specimen identifying the neoplasm that can also be measured and described [9, 10].

Total or Partial Penectomy

Although penile tumor can arise from any compartment of the penis, the glans is the most frequent site of origin, followed by the foreskin, the coronal sulcus, and the shaft. Penile tumor may be multifocal: the involvement of more than one site is possible depending on the geographical area of the report [11].

Penile squamous cell carcinomas (SCCs) generally originate from the epithelial tissues in the extremity of the penis (glans, coronal sulcus, and mucosal surface of the prepuce). If included in the specimen, the foreskin should be classified, according to the length, as short, medium, long, and/or phimotic [12]. The proximal margin of resection is removed and the whole urethral circumference is submitted. It is advisable to cut the proximal margin of the resection en face to include the entire circumference of the urethra. In the case of a retracted urethra, the resection margin has to be defined and enclosed completely.

The margin of the resection is composed of the following three parts that should be analyzed:

- Skin covering the shaft together with the underlying tissues (dartos and penile fascia)
- Corpora cavernosa with the tunica albuginea
- Urethra with the surrounding tissues including the lamina propria, corpus spongiosum, albuginea, and penile fascia

It is feasible to process the urethra and the periurethral cylinder in the same tissue cassette; the skin of the shaft and the tissues beneath it can be placed together with the corpora cavernosa. As the specimen is usually large, more than one cassette can be used to include the entire resection margin. The remaining part has to be fixed in formalin overnight. In the case of large cancers (spreading to most of the glans), when fixation is completed, the block can be cut longitudinally and centrally taking the meatus and the proximal urethra as reference (Fig. 14.1, upper and lower panels). The urethra does not need to be examined. The specimen should be divided into the left and right halves, each of which is then cut into 2–6 serial sections. In small or asymmetric tumors, located on the dorsal or ventral surface of the penis, it is possible to use the central part of the neoplasm itself as the axis of sectioning. If the neoplasm is widespread and involves different compartments (glans, sulcus, and foreskin), the foreskin should not be separated so that the specimen is intact for sectioning.

In the case of small cancers sited solely in the glans, the foreskin can be removed making sure that a 3-mm edge is left around the coronal

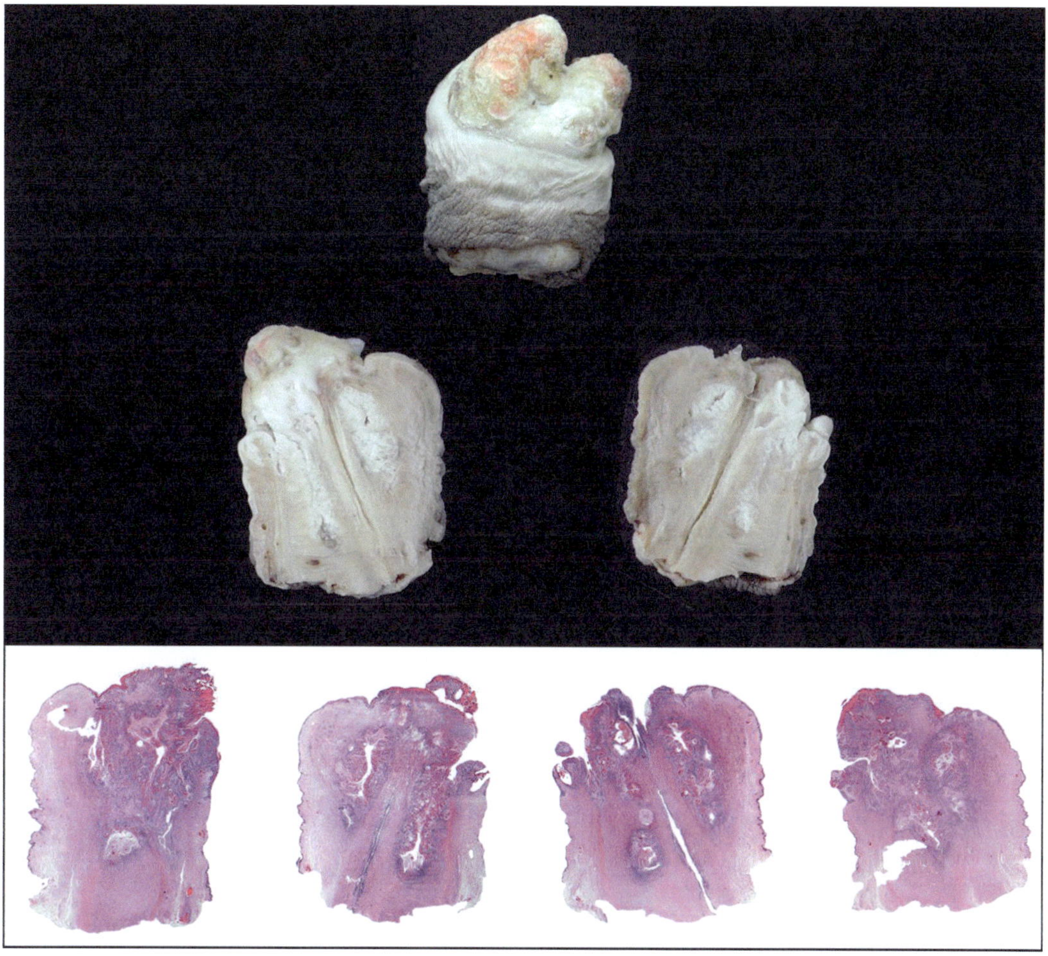

Fig. 14.1 *Upper panel* – In the case of large cancer (spreading to most of the glans), the specimen is cut longitudinally and centrally taking the meatus and the proximal urethra as reference point. *Lower panel* – Whole mount sections of the glans with tumor

sulcus. The foreskin should be cut as shown in the circumcision specimen and labeled from 1 to 12 clockwise serially and systematically (even though the primary carcinoma is in the glans). The remaining part of the specimen should be processed as described above [9].

Lymphadenectomy and/or Sentinel Lymph Node

Lymph nodes without evident metastasis, if larger than 5 mm, are cut across the hilus into parallel slices of 2 mm. On the contrary, if the longitudinal axis is shorter than 5 mm, they are processed entirely. One or two sections are generally sufficient for lymph nodes that contain an overt metastasis [13].

Sentinel lymph nodes, usually identified by lymphoscintigraphy, are marked with radioactive colloid. Negative lymph nodes are processed entirely (steps of 250 μm). Immunocytochemistry can be used to evaluate each second section [13].

TNM Staging, Including the Resection Margins

The TNM staging system is nowadays accepted worldwide [14]. A revision of the current TNM expected later in 2015. The T parameter is assigned to the primary tumor that has never been treated before. The prefix modifier "p" stands for a pathological rather than a clinical ("c") classification. Pathological classification is based on histological evidence: pT requires either the excision of the primary tumor or a biopsy suitable for determining the highest pT class, pN implies the resection of lymph nodes adequate to identify metastasis, and pM involves the evaluation of distant secondary deposits. As a consequence, pathological staging is designed after the surgical removal of primary tumors. Finally it is essential to remember that a positive resection margin is related to the worst prognosis. In partial penectomy, according to the TNM staging system (Table 14.1), the pathology report should provide information about:

- The proximal urethra and the periurethral cylinder including epithelium, subepithelial connective tissue, corpus spongiosum, and penile fascia
- The proximal shaft with corpora cavernosa separated and surrounded by the tunica albuginea and Buck's fascia
- The skin of the shaft with the corporal dartos

In circumcision specimens the coronal sulcus and cutaneous margin need to be evaluated entirely.

If present, lymph nodes (LNs) should be counted and measured: the total number and size of each node should be reported along with the number and localization (e.g., inguinal vs. pelvic) of positive nodes or the presence of extracapsular extensions.

Table 14.1 TNM staging system: primary tumor (pT)

pTX:	Primary tumor cannot be assessed
pT0:	No evidence of primary tumor
pTis:	Carcinoma in situ
pTa:	Noninvasive verrucous carcinoma
pT1a:	Tumor invades subepithelial connective tissue without lymph vascular invasion and is not poorly differentiated
pT1b:	Tumor invades subepithelial connective tissue with lymph vascular invasion or is poorly differentiated
pT2:	Tumor invades corpus spongiosum or cavernosum
pT3:	Tumor invades urethra
pT4:	Tumor invades other adjacent structures

Depth of Invasion (i.e., Tumor Thickness)

In small cancers, tumor thickness is easily measured in sections made by a perpendicular cut along the tumor central axis. In wider tumors, such as large glans neoplasms, it is suggested to cut the specimen into two halves longitudinally and subsequently to obtain parallel sections from each half. The depth of invasion of SCCs is the distance in millimeters from the epithelial-stromal junction of the adjacent benign epithelium to the deepest part in the invasive front. This system is applied to all cancer types with the exception of verruciform tumors. In these cases measuring the depth from the surface (excluding the keratin layer) to the deepest point of invasion is suggested. The risk of secondary deposits is minimal when the tumor thickness is less than 5 mm and increases (with a higher risk of nodal involvement) when the infiltration reaches deeper anatomical layers [15]. Tumors that invade the corpus cavernosum entail a higher risk of nodal metastases than those invading exclusively the corpus spongiosum. For these reasons the final pathology report should state the deepest erectile tissue infiltrated. Deeper infiltration correlated with higher histological grade, even if some exceptions are known [16].

Lymphovascular Invasion (LVI)

Lymphovascular invasion unfavorably affects prognosis [17, 18]. The importance of LVI is proved by the seventh edition of the TNM staging that divides T1 tumors into T1a and T1b according to the absence or presence of LVI or poorly differentiated components [14]. LVI is commonly seen in the invasive tumor front, but it may also occur at a certain distance from the tumor in different anatomical compartments including the lamina propria, the penile fascia, and above all, in the lamina propria of the surrounding the penile urethra. Venous invasion suggests an advanced stage and is easily associated with the involvement of the corpora spongiosa and cavernosa.

Perineural Invasion (PI)

The predictive models, which have recently been proposed to better assess clinical and pathological features and are included in the nomograms for the clinical evaluation of lymph nodes, take into consideration histologic growth pattern, tumor grade, and vascular and urethral infiltration, including the invasion of the corpora spongiosa and cavernosa. PI and histological grade are strongly related (as independent factors) to mortality in tumors with a depth of 5 to 10 mm. The classification of patients into risk categories is applied to predict the probability of LN involvement in order to guide the therapeutic approach. The risk group is defined on the basis of the histological grade and pT stage. The predictive power increases if the combination of histological grade, deepest anatomical level of infiltration, and the presence of PI is considered. The abovementioned factors are used to contrive a prognostic index [19].

Frozen Section (FS)

FSs may be employed to examine the resection margins and the sentinel lymph nodes [10, 13]. When the urethra, periurethral vessels, and soft tissue are infiltrated (as usually occurs), these tissues should be frozen for evaluation. In circumcision specimens, the circumference and the full thickness of the surgical margin have to be evaluated. In order to avoid unnecessary section, the surgeon is advised to mark the area of concern with a suture. When FS examination is requested, the lymph node should be bisected, and one section should be made from each cut surface. After both halves are embedded, the first slides are examined microscopically.

References

1. Pow-Sang MR, Ferreira U, Pow-Sang JM, Nardi AC, Destefano V. Epidemiology and natural history of penile cancer. Urology. 2010;76:S2–6.
2. Pow-Sang MR, Benavente V, Pow-Sang JE, Morante C, Meza L, Baker M, Pow-Sang JM. Cancer of the penis. Cancer Control. 2002;9:305–14.
3. Calmon MF, Tasso Mota M, Vassallo J, Rahal P. Penile carcinoma: risk factors and molecular alterations. Scientific World J. 2011;11:269–82.
4. Madsen BS, van den Brule AJ, Jensen HL, Wohlfahrt J, Frisch M. Risk factors for squamous cell carcinoma of the penis – population-based case–control study in Denmark. Cancer Epidemiol Biomarkers Prev. 2008;17:2683–91.
5. Chaux A, Cubilla AL. Advances in the pathology of penile carcinomas. Hum Pathol. 2012;43:771–89.
6. Young RH, Srigley JR, Amin MB, Ulbright TM, Cubilla AL. Tumors of the prostate gland, seminal vesicles, male urethra, and penis. AFIP atlas of tumor pathology. 3rd series. Fascicle 28. Washington, DC: AFIP; 2000.
7. Deem S, Keane T, Bhavsar R, El-Zawahary A, Savage S. Contemporary diagnosis and management of squamous cell carcinoma (SCC) of the penis. BJU Int. 2011;108:1378–92.
8. Solsona E, Bahl A, Brandes SB, Dickerson D, Puras-Baez A, van Poppel H, Watkin NA. New developments in the treatment of localized penile cancer. Urology. 2010;76:S36–42.
9. Velazquez EF, Amin MB, Epstein JI, Grignon DJ, Humphrey PA, Pettaway CA, Renshaw AA, Reuter VE, Srigley JR, Zhou M, Cubilla AL; Members of the Cancer Committee, College of American Pathologists. Protocol for the examination of specimens from patients with carcinoma of the penis. CAP Protocol, web posting date: October 2013.
10. Chaux A, Velazquez EF, Algaba F, Ayala G, Cubilla AL. Developments in the pathology of penile squamous cell carcinomas. Urology. 2010;76:S7–14.
11. Cubilla AL, Piris A, Pfannl R, Rodriguez I, Agüero F, Young RH. Anatomic levels: important landmarks in penectomy specimens: a detailed anatomic and histologic study based on examination of 44 cases. Am J Surg Pathol. 2001;25:1091–4.
12. Velazquez EF, Bock A, Soskin A, Codas R, Arbo M, Cubilla AL. Preputial variability and preferential association of long phimotic foreskins with penile cancer: an anatomic comparative study of types of foreskin in a general population and cancer patients. Am J Surg Pathol. 2003;27:994–8.
13. Mikuz G, Winstanley AM, Schulman CC, Debruyne FM, Parkinson CM. Handling and pathology reporting of circumcision and penectomy specimens. Eur Urol. 2004;46:434–9.
14. Edge SB, Byrd DR, Carducci MA, Compton CC, editors. AJCC cancer staging manual. 7th ed. New York: Springer; 2009.
15. Velazquez EF, Ayala G, Liu H, Chaux A, Zanotti M, Torres J, Cho SI, Barreto JE, Soares F, Cubilla AL. Histologic grade and perineural invasion are more important than tumor thickness as predictor of nodal metastasis in penile squamous cell carcinoma invading 5 to 10 mm. Am J Surg Pathol. 2008;32:974–9.
16. Guimarães GC, Cunha IW, Soares FA, Lopes A, Torres J, Chaux A, Velazquez EF, Ayala G, Cubilla

AL. Penile squamous cell carcinoma clinicopathological features, nodal metastasis and outcome in 333 cases. J Urol. 2009;182:528–34.
17. Novara G, Galfano A, De Marco V, Artibani W, Ficarra V. Prognostic factors in squamous cell carcinoma of the penis. Nat Clin Pract Urol. 2007;4:140–6.
18. Emerson RE, Ulbright TM, Eble JN, Geary WA, Eckert GJ, Cheng L. Predicting cancer progression in patients with penile squamous cell carcinoma: the importance of depth of invasion and vascular invasion. Mod Pathol. 2001;14:963–8.
19. Chaux A, Caballero C, Soares F, Guimarães GC, Cunha IW, Reuter V, Barreto J, Rodríguez I, Cubilla AL. The prognostic index: a useful pathologic guide for prediction of nodal metastases and survival in penile squamous cell carcinoma. Am J Surg Pathol. 2009;33:1049–57.

Index

M. Colecchia (ed.), *Pathology of Testicular and Penile Neoplasms*,
DOI 10.1007/978-3-319-27617-5

T

Y

MIX
Papier aus verantwortungsvollen Quellen
Paper from responsible sources
FSC® C105338

If you have any concerns about our products,
you can contact us on
ProductSafety@springernature.com

In case Publisher is established outside the EU,
the EU authorized representative is:
Springer Nature Customer Service Center GmbH
Europaplatz 3, 69115 Heidelberg, Germany

Printed by Libri Plureos GmbH
in Hamburg, Germany